ATLAS OF CLINICAL NEUROLOGY

Project Editor
David Bennett

Design
Madeleine Hall
David Buss
Glenn Davidson
Julian Dorr
Max Dyson
Sharon Hayles
Mehmet Hussein

Illustration
(Diagrams)
Pam Corfield
Edwina Hannam
Lydia Malim
(Linework)
Jeremy Cort
Maurizia Merati
Andrew Park

Index
Doreen Blake

ATLAS OF CLINICAL NEUROLOGY

G David Perkin

BA MB FRCP

Consultant Neurologist   Charing Cross and
Hillingdon Hospitals   London UK

Frank Clifford Rose

FRCP

Director Academic Unit of Neuroscience
Charing Cross and Westminster Medical School,
University of London   London UK

William Blackwood

MB ChB FRCSE FRCPE FRCPath

Emeritus Professor of Neuropathology
University of London   London UK

Harry H Shawdon

MA MB BChir MRCP FRCR

Consultant Radiologist
Charing Cross and Westminster Medical School
University of London   London UK

J B Lippincott Company · Philadelphia

Gower Medical Publishing · London · New York

Distributors of English Editions:

All countries (except USA, Canada and Japan):
Baillière Tindall,
1 St Anne's Road,
Eastbourne,
East Sussex,
BN21 3UN
England

USA and Canada:
J.B. Lippincott Company,
East Washington Square,
Philadelphia PA 19105 USA

Japan:
Nishimura Co., Ltd.;
1-754-39 Asahimachi-dori,
Niigata-shi 951,
Japan

ISBN 0-397-58299-4 (Lippincott)
     0-906923-25-5 (Gower)

Library of Congress Catalog Card Number: 85-82196

Library Cataloging in Publication Data is available

Printed in Italy by Federico Motta Editore Spa.
Origination by Mandarin Offset Ltd., Hong Kong.

Contents

13. Non-Metastatic Neurological Syndromes and Neurological Complications of Systemic Disease

Acknowledgements

We wish to thank the following individuals for their kind contributions:

Dr A Ameen, University Hospital, Basrah, Iraq. (Fig. 9.30)
Dr J Ambrose, Consultant Neuroradiologist, The Atkinson Morley Hospital, Wimbledon, London, UK. (Fig. 5.20)
Dr Professor J E Banatvala, Department of Virology, St. Thomas's Hospital, London, UK. (Fig. 9.50)
Dr R O Barnard, Department of Neuropathology, Maida Vale Hospital, London, UK.
(Figs. 6.8, 7.13, 7.19, 7.20, 7.22, 7.23, 7.26, 7.27 (left), 7.48 (right), 9.16, 9.46, 10.1 (right), 10.2, 10.3, 10.4, 10.26 (lower), 10.29, 10.30 and 10.31).
Dr R St. C Barnetson, Consultant Dermatologist, Department of Dermatology, Edinburgh Royal Infirmary, Edinburgh, UK. (Figs. 2.8, 2.9, and 12.43)
Professor A E Becker, Wilhelmina Gasthuis, Amsterdam, Netherlands. (Fig. 4.49)
Dr P O Behan, Reader in Neurology, Institute of Neurological Sciences, Glasgow, UK. (Figs. 2.11, 3.23, 3.29 and 3.30)
Professor J A N Corsellis, Runwell Hospital, Wickford, Essex, UK. (Fig. 6.17)
Mr B Crymble, Consultant Neurosurgeon, Hurstwood Park Neurological Centre, Haywards Heath, UK. (Fig. 11.37)
Dr M E Edmonds, Lecturer in Medicine, Diabetic Department, King's College Hospital, London, UK. (Fig. 2.16)
Dr M Erdohazi, Late Consultant Neuropathologist, Hospital for Sick Children, London, UK. (Fig. 8.5)
Dr M Gawel, Consultant Neurologist, Sunnybrook Hospital, Toronto, Ontario, Canada. (Figs. 3.11, 3.32, 3.33, 9.20 and 9.24)
Mr D N Grant, Consultant Neurosurgeon, The National Hospital, London, UK. (Fig. 11.31)
Dr D G F Harriman, Department of Neuropathology, The General Infirmary, Leeds. (Figs. 10.33 and 10.34)
Drs L Henriksen, O B Paulson and N A Lassen, Department of Neuromedicine, Rigshospitalet, Copenhagen, Denmark. (Fig. 4.11)
Dr I Janota, Department of Neuropathology, Institute of Psychiatry, London, UK. (Figs. 6.1, 6.2 (right), 6.22, 6.23, 6.24, 6.29 and 6.30)
Dr B Kendall, Department of Neuroradiology, The National Hospital, London, UK. (Figs. 11.18 and 11.56)
Dr R S Kocen, Consultant Neurologist, The National Hospital, London, UK. (Fig. 11.45 (right))
Professor V Logue, Emeritus Professor of Neurosurgery, The National Hospital, London, UK. (Figs. 2.21, 2.24, 7.53 (left), 11.51, and 12.4)
Professor W I McDonald, Consultant Neurologist, The National Hospital, London, UK. (Fig. 3.16)
Dr J Payan, Consultant Neurophysiologist, Guy's and King's College Hospitals, London, UK. (Fig. 3.31)
Dr R W Ross Russell, Consultant Neurologist, The National Hospital, London, UK. (Figs. 11.38, 11.39 and 11.55)
Dr P Rudge, Consultant Neurologist, The National Hospital, London, UK. (Fig. 11.45 (left))
Mr M Sanders, Consultant Neuro-ophthalmologist, The National Hospital, London, UK. (Fig. 4.36)
Dr C L Scholtz, Department of Histopathology, The London Hospital, London, UK. (Figs. 13.3 (right) and 13.8 (lower))
Mr D Spalton, Consultant Ophthalmic Surgeon, Medical Eye Unit, St. Thomas's Hospital, London, UK. (Fig. 12.1)
Dr P E Sylvester, Consultant Psychiatrist, St. Lawrence's Hospital, Caterham, UK. (Figs. 8.8 and 8.9)
Mr K Till, Honorary Consultant Neurosurgeon, The Hospital for Sick Children, London, UK. (Fig. 11.37)
Mr L S Walsh, Emeritus Consultant Neurosurgeon, The National Hospital, London, UK. (Figs. 10.38 and 11.20)
Professor R O Weller, Department of Neuropathology, Southampton General Hospital, Southampton, UK. (Figs. 6.2 (left), 6.3, 7.42, 7.47, 10.22 and 10.29 (right))
Dr R J Wise, MRC Cyclotron Unit, Hammersmith Hospital, London, UK. (Fig. 4.13)

In addition:

Fig. 4.6 is redrawn from Figures 5 and 6 in 'Variation in Form of Circle of Willis'. *Archives of Neurology* **8**, 8-14, 1963, by H E Riggs and C Rupp.
Fig. 4.16 is redrawn from Figure 3 in 'Swelling of the Brain Following Ischaemic Infarction with Arterial Occlusion'. *Archives of Neurology* **1**, 161-177, by C M Shaw, E C Alvord Jnr. and R G Berry.
Fig. 4.35 is reproduced from Figure 3 in 'Recurrent Cholesterol Embolism as a Cause of Fluctuating Cerebral Symptoms'. *Journal of Neurology, Neurosurgery and Psychiatry* **30**, 489-496, 1967, by W I McDonald.
Fig. 4.29 is redrawn from Figure 11.10c in 'Neurological Differential Diagnosis', by J Patten, Springer Verlag, 1977.
Figs. 5.3 and 5.4 are redrawn from Figures 5 and 6, and Figure 11 respectively, in 'The Occurrence and Significance of Intracerebral Micro-aneurysms'. *Journal of Pathology and Bacteriology* **93**, 393-411, 1967, by F M Cole and P Q Yates.
Figs. 5.14 and 5.15 are from 'Computer Tomographic Features of Giant Intracranial Aneurysms'. *Clinical Radiology* **31**, 41-48, 1980 (Figure 5, and Figures 1 and 3 respectively). R Golding, R C Peatfield, H H Shawdon and J H Rice Edwards.
Fig. 6.1 is reproduced from Figure 2 in 'Alzheimer's Disease in a Mother and Identical Twin Sons'. *Psychological Medicine* **9**, 771-774, 1979, by M G Sharman, D C Watt, I Janota and L H Carrasco.
Fig. 6.2 (right) is reproduced from Figure 4.1b in 'Recent Advances in Histopathology Number 11', edited by P P Anthony and R N M MacSween, Churchill Livingstone, 1981.
Figs. 6.22 and 6.24 are reproduced from Figures 3 and 1a respectively in 'Progressive Supranuclear Palsy - Clinico-pathological Study of Four Cases'. *Brain* **92**, 663-678, 1969, by S Behrman, J D Carroll, I Janota and W B Matthews.
Figs. 9.14 and 9.15 are reproduced from Figures 11 and 14 in 'Torulosis of the Central Nervous System in Britain'. *Brain* **81**, 542-555, 1958, by F Clifford Rose, H C Grant and A L Jeanes.
Figs 13.1 and 13.2 are from 'Polioencephalite Diffuse et Neoplasme Visceral'. *Acta Neurol Belg.* **78**, 167-173, 1978, by J P Mullier, M Duret, P Khoubesserian and J J Vanderhaeghen.
Fig. 13.3 (left) is from 'Etude Clinique et Anatomique de Deux Cas de Degenerescence Cerebelleuse Subaigue'. *Acta. Neurol. Belg.* **71**, 324-344, 1971, by J J Vanderhaeghen *et al.*
Figs. 13.7 and 13.8 (upper) are from 'Leuco-encephalite Multifocale Progressive'. *Acta. Psych. Neruol. Belg.* **65**, 816-837, 1965, by J J Vanderhaeghen *et al.*
Fig. 13.9 is from 'Ocular Toxoplasmosis, Trigeminal Herpes Zoster and Pulmonary Tuberculosis in a Patient with Hodgkin's Disease', *Ophthalmologia*, Basel **171**, 237-243, 1975, by D Toussant and J J Vanderhaeghen.

Preface

Despite the introduction of increasingly sophisticated investigative techniques, the practice of Neurology remains essentially clinical, depending on meticulous history-taking and physical examination. An atlas is an excellent means for presenting this approach.

The atlas is divided into thirteen chapters, the titles of which are arbitrary, since some cover a diverse range of conditions. Clinical, electrophysiological, radiological and pathological material has been incorporated, the balance depending on how well the particular condition lends itself to illustration. An atlas of this nature cannot cover the subject with equal detail, since clinical illustration has limited application for certain disorders, for example, those of higher cortical function. There are also particular problems in presenting disorders of movement so that pictures taken from video recordings have been used to capture particular postures. The atlas is not intended as a comprehensive account of Neurology. The accompanying text serves as background information to supplement the illustrative material which is complemented, where appropriate, by a brief clinical history.

It is a pleasure to thank our numerous colleagues at the Charing Cross Hospital who provided pictures from their personal collection. Acknowledgements to individuals and Institutes outside Charing Cross appear separately.

We gratefully acknowledge the secretarial services of Ms. Julia Bavington.

G.D.P.
F.C.R.
W.B.
H.H.S.

1. Neurological Investigations

Whilst history taking and examination remain of cardinal importance in the assessment of the patient presenting with a neurological disorder, various investigative techniques may be required to establish a correct diagnosis. A brief description of these methods will be given here, many of which remain of relevance despite the availability of computerised axial tomography.

The Cerebrospinal Fluid

The cerebrospinal fluid (CSF) is formed partly from the choroid plexuses of the ventricular system, and partly by diffusion through the pial lining of the ventricles. The total volume is around 120 ml and it is produced at a rate of around 0.3–0.4 ml/minute. Having left the fourth ventricle via the median and lateral recesses, the fluid circulates over the surface of the spinal cord and cerebral hemispheres prior to its reabsorption through the arachnoid villi of the superior sagittal sinus (Fig. 1.1).

CSF may be obtained by insertion of a needle into the lateral ventricle, for example during ventriculography, but more usually by puncture of the cisterna magna, or the lumbar subarachnoid space. Although the spinal cord terminates at the lower border of the first lumbar vertebra in adults, the subarachnoid space continues to the level of the second or third sacral vertebra. This space, containing only nerve roots and CSF, can be entered by insertion of a needle between adjacent lumbar vertebrae, usually the second and third, or the third and fourth (Fig. 1.2).

The bevelled hollow needle, with stylet, is introduced having infiltrated the skin and subcutaneous tissues with a local anaesthetic. The fluid pressure, normally between 60 and 150 mm of water, is measured with a manometer

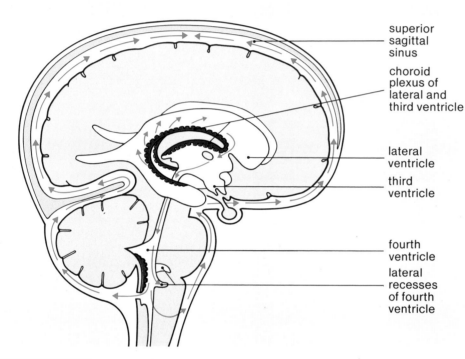

Fig 1.1 Diagram showing the sites of formation and the circulation of cerebrospinal fluid.

superior sagittal sinus

choroid plexus of lateral and third ventricle

lateral ventricle

third ventricle

fourth ventricle

lateral recesses of fourth ventricle

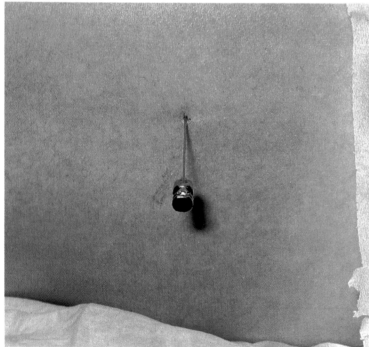

Fig 1.2 Lumbar puncture.

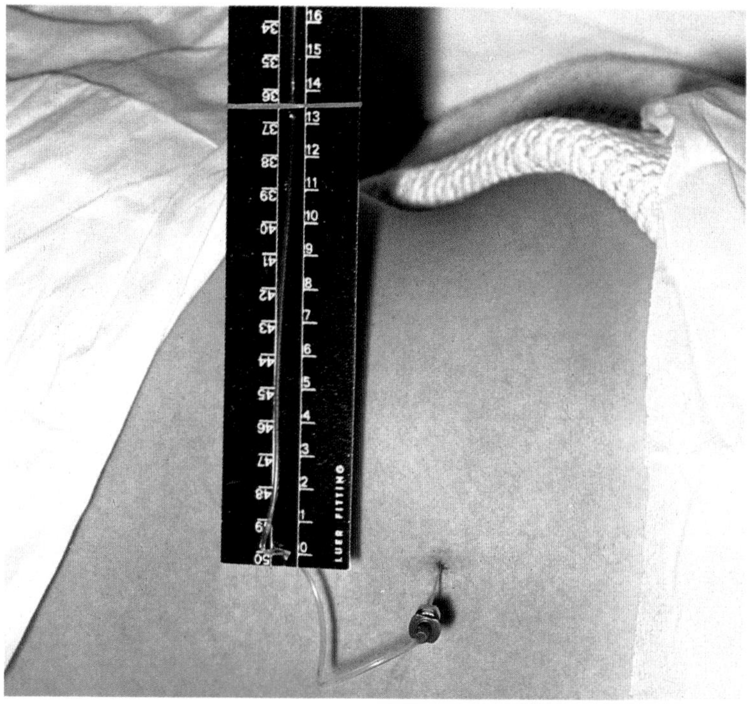

Fig 1.3 CSF manometry. The recorded pressure is approximately 135 mm.

(Fig. 1.3). Rather higher pressures may be found in anxious individuals, and transiently during coughing. The procedure is potentially hazardous in patients with raised intracranial pressure due to a space-occupying lesion, when removal of fluid may be followed by herniation of the cerebellar tonsils and acute medullary compression. Where the raised pressure is due to benign intracranial hypertension however, lumbar puncture may have a transient therapeutic benefit (Fig. 1.4).

The constituents of the CSF routinely examined include protein, glucose and cells. The normal cell count does not exceed 5 lymphocytes/mm^3, whilst the normal upper limit for the protein concentration (with some variation from laboratory to laboratory) is 0.45 g/l. Certain laboratories have the facility for examination of the IgG concentration, and for performing electro-phoresis of the fluid (Fig. 1.5). Analysis of the Lange curve, performed by adding serial dilutions of CSF to a colloidal gold solution, is a qualitative estimation of IgG concentration now seldom performed.

RIHSA Scanning

In RIHSA scanning human serum albumin labelled most commonly with radioactive technetium (99m Tc) is injected into the lumbar subarachnoid space or the cisterna magna. Serial scans allow observation of the passage of radioactivity over the surface of the brain (Fig. 1.6). Normally, activity reaches the basal cisterns and inferior Sylvian fissures within 4 hours, and concentrates over the vertex by 24 hours. The investigation is of limited value in the assessment of patients suspected of having 'low-pressure' hydrocephalus.

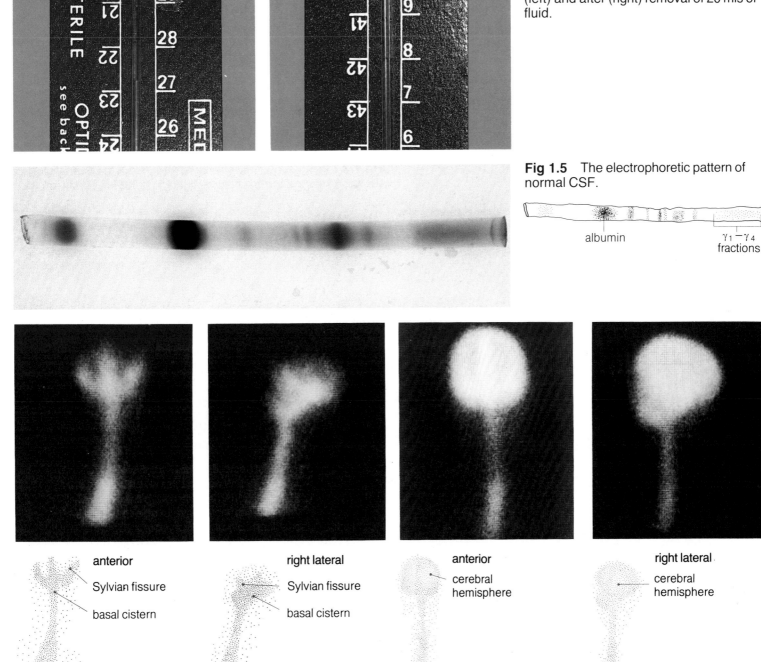

Fig 1.4 CSF pressure recordings in benign intracranial hypertension: before (left) and after (right) removal of 20 mls of fluid.

Fig 1.5 The electrophoretic pattern of normal CSF.

albumin $\gamma_1 - \gamma_4$ fractions

anterior
Sylvian fissure
basal cistern

right lateral
Sylvian fissure
basal cistern

anterior
cerebral hemisphere

right lateral
cerebral hemisphere

Fig 1.6 Normal RIHSA scans. These views show the radioactivity detected at 4 hours in the Sylvian fissures and basal cisterns (left) and at 24 hours extending over the cerebral hemispheres towards the vertex (right).

Skull Radiography

Whilst the skull radiograph may, on occasions, provide information of diagnostic importance, for example in the case of bone destruction, its role in routine neurological investigation is slight. The lateral view is of particular importance in the assessment of the size and shape of the pituitary fossa (Fig. 1.7).

The inclined posteroanterior projection permits identification, amongst other structures, of the posterior wall of the orbits, including the superior orbital fissures (Fig. 1.8). The inclined anteroposterior view (or Towne projection) displays particularly the petrous temporal bones and the dorsum sellae (Fig. 1.9). A vertico-submental view demonstrates the skull base, of relevance

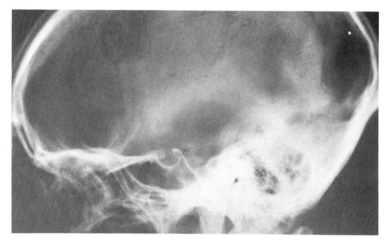

Fig 1.7   Lateral radiograph of the normal skull.

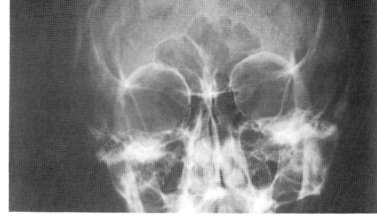

Fig 1.8   Inclined posteroanterior radiograph of the normal skull showing the structures comprising the posterior wall of the orbits.

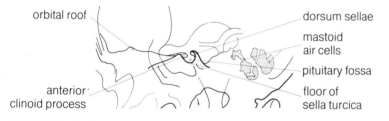

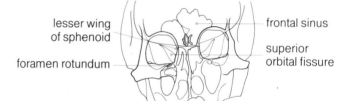

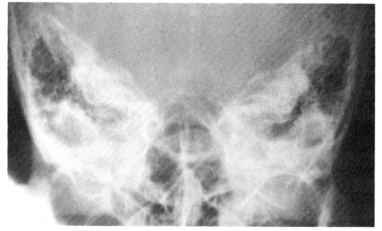

Fig 1.9   Inclined anteroposterior radiograph of the normal skull showing the petrous temporal bones and the dorsum sellae.

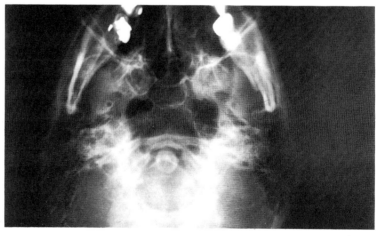

Fig 1.10   Verticosubmental radiograph of the normal skull.

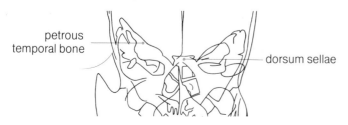

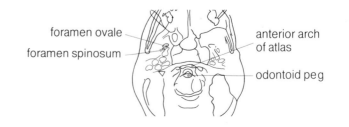

when bone destruction by an expanding nasopharyngeal carcinoma is suspected (Fig. 1.10).

Spinal Radiography

Spinal radiography is most commonly performed where there are symptoms suggesting cervical or lumbar root compression. Lateral and anteroposterior views of the lumbar spine allow identification of the components of the neural arch, together with the shape and size of the intervertebral foramina (Fig. 1.11). In the cervical region, additional oblique views are necessary to accurately define these foramina, which characteristically may show encroachment in patients with cervical root compression due to spondylitic disease (Figs. 1.12 & 1.13).

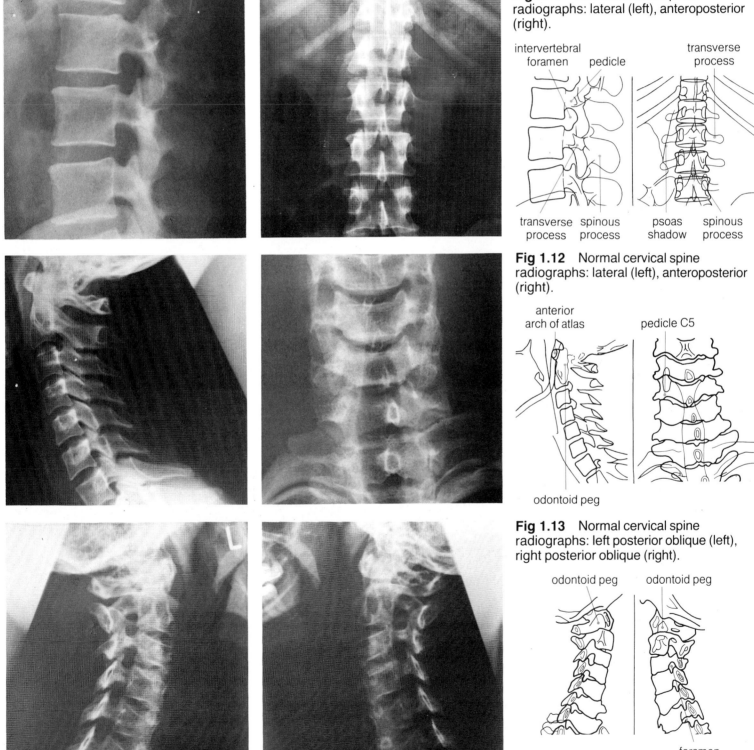

Fig 1.11   Normal lumbar spine radiographs: lateral (left), anteroposterior (right).

Fig 1.12   Normal cervical spine radiographs: lateral (left), anteroposterior (right).

Fig 1.13   Normal cervical spine radiographs: left posterior oblique (left), right posterior oblique (right).

1.5

Myelography

A number of different contrast media have been used for injection into the lumbar subarachnoid space in order to demonstrate radiologically the configuration of the spinal cord and its nerve roots. Although both air and oil-soluble agents can be used for this purpose, a water-soluble medium is the agent generally favoured in the United Kingdom.

The injection is usually performed between the third and fourth lumbar vertebrae, the volume of contrast medium required varying according to the part of the spinal canal to be assessed. CSF samples are taken before the myodil is injected, since a pleocytosis with an elevation of protein concentration commonly follows the procedure.

The procedure allows ready identification of the lumbar and cervical root pouches (those in the thoracic region are

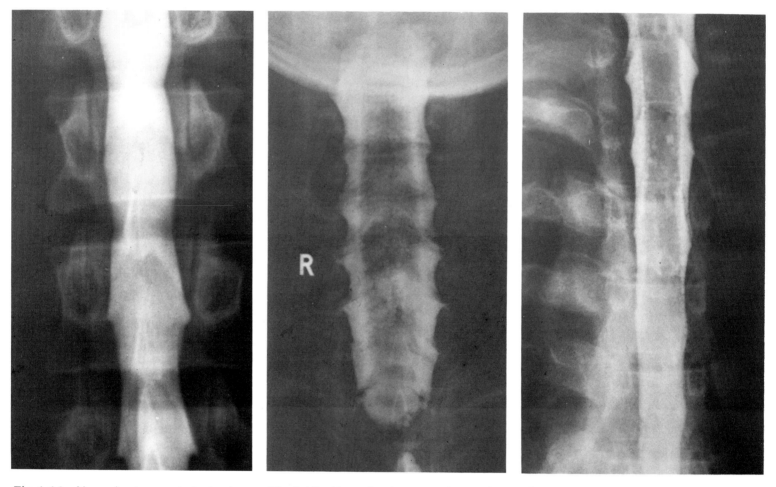

Fig 1.14 Normal anteroposterior lumbar myelogram showing the root pouches.

Fig 1.15 Normal anteroposterior cervical myelogram showing the root pouches and the anterior spinal artery.

Fig 1.16 Normal anteroposterior thoracic myelogram.

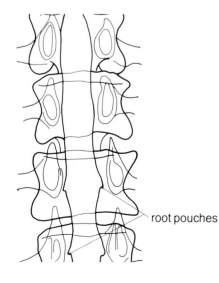

root pouches

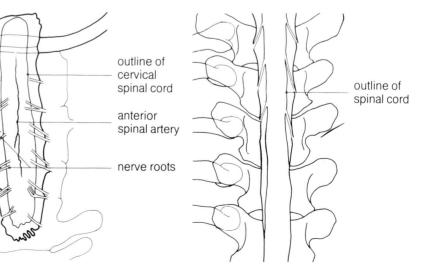

outline of cervical spinal cord

anterior spinal artery

nerve roots

outline of spinal cord

less well defined), together with the shape and size of the spinal cord (Figs. 1.14–1.16). By appropriate positioning, the contrast medium can be manoeuvred into the posterior fossa in order to delineate the basal cisterns, the fourth ventricle and the aqueduct (Fig. 1.17). Where oil-soluble media are used, they are removed at the end of the procedure to lessen risk of a post-myelogram reaction with arachnoiditis.

Air Encephalography

In this procedure air, introduced by the lumbar route, is used to outline the ventricular system, the basal cisterns and the cortical spaces (Figs. 1.18 & 1.19). The examination is normally performed under a general anaesthetic and may be followed by a considerable headache. The information so obtained is available, with considerably less morbidity, using computerised axial tomography, and as a consequence air encephalography has become a largely obsolete procedure.

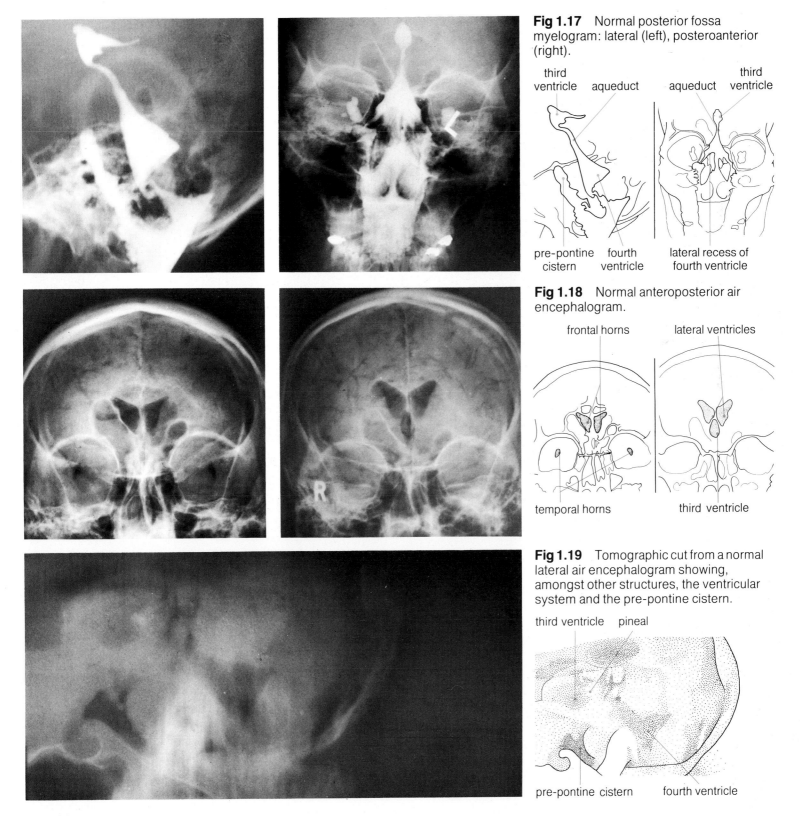

Fig 1.17 Normal posterior fossa myelogram: lateral (left), posteroanterior (right).

third ventricle   aqueduct   aqueduct   third ventricle

pre-pontine cistern   fourth ventricle   lateral recess of fourth ventricle

Fig 1.18 Normal anteroposterior air encephalogram.

frontal horns   lateral ventricles

temporal horns   third ventricle

Fig 1.19 Tomographic cut from a normal lateral air encephalogram showing, amongst other structures, the ventricular system and the pre-pontine cistern.

third ventricle   pineal

pre-pontine cistern   fourth ventricle

1.7

Cerebral Angiography

Visualisation of the cerebral vessels can be obtained either by injection of contrast medium directly into the carotid or vertebral arteries, or alternatively through a catheter introduced via the aortic arch. Direct carotid or vertebral puncture is now less commonly performed. Most recently a technique involving intravenous injection of contrast and computerised subtraction of the arterial phase has been introduced (digital subtraction angiography).

For arch angiography, an introducer for the catheter is inserted, usually into the femoral artery (Figs. 1.20 & 1.21). The catheter is manipulated into the appropriate position for arch injection using radiological screening to verify the catheter's position (Figs. 1.22–1.24).

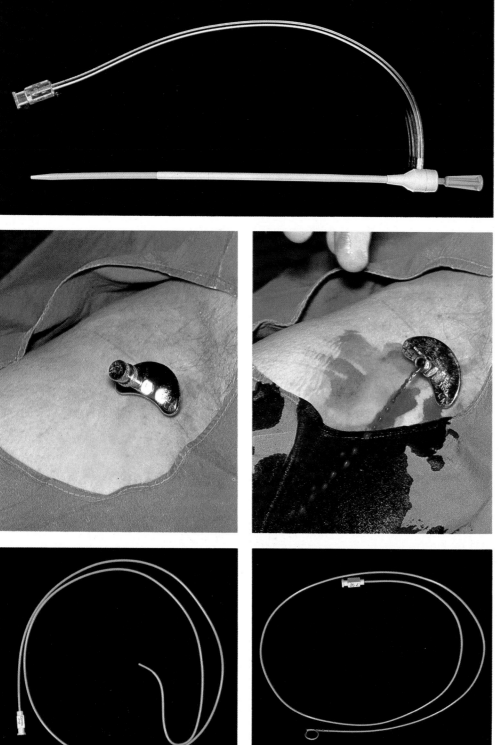

Fig 1.20 The introducer for the catheter used in angiography.

Fig 1.21 The introducer in the femoral artery (left) showing free flow on removal of the stylet (right).

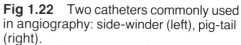

Fig 1.22 Two catheters commonly used in angiography: side-winder (left), pig-tail (right).

The catheter can be manipulated into whichever carotid or vertebral vessel requires examination following demonstration of the aortic arch and its branches (Fig. 1.25). The procedure is not without risk. Persisting neurological deficit has been said to be rare, occurring in less than one per cent of patients, or to be encountered as frequently as in every tenth examination. The factors possibly influencing this morbidity are not clear.

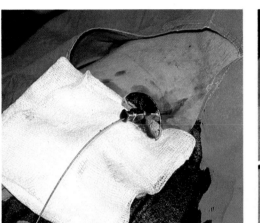
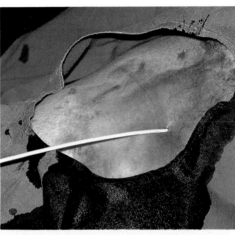

Fig 1.23 Insertion of the guide wire (left) and the final catheter position (right) in the femoral artery for arch angiography.

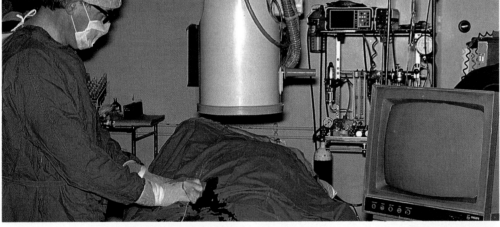

Fig 1.24 Screening in arch angiography.

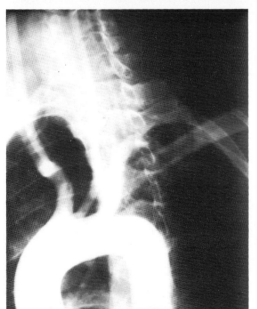
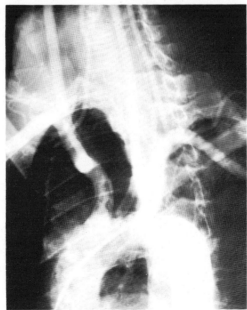

Fig 1.25 Arch angiogram showing separate phases after injection of contrast medium into the aortic arch: early (left) and late (right).

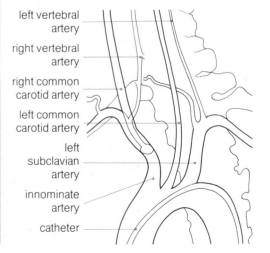

left vertebral artery

right vertebral artery

right common carotid artery

left common carotid artery

left subclavian artery

innominate artery

catheter

Computerised Axial Tomography

The introduction of this technique has revolutionised neurological practice. It allows the ready identification of many intracranial disorders with a procedure which presents little hazard to the patient.

With the introduction of faster scanning times, problems of movement artefact have lessened, and it is unusual for sedation to be necessary and even less common for anaesthesia to be contemplated except in the very young.

With the patient appropriately positioned scans are displayed prior to print out (Figs. 1.26 & 1.27). Most patients are then injected with Conray to improve visualisation of certain pathological structures, particularly tumours. An understanding of neuroanatomy is essential in the interpretation of the findings (Figs. 1.28 & 1.29). The procedure has almost completely replaced air encephalography. Cerebral

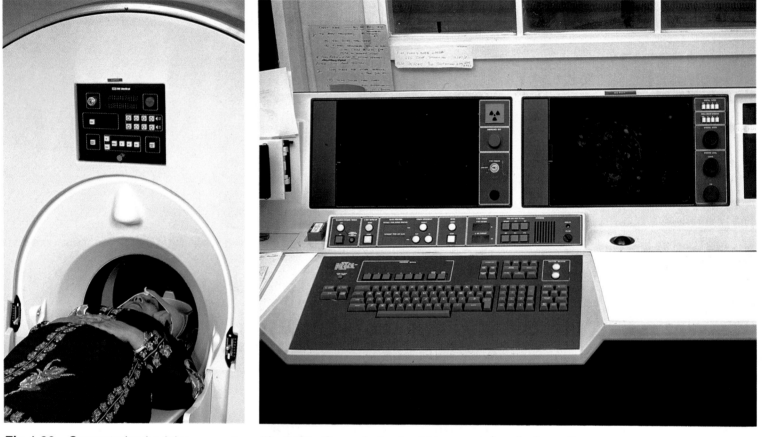

Fig 1.26 Computerised axial tomography: subject positioned in the scanner.

Fig 1.27 Computerised axial tomography: display unit.

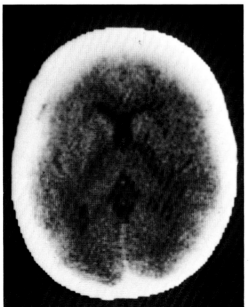

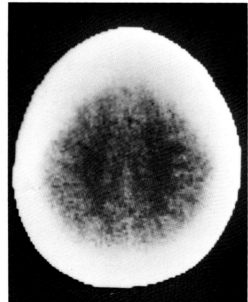

Fig 1.28 Normal CT scans at two levels showing the frontal horns (left) and central white matter (right).

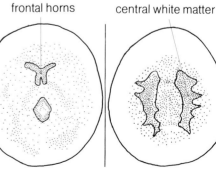

frontal horns   central white matter

angiography remains essential in the investigation of extracranial atheromatous disease and of intracranial aneurysm, whilst myelography continues to be widely used for the assessment of spinal cord and nerve root disorders.

Magnetic Resonance Imaging

Using this technique protons of hydrogen nuclei within the body system are first aligned in a magnetic field and then excited by radiofrequency radiation from a coil surrounding the head. The signals so triggered are detected in a receiver lying within the transmitter system.

In comparison to conventional CT scanning, MRI allows differentiation of grey and white matter, both in the normal scan and in the presence of a number of pathological processes (Figs. 1.30 & 1.31). It promises to be particularly valuable in the evaluation of spinal cord disease.

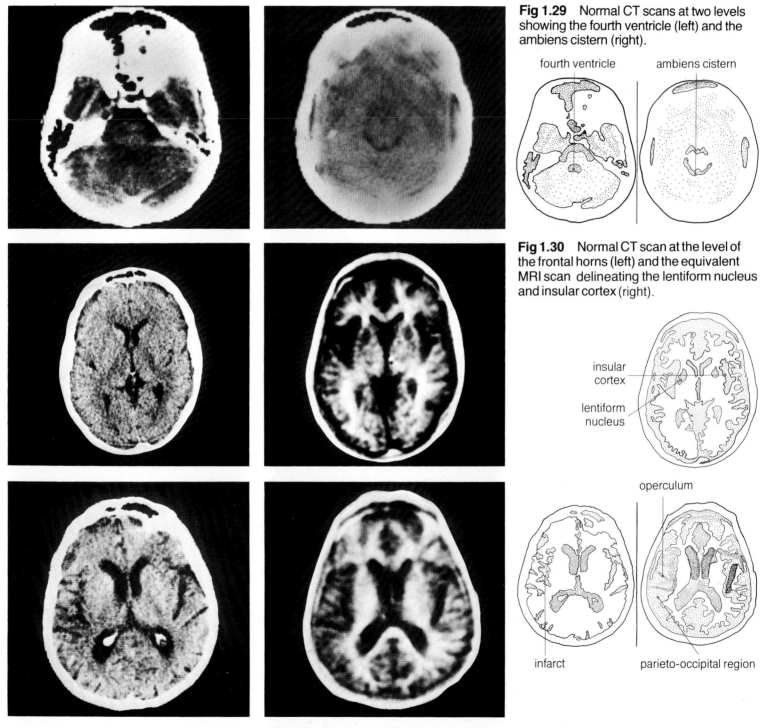

Fig 1.29 Normal CT scans at two levels showing the fourth ventricle (left) and the ambiens cistern (right).

fourth ventricle   ambiens cistern

Fig 1.30 Normal CT scan at the level of the frontal horns (left) and the equivalent MRI scan delineating the lentiform nucleus and insular cortex (right).

insular cortex

lentiform nucleus

operculum

infarct   parieto-occipital region

Fig 1.31 CT and MRI scans showing cerebral infarction. The infarct is revealed on the CT scan as an ill-defined, low-density dark area (left). The equivalent MRI scan shows a loss of white matter in the operculum and parieto-occipital region lateral to the posterior horn of the lateral ventricle (right).

Electroencephalography

Eight or sixteen channel EEG recorders are used to measure cerebral potentials via scalp electrodes (Fig. 1.32). A standard system of electrode placement is used and the signals, first amplified, are then recorded on paper (Fig. 1.33). Bipolar recording measures the potential difference between two electrodes, unipolar the difference between a single electrode and, most commonly, an average reference electrode which summates potentials from all the measuring sites.

With maturation of the human brain, the basic EEG rhythms accelerate from the initially predominant theta and delta activity to the normal adult record, in which the dominant rhythm is designated alpha, at 8–13 Hz, and is most conspicuous in the post-central areas (Fig. 1.34).

As a routine part of the recording, the patient is asked to hyperventilate and is exposed to a photic stimulus consisting of a flashing light source at a frequency up to 20/second. The EEG is of particular value in the investigation of epilepsy. With the advent of CT scanning, the role of the EEG in the investigation and management of other neurological disorders has diminished. It is no longer considered an essential part of the assessment of brain death, and its value in diagnosis, outside epilepsy, is largely confined to such conditions as Creutzfeld-Jakob disease and subacute sclerosing panencephalitis.

Visually Evoked Responses

Stimulation of the visual pathway by an alternating

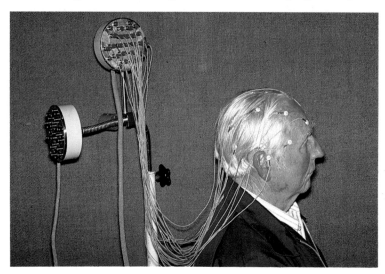

Fig 1.32   EEG electrodes positioned on the scalp.

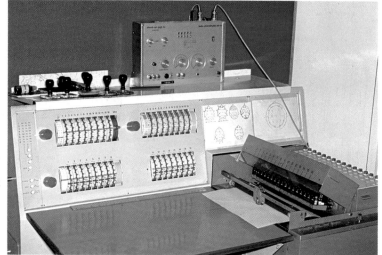

Fig 1.33   The EEG recording apparatus.

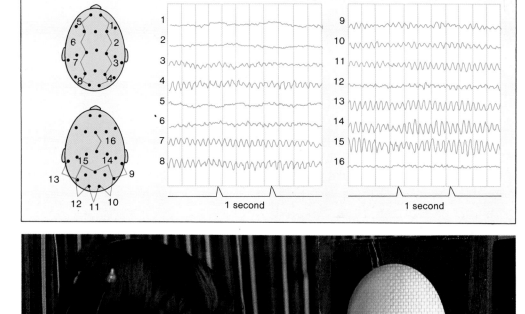

Fig 1.34   A normal 16 channel EEG record (position 6).

Fig 1.35   Subject being tested for visually evoked responses using a screen of alternating light and dark squares.

pattern of light and dark squares produces a well-defined positive potential, recorded with occipital electrodes (Figs. 1.35–1.37). The amplitude of the response is dependent on a number of factors, including visual acuity, whereas the latency is independent of acuity.

Abnormal responses, particularly with respect to latency, have been identified most commonly in multiple sclerosis. A wide variety of other neurological disorders, including Freidreich's ataxia and Parkinson's disease, have a similar effect, though usually to a lesser degree in terms of prolongation of the latency. The procedure is of particular value in the diagnosis of multiple sclerosis, allowing the identification of more widespread, though subclinical, involvement of the nervous system than the patient's presenting symptoms might have suggested.

Auditory Evoked Responses

By an analogous technique, using a click stimulus, and recording with electrodes over the skull, early, middle and late responses have been identified, which are thought to arise from specific parts of the auditory pathway. The five early components occur within 8 ms of the stimulus and arise successively from the auditory nerve, the cochlear nucleus, the superior olivary nucleus, the lateral lemniscus and the inferior colliculus.

Of the early components, the fifth is the only one which is recordable in all normal subjects (Fig. 1.38). Its latency, in the region of 6 ms for a stimulus strength of 70 dB, becomes longer as the stimulus strength is reduced.

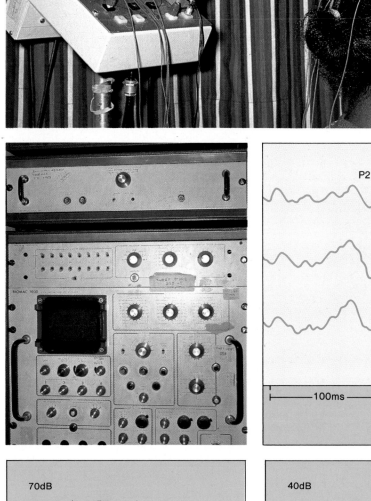

Fig 1.36 Electrode placement for visually evoked responses.

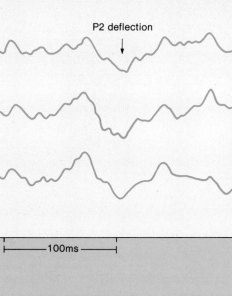

Fig 1.37 The recording apparatus used in the visually evoked response test (left), and normal potentials (right).

P2 deflection

├─── 100ms ───┤

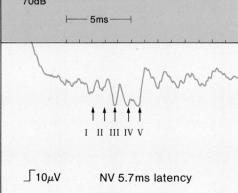

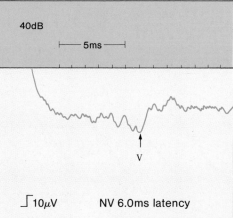

70dB

├─ 5ms ─┤

↑ ↑ ↑ ↑ ↑
I II III IV V

⌐10μV   NV 5.7ms latency

40dB

├─ 5ms ─┤

↑
V

⌐10μV   NV 6.0ms latency

Fig 1.38 Normal auditory evoked response using the two stimuli of different amplitudes: 70dB (left) and 40 dB (right). At 40 dB only the fifth component of the early response is readily detectable.

The technique is again of value in detecting clinically silent brain stem lesions. For example the NV response may be abnormal in some fifty per cent of multiple sclerosis cases without evidence of brain stem abnormalities on neurological examination.

Somatosensory Evoked Potentials
Here the median nerve, for example, is stimulated at the wrist and recordings made with disc electrodes over the cervical spine. The investigation has mostly been applied to the assessment of patients with multiple sclerosis.

Electromyography
Modern electromyography includes both the sampling of muscle to analyse spontaneous activity and the shape of units activated voluntarily, as well as the measurement of sensory and motor conduction (Fig. 1.39).

For sensory conduction in the upper limbs, ring electrodes are applied to median or ulnar innervated fingers, and the potential recorded at the wrist (Fig. 1.40). The potential so obtained can be analysed in terms of its amplitude, and the latency from stimulus to potential peak (Fig. 1.41). In the lower limbs, the only pure sensory nerve commonly studied is the sural nerve, stimulated usually in the calf and the antidromic potential measured at the ankle.

Motor conduction studies can be made using either surface or needle electrodes. The velocity of conduction in a given segment of the nerve can be measured by stimulating the nerve at two separate points, and

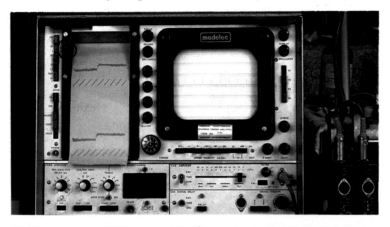

Fig 1.39 The apparatus used in electromyography and nerve conduction studies.

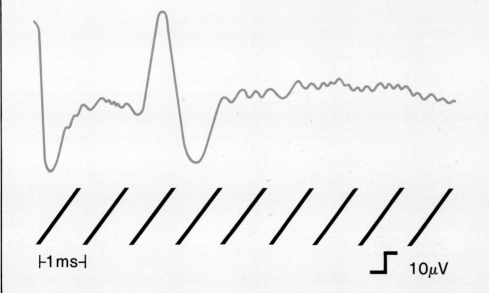

Fig 1.40 Ring electrodes on the index finger for the recording of the median sensory action potential.

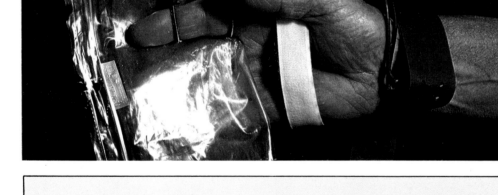

Fig 1.41 Normal median sensory action potential.

|–1 ms–| 10μV

1.14

measuring the time difference in the latencies of the muscle action potential so evoked. For example for the ulnar nerve, surface electrodes are positioned over the hypothenar eminence, and the nerve stimulated first at the wrist and then at the elbow (Fig. 1.42). In the lower limb, electrodes can be placed in or on extensor digitorum brevis and the lateral popliteal nerve stimulated at the knee, followed by the anterior tibial nerve at the ankle. Other peripheral nerves can be studied in a similar fashion (Fig. 1.43).

Sampling of muscle fibre activity requires the use of a concentric needle electrode (CNE) (Fig. 1.44). Spontaneous activity, outside the area of the end-plate, is absent in normal muscle. With voluntary activation of the muscle in question, motor unit potentials can be recorded, and their size and duration measured. With increasing activation individual units merge into an interference pattern which is influenced not only by a number of different pathological processes which can affect muscle, but also by the patient's motivation.

Muscle and Nerve Biopsy

Muscle biopsy can be performed either under direct vision, or by a needle. The former has the advantage of allowing a larger, and hopefully more representative, specimen to be obtained. The latter procedure is less traumatic and can, theoretically, be repeated if necessary to follow the progress of a particular condition.

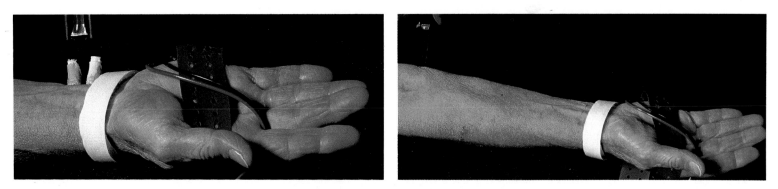

Fig 1.42 Ulnar motor nerve conduction studies: stimulation at the wrist (left) and at the elbow (right).

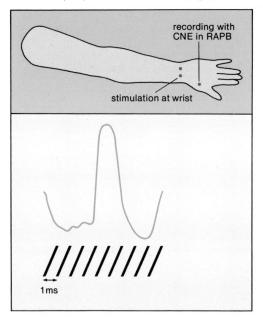
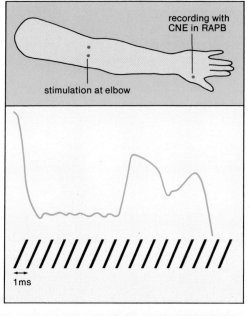

Fig 1.43 Median motor conduction studies with a concentric needle electrode in right abductor pollicis brevis (RAPB) and median nerve stimulation at the wrist and elbow. By measuring the distance between the two points of stimulation and the time difference in the latencies of the muscle action potentials recorded, the speed of conduction may be calculated.

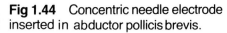

Fig 1.44 Concentric needle electrode inserted in abductor pollicis brevis.

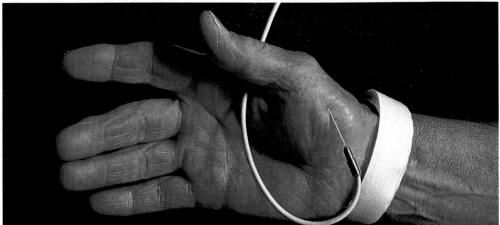

In normal muscle, the fibres lie in close relationship to each other, with one or more peripheral nuclei. Fibre size increases with age until adulthood, and may show some variation within the same biopsy specimen (Fig. 1.45).

Specific staining techniques allow separation of muscle fibres into two main types, Type I or slow reacting, and Type II or fast reacting fibres. Type II is divided into two or even three subcategories considered by some to reflect variations in the fibre's capacity to show resistance to fatigue. Staining with myofibrillar adenosine triphosphate (ATPase) at pH 9.4, produces a dark staining reaction in Type II and a light reaction in Type I fibres (Fig. 1.46). Using nicotine adenine dinucleotide tetrazolium reductase (NADH –tr) the reverse staining is encountered, with some difference also between Type II A and II B fibres.

There is considerable variation in normal muscle in the distribution of fibre type. In biceps, there are approximately equal numbers of Type I, Type IIA and Type IIB fibres. An increased proportion of one fibre type, or a selective atrophy, are recognised consequences of certain muscle disorders.

Nerve biopsy is rarely performed. Usually the sural nerve is chosen, leading consequently to some alteration in sensation along the lateral border of the foot. Examination of the specimen may allow better classification of a neuropathic process, and occasionally provides diagnostic information (eg.with amyloidosis).

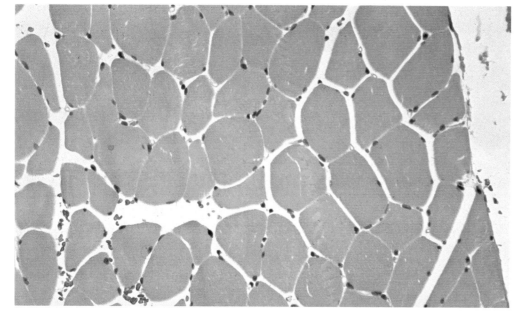

Fig 1.45 Histology of normal muscle. H & E stain, × 600.

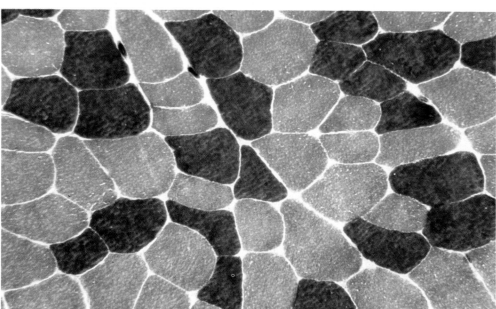

Fig 1.46 Histology of normal muscle: Type 1, lightly staining and Type 2, darkly staining. ATPase stain (at pH 9.4), × 600.

2. Peripheral Nerve Disease

Diffuse disturbance of peripheral nerve function causes the syndrome of peripheral neuropathy, or neuritis. Involvement of more than one peripheral nerve, but not in a diffuse pattern, is entitled mononeuritis multiplex, whilst a single nerve disturbance can be designated as a mononeuropathy.

PERIPHERAL NEUROPATHY

Typically this manifests clinically as distal weakness, sometimes with wasting, distal sensory loss and hypo- or areflexia. The causes of this clinical syndrome are legion, including both familial and acquired disorders. A clinical classification which divides the condition into sensory, motor or mixed neuropathies is of limited value, since the same condition, for example diabetes, may present in a number of clinical guises. A system based on metabolic dysfunction of the axon is limited to certain axonal neuropathies, whilst a pathological classification into axonal and demyelinating neuropathies leaves a large number of cases in which both elements are to be found. In the end, despite its limitation, a method using the underlying disease process as its basis provides the most acceptable classification.

Familial Disorders
CHARCOT-MARIE-TOOTH DISEASE

This condition is subdivided into a hypertrophic form (Type I) where demyelination is prominent and a neuronal form (Type II) where axonal degeneration is more conspicuous. Rarely, spinal muscular atrophy, a disease of the anterior horn cell, may produce a similar clinical picture.

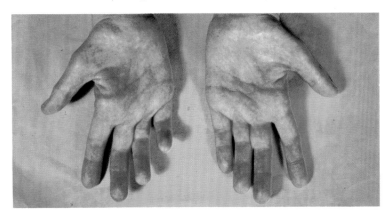

Fig. 2.1. Charcot-Marie-Tooth disease: wasting of small hand muscles.

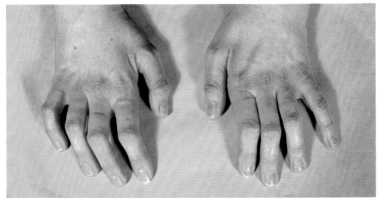

Onset of distal weakness occurred at age 9. Examination, aged 38, revealed gross distal weakness of upper and lower limbs with absent ankle jerks and depressed vibration sense in the feet. The peripheral nerves were thickened.

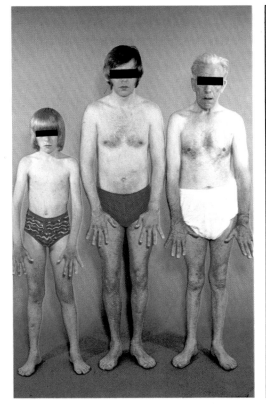

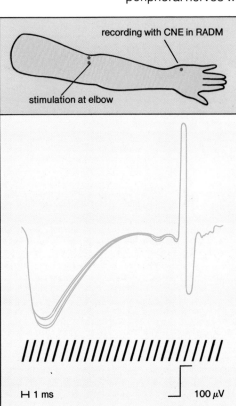

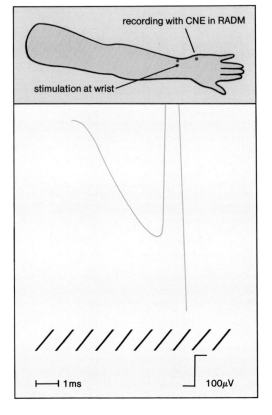

Fig. 2.2. Charcot-Marie-Tooth disease in three generations: distal wasting is most evident in the propositus (right).

Fig. 2.3. Charcot-Marie-Tooth disease. Conduction velocity in the ulnar nerve in the forearm, with concentric needle electrode (CNE) in right abductor digiti minimi (RADM) and nerve stimulation at elbow and wrist. Motor conduction velocity in the forearm is 19 m/sec with a distal motor latency of 6.3 ms.

In the hypertrophic form pes cavus is usual, combined with gross distal weakness and wasting of the lower limbs, predominantly affecting tibialis anterior, the peronei and the small foot muscles. There is weakness and wasting of the small hand muscles (Fig. 2.1). Sensory changes are less conspicuous. Many patients in this group will have nerve hypertrophy. The condition is inherited as an autosomal dominant (Fig. 2.2). Involvement of non-neuronal structures is uncommon. The neuronal form (Type II) has a similar clinical picture but appears later, affects the hands less severely, but the plantar flexors of the feet more so than in the hypertrophic form. Pes cavus is the rule in this group.

Nerve conduction studies in the hypertrophic form show marked slowing of conduction velocity with prolongation of distal motor and sensory latencies (Fig. 2.3).

DEJERINE-SOTTAS DISEASE (Type III)

This condition, an autosomal recessive, presents in childhood with severe distal weakness, wasting and sensory loss. The peripheral nerves are enlarged. Pathological changes include Schwann cell proliferation, endoneurial fibrosis and segmental demyelination (Fig. 2.4).

HEREDITARY SENSORY NEUROPATHY

Patients with this condition, inherited as a dominant (Type I) or recessive (Type II), present with distal sensory loss, trophic ulcers and lancinating pains, mainly in the lower limbs. In Type I, pain and temperature sensation are selectively involved whereas touch is more affected in Type II. Histological changes include loss of fibres in the dorsal roots with corresponding degeneration of the posterior columns of the spinal cord (Fig. 2.5).

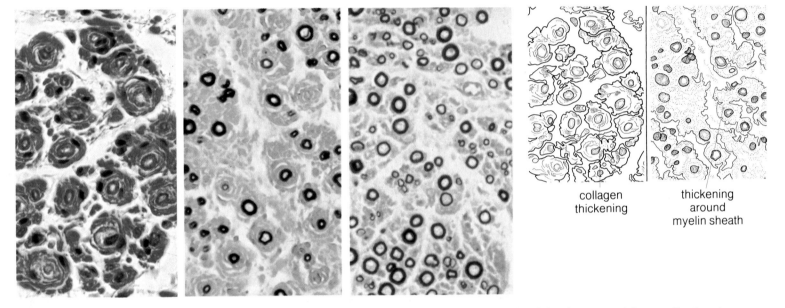

collagen
thickening

thickening
around
myelin sheath

Fig. 2.4. Dejerine-Sottas disease. Nerve histology showing collagen as blue-green with Masson's trichrome stain (left, x 350); and with osmic acid stain showing reduction in the number of myelinated fibres with thickening around the myelin sheaths, composed of collagen and Schwann cells (middle, x 375). A control section is shown on the right.

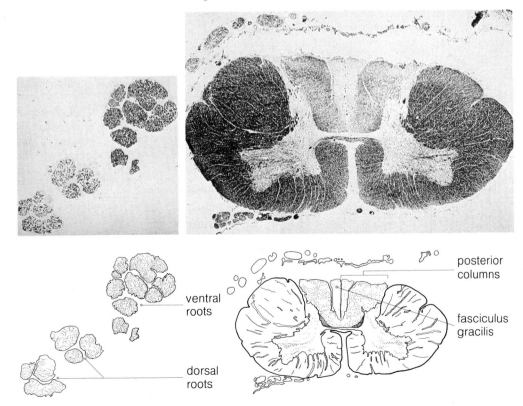

Fig. 2.5. Hereditary sensory neuropathy. Root and spinal cord histology showing fibre fall out in dorsal roots, (left, x 25) and degeneration of posterior columns at the cervical level, maximal in fasciculus gracilis (right, x 6).

From childhood, loss of pain sensation below the knees occurred, followed by infected foot ulcers, and loss of distal sensation in the upper limbs. The patient died from a chest infection, aged 39. His father's feet were insensitive to tickle.

ventral
roots

dorsal
roots

posterior
columns

fasciculus
gracilis

METACHROMATIC LEUCODYSTROPHY

In this condition, deficiency of one of the enzymes, arylsulphatase A, (B, C) is associated with the accumulation of sulphatides and the development of demyelination in the central and peripheral nervous systems. Peripheral nerve sections show loss of large myelinated fibres, widespread demyelination, infiltration by phagocytes, and deposition of metachromatic (sulphatide) granules (Fig. 2.6).

AMYLOID NEUROPATHY

Various types of amyloid disease may be associated with a peripheral neuropathy, including the forms inherited as an autosomal dominant and the non-familial type. A generalised neuropathy is usual, sometimes with a predilection for particular sites, for example in or around the median nerve in the carpal tunnel. Pain and temperature fibres may be predominantly affected and the process sometimes extends to involve autonomic fibres. Peripheral nerve may show amyloid deposition (Fig. 2.7) together with evidence, particularly in the Portugese type described by Andrade, of loss of unmyelinated nerve fibres (Fig. 2.7).

Other forms of hereditary neuropathy include those associated with porphyria, Refsum's disease and Friedreich's ataxia.

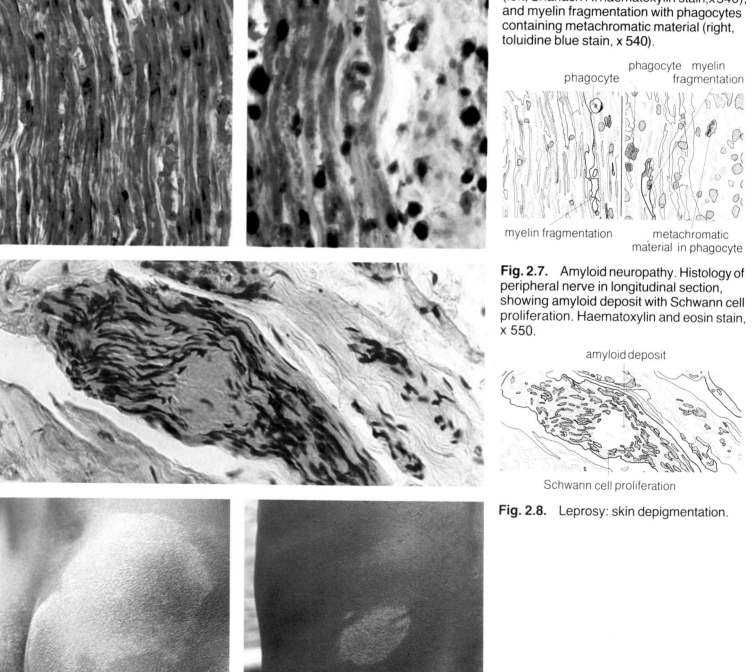

Fig. 2.6. Metachromatic leucodystrophy. Peripheral nerve histology showing myelin fragmentation with phagocytic infiltration (left, Sharlach R. haematoxylin stain, x 540), and myelin fragmentation with phagocytes containing metachromatic material (right, toluidine blue stain, x 540).

phagocyte
phagocyte   myelin
fragmentation
myelin fragmentation
metachromatic
material in phagocyte

Fig. 2.7. Amyloid neuropathy. Histology of peripheral nerve in longitudinal section, showing amyloid deposit with Schwann cell proliferation. Haematoxylin and eosin stain, x 550.

amyloid deposit

Schwann cell proliferation

Fig. 2.8. Leprosy: skin depigmentation.

Acquired Neuropathies

Major groups of conditions associated with a peripheral neuropathy include infective diseases, collagen vascular disease and metabolic disorders.

Perhaps the commonest worldwide cause of peripheral neuropathy is leprosy. Differing types of this condition are partly related to variations in host resistance to the causative agent, mycobacterium leprae. Hypopigmented anaesthetic areas occur in tuberculoid leprosy whilst enlarged peripheral nerves occur in both tuberculoid and lepromatous forms (Figs. 2.8 & 2.9). In tuberculoid leprosy, nerve biopsy (Fig. 2.10) reveals infiltration by granulomata sometimes with giant cell formation, together with segmental demyelination. In lepromatous leprosy, the perineurium and Schwann cells show infiltration by lepromatous bacilli (Fig. 2.10).

Guillain-Barré syndrome is known under a number of synonyms. It manifests as an acute, predominantly motor, polyneuropathy, often with facial and bulbar involvement. Some fifty per cent of patients give a history of a prodromal illness, particularly of the upper respiratory tract. Incomplete recovery is encountered in some 10 per cent of patients. Segmental demyelination is the predominant pathological process, but axonal involvement is not infrequent, resulting in muscle wasting which may persist (Fig. 2.11)

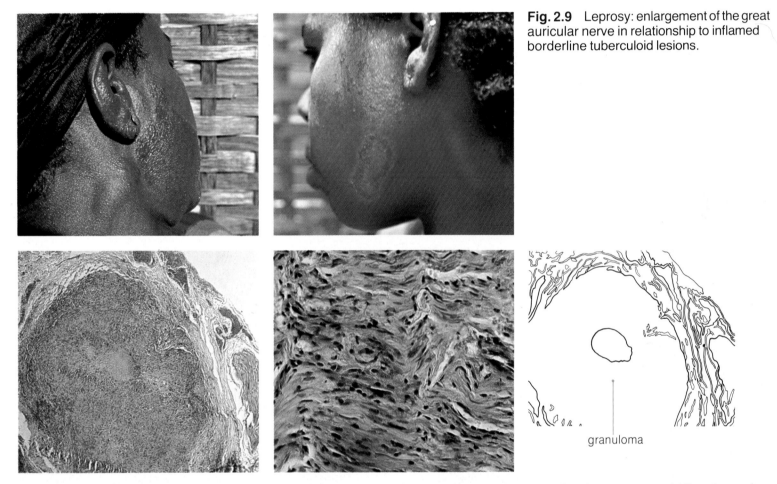

Fig. 2.9 Leprosy: enlargement of the great auricular nerve in relationship to inflamed borderline tuberculoid lesions.

granuloma

Fig. 2.10. Nerve histology in tuberculoid and lepromatous leprosy. Nerve section in tuberculoid leprosy showing granuloma (left, H&E stain, x 150), and a section of ulnar nerve in lepromatous leprosy showing infiltration by bacilli (red) (right, Ziehl-Neelsen stain, x 450).

The right hand section was taken from a 20 year old Egyptian male with lepromatous leprosy who gave a three year history of peripheral wasting, sensory loss and enlarged peripheral nerves.

Fig. 2.11. Guillain-Barré syndrome: limb wasting.

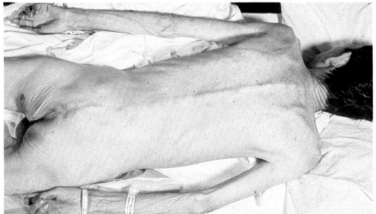

Peripheral neuropathy can occur in any of the collagen vascular diseases, usually as a consequence of a vasculopathy affecting the vasa nervorum (Figs. 2.12 & 2.13). In rheumatoid arthritis a variety of clinical syndromes are described, including sensory neuropathy, a digital neuropathy and a mixed sensorimotor neuropathy (Figs. 2.14 & 2.15). Peripheral neuropathy is common in polyarteritis nodosa, which may also present with mononeuritis multiplex.

Diabetes is similarly associated with a number of differing neuropathic complications. A generalised neuropathy, predominantly sensory, is seen, sometimes with involvement of autonomic fibres. Mononeuritis multiplex occurs, as do isolated cranial nerve palsies. When distal sensory loss is severe, trophic ulcers develop along with painless fractures and Charcot joints (Fig. 2.16). The neuropathy is of the demyelinating type though accompanied in some instances by axonal

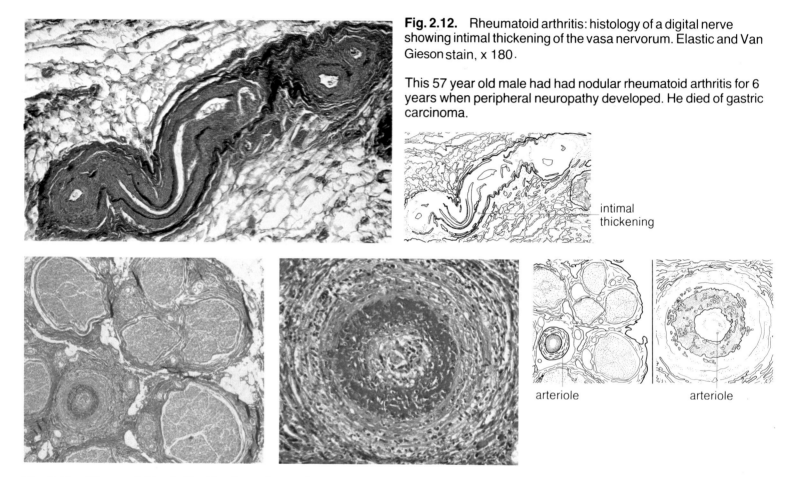

Fig. 2.12. Rheumatoid arthritis: histology of a digital nerve showing intimal thickening of the vasa nervorum. Elastic and Van Gieson stain, x 180.

This 57 year old male had had nodular rheumatoid arthritis for 6 years when peripheral neuropathy developed. He died of gastric carcinoma.

intimal thickening

arteriole   arteriole

Fig. 2.13. Rheumatoid arthritis: histology of a sural nerve showing fibrinoid arteritis. An eosinophilic deposit (staining bright red) involves the media with destruction of the intima and occlusion of the lumen of a large arteriole. There is perineurial fibrosis of the nerve bundles. Trichrome stain: x 30 (left), x 180 (right).

This 68 year old female presented with a long history of rheumatoid arthritis and developed a severe vasculitis with sensorimotor neuropathy, skin ulceration and visceral involvement.

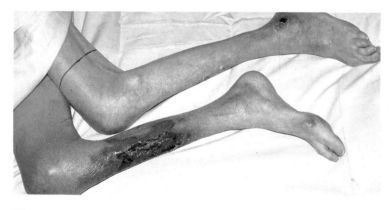

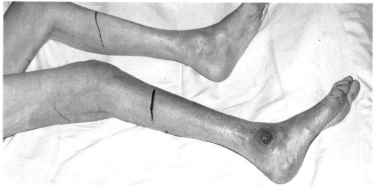

Fig. 2.14. Rheumatoid arthritis: sensorimotor neuropathy. The black lines indicate the margins of distal sensory impairment.

This 60 year old woman had a nodular seropositive rheumatoid arthritis, complicated by a severe mixed peripheral neuropathy.

2.6

degeneration. Slowing of conduction velocity, particularly in sensory nerves, may be prominent. In diabetic amyotrophy, weakness and wasting of the thighs are accompanied by depression of the knee reflexes but relatively minor sensory abnormalities. There is some evidence that careful diabetic control hinders the development of these complications, and improves the prognosis for recovery.

Though numerous other causes of peripheral neuropathy are recognised, for example alcoholism, toxic and deficiency disorders and malignant disease, it has to be acknowledged that in a substantial proportion of patients presenting with this clinical syndrome the underlying cause remains unidentified (Fig. 2.17).

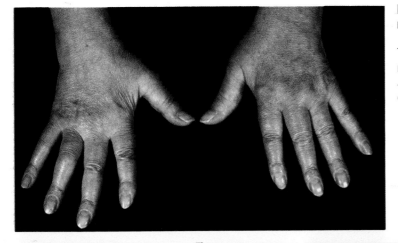

Fig. 2.15. Rheumatoid arthritis: wasting of the small hand muscles.

This 61 year old female had longstanding rheumatoid arthritis. Her main neurological complaint was of paroxysmal lower limb pain and numbness, precipitated by exercise, due to intermittent claudication of the cauda equina.

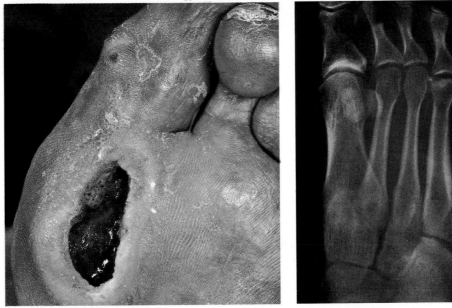

Fig. 2.16. Diabetes: perforating ulcer surrounded by callous tissue under first metatarsal head (left) and fractures at the bases of the fourth and fifth metatarsals and the head of the fourth metatarsal (right).

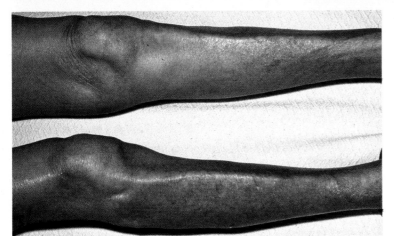

Fig. 2.17. Peripheral neuropathy. Distal lower limb wasting in peripheral neuropathy of unknown cause.

The patient, aged 84, had evidence of a mixed neuropathy with severe wasting, depressed reflexes and reduced sensation peripherally in the lower limbs.

THE MONONEUROPATHIES

These may occur as a result of the entrapment of a nerve in a confined space, for example the median nerve in the carpal tunnel or as a result of direct injury to the nerve, for example the radial nerve as it crosses the spiral groove of the humerus. Alternatively a nerve may become stretched over a bony or tendonous point, for example, with the ulnar nerve in the ulnar groove. Sometimes a mononeuropathy may reflect a systemic disease such as polyarteritis nodosa.

Carpal Tunnel Syndrome

This is the commonest of the entrapment or compressive neuropathies. The condition occurs more often in women and correlates with the dimensions of the carpal tunnel as assessed by computerised tomography. Several disorders predispose to its development, either by influencing the configuration of the canal (for example, myxoedema or previous bony injury), or by enlarging the nerve itself (for example leprosy).

Most patients present with pain or paraesthesiae. The pain is often rather diffusely distributed in the limb, and occurs predominantly at night. Sensory signs may be rather nebulous, though some discrete alteration of sensation between median and ulnar innervated digits is likely. Weakness of abductor pollicis brevis develops, eventually with wasting of the thenar eminence and failure of opposition produces a lack of thumb rotation when it is opposed to the base of the little finger (Fig. 2.18). In some patients, the syndrome may be precipitated by deformity of the canal consequent to previous wrist fracture (Fig. 2.19).

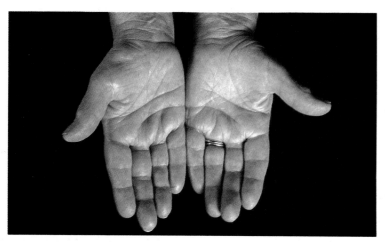

Fig. 2.18. Carpal tunnel syndrome: wasting of the thenar eminence (left); failure of opposition (right).

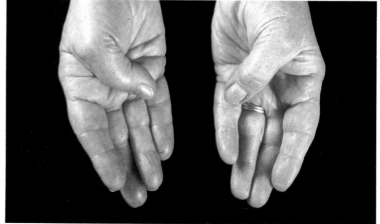

This 74 year old female presented with a longstanding right carpal tunnel syndrome.

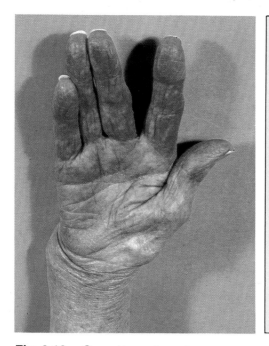

Fig. 2.19. Carpal tunnel syndrome: wasting of the thenar eminence and wrist deformity due to previous fracture.

The patient, an 87 year old female, had been referred following a cerebrovascular accident. She had fractured her wrist 10 years before and the median nerve lesion had been present since.

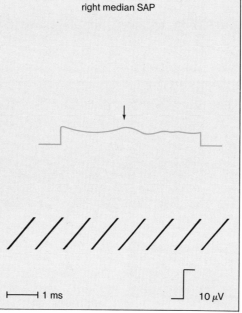

Fig. 2.20. Carpal tunnel syndrome: nerve conduction studies. Depressed, dispersed and delayed median sensory action potential (left); prolonged distal motor latency to abductor pollicis brevis (right).

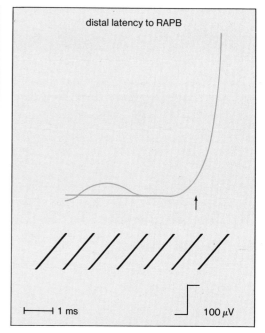

This 63 year old female had a 9 month history of nocturnal paraesthesiae in both hands. Her thyroid function tests suggested early hypothyroidism.

Electrophysiological assessment is vital in the diagnosis. Reduction of the median sensory action potential amplitude (sometimes from a single digit) may occur with or without prolongation of its latency (Fig. 2.20). Alteration of the median/ulnar sensory amplitude ratio may be a more sensitive test of early median involvement. Prolongation of the distal motor latency to abductor pollicis brevis is common (Fig. 2.20). Comparison with the unaffected hand (though the condition is more often bilateral than symptoms suggest) may be of value. In more advanced cases there may be evidence of denervation in abductor pollicis brevis. If surgery is undertaken, the site of constriction of the nerve within the carpal tunnel can often be identified (Fig. 2.21).

Ulnar Nerve Compression

This occurs most commonly at the level of the elbow and produces both sensory and motor abnormalities. In advanced cases, a characteristic hand posture (claw-hand) develops with hyperextension of the fourth and fifth digits at the metacarpophalangeal joints and flexion at the interphalangeal joints due to loss of lumbrical action (Fig. 2.22). With prolonged compression, the nerve becomes thickened at the elbow, sometimes with a positive Tinel sign. Acute compression, for example during a drug or alcohol induced stupor, may be deducible from the presence of pressure marks (Fig. 2.23). Though proximal lesions may involve all ulnar innervated muscles, adductor pollicis and the interossei tend to be predominantly affected (Fig. 2.24).

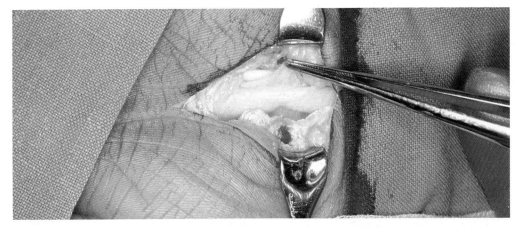

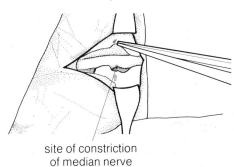

Fig. 2.21. Carpal tunnel syndrome. Operative view showing a constricted nerve within the carpal tunnel.

site of constriction
of median nerve

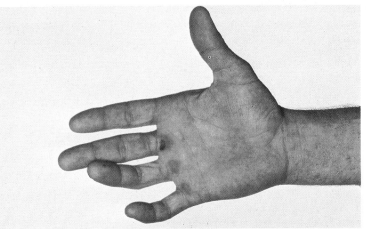

Fig. 2.22. Ulnar nerve palsies: flexion deformity of the fourth and fifth digits.

The patient, a 20 year old drug addict, developed sciatic and bilateral ulnar nerve palsies following a prolonged sleep, induced by drugs, whilst sitting in a hard chair.

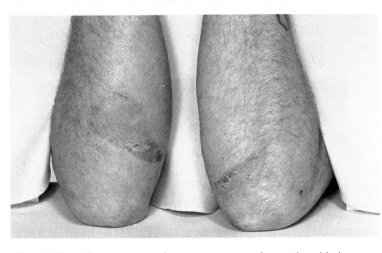

Fig. 2.23. Ulnar nerve palsy: pressure marks on the skin in bilateral acute ulnar nerve compression (the patient shown in figure 2.22).

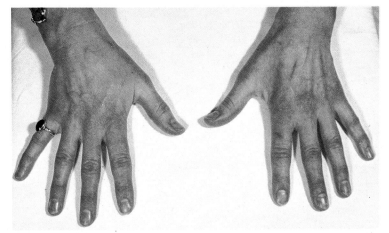

Fig. 2.24. Left ulnar nerve palsy showing wasting of the interossei, hypothenar eminence and adductor pollicis.

2.9

Fractures in the region of the elbow may result in a bony deformity which in turn predisposes to ulnar nerve stretching (Figs. 2.25 & 2.56).

Electrophysiological investigation is likely to show a depressed ulnar sensory action potential (Fig. 2.27), often with slowing in the elbow or forearm segment, with a corresponding slowing of motor conduction velocity, particularly across the elbow. Decrement of the muscle action potential amplitude from abductor digit minimi may be encountered when comparison is made between stimulation at the elbow, and at the wrist (Fig. 2.27).

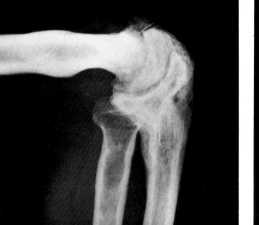 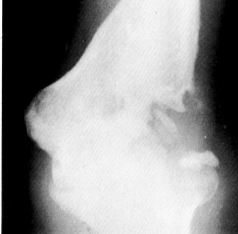 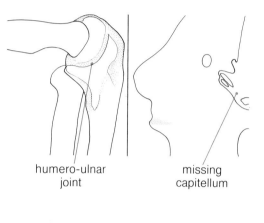

humero-ulnar joint   missing capitellum

Fig. 2.25. Two plane radiographs of the right elbow showing valgus deformity, missing capitellum and irregularity of the articular surfaces of the humero-ulnar joint.

The patient, a 30 year old male, was referred with migrainous neuralgia. Nine years previously a road traffic accident had led to an injury of the right elbow. An ulnar neuropathy developed and the nerve had been transposed.

Fig. 2.26. Ulnar neuropathy. Flexion deformity of the right elbow in the same patient as in figure 2.25.

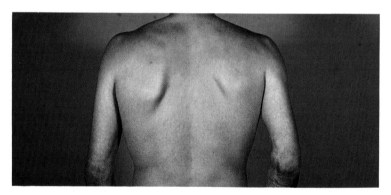

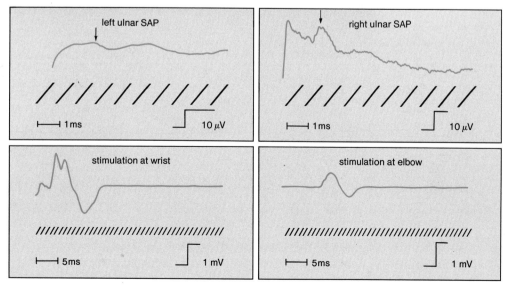

Fig. 2.27. Ulnar neuropathy. Nerve conduction studies: depressed left ulnar sensory action potential (left, upper); slowing of ulnar motor conduction velocity in the forearm (42 m/sec) with 62% decrement of muscle action potential amplitude between elbow and wrist (lower) The right ulnar SAP was normal (right, upper).

This 61 year old male presented with deadness of the ulnar border of the left hand, little and ring fingers for one year. Weakness of the hand developed over a similar period. Examination showed wasting and weakness of the ulnar innervated small hand muscles with reduced sensation in an ulnar distribution and a thickened nerve at the elbow.

Radial Nerve Compression

Typically the nerve is injured as it crosses the spiral groove of the humerus, often as the patient, in an alcohol induced stupor, sleeps with the arm extended over a firm support. The triceps muscle is spared, but there is weakness of brachioradialis and supinator, and of the extensors of the wrist and fingers. The brachioradialis component of the supinator reflex is absent. The fingers and wrist assume a characteristic posture (Figs. 2.28 & 2.29). Sensory changes are often slight, frequently confined to a small zone of reduced sensation in the region of the anatomical snuff box.

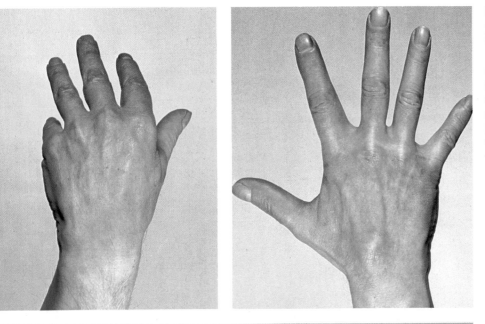

Fig. 2.28. Radial palsy. Hand and wrist posture (left) compared to the normal right hand (right).

Eleven days previously, this 57 year old male had drunk excessively. He fell asleep after reaching home and subsequently noticed difficulty in rolling a cigarette with his left hand. Examination showed weakness of finger and wrist extensors with slight reduction of the pin prick response at the base of the thumb.

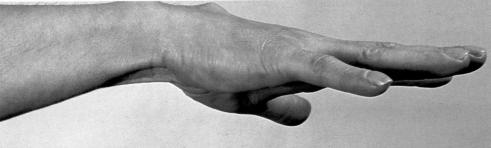

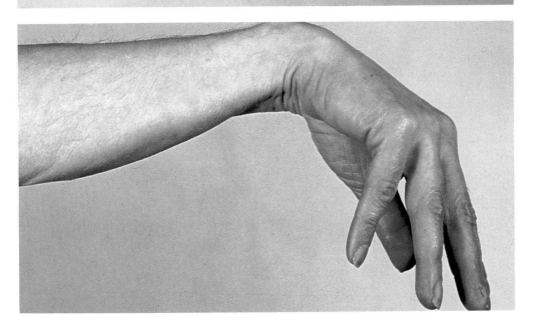

Fig. 2.29. Radial palsy. The hand and wrist postures of the same patient in figure 2.28.

Cervical Rib Syndrome

This condition is more common in women and is due to stretching of the C8 and D1 nerve roots, or the inferior trunk of the brachial plexus, over a fibrous band passing from the C7 transverse process to the first rib. Sensory symptoms, either pain or paraesthesiae, usually antedate motor involvement, and tend to be distributed along the ulnar border of the forearm and hand. Wasting and weakness predominantly affect the thenar eminence, though in longstanding cases, wasting of the small hand muscles becomes generalised (Figs. 2.30 & 2.31). Radiological changes, which unlike the symptomatology are usually bilateral, are more likely to show elongation and beaking of the transverse process of the seventh cervical vertebra than a defined cervical rib (Fig. 2.32). Electromyographic abnormalities include depression or absence of the ulnar sensory action potential, and reduction of the interference pattern in the small hand muscles, sometimes with occasional giant units (Fig. 2.33).

Femoral Neuropathy

Isolated femoral nerve lesions are rather uncommon. They result in weakness and wasting of the quadriceps

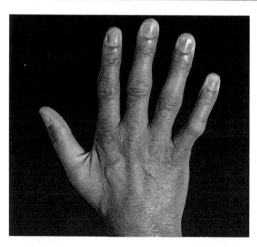

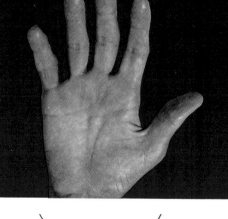

Fig. 2.30. Cervical rib syndrome: wasting of the right thenar eminence.

This 37 year old man had a two year history of weakness of the right thumb with periodic pain along the ulnar border of the forearm. Examination showed gross wasting of the right thenar eminence with moderate weakness of the ulnar innervated small hand muscles. Radiography revealed beaking of the C7 transverse processes. The patient refused surgery.

Fig. 2.31. Cervical rib syndrome: wasting of the small hand muscles.

This 39 year old man gave a 5 year history of wasting of the right hand. Examination showed thinning of the forearm and of all the small hand muscles. There was reduction in the pin prick response over the ulnar border of the hand. Electrophysiological and radiological investigation suggested a cervical rib syndrome and a cervical band was subsequently resected.

Fig. 2.32. Cervical rib syndrome. Radiograph of the thoracic inlet of the patient in figure 2.31 showing beaking of the right C7 transverse process and a rudimentary left cervical rib.

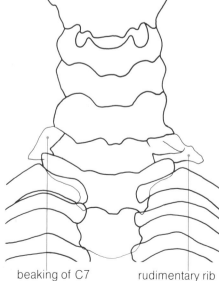

beaking of C7 transverse process

rudimentary rib

muscle with loss of the knee reflex (Fig. 2.34). Sensory abnormalities are variable, usually occupying the thigh, and the medial part of the leg below the knee if the saphenous branch of the nerve is affected.

Sciatic Nerve Lesions
The sciatic nerve may be damaged by a perforating injury, by fractures of the pelvis or femur, and by dislocation of the hip. The nerve may also be damaged by injections into the buttock. A complete sciatic palsy is seldom seen and, even then, the peroneal group of muscles tends to be predominantly affected.

Theoretically there may be weakness of knee flexors, ankle and toe plantar- and dorsiflexors and eversion and inversion (Fig. 2.35 & 2.36). The ankle jerk is depressed or absent and sensation affected over most of the leg below the knee except for the medial part supplied by the saphenous nerve.

Of the other mononeuropathies, the one most frequently seen is lateral popliteal palsy. The nerve is particularly susceptible to trauma as it winds round the neck of the fibula. Though involvement of the peronei, tibialis anterior and the extensors might be expected to be uniform, extensor hallucis longus is often most severely affected.

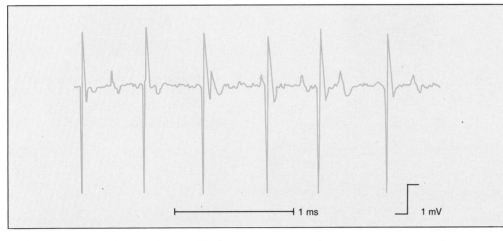

Fig. 2.33. Cervical rib syndrome. EMG of abductor digiti minimi showing large units (same patient as in figure 2.31).

1 ms   1 mV

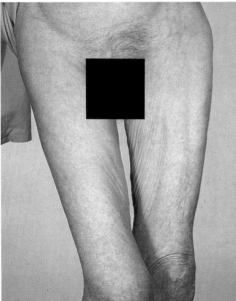

Fig. 2.34. Femoral neuropathy: wasting of the quadriceps muscle.

This female patient, aged 80, had a long history of rheumatoid arthritis. Following a deep vein thrombosis she was anticoagulated but developed a haematoma in the right thigh, with subsequent weakness of the quadriceps muscle. Examination showed wasting of both thighs, more marked on the right, an absent right knee jerk and reduced sensation over the thigh extending onto the anteromedial part of the calf.

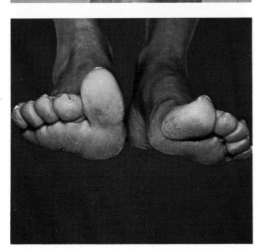

Fig. 2.35. Sciatic palsy. The patient is attempting to dorsiflex the big toes. There is a reduced range of movement on the left.

Following excessive alcohol intake, this 51 year old woman had carried out yoga exercises comprising squatting with trunk flexion. On completing the exercises she found the left foot was limp. Examination 3 weeks later showed wasting of the left calf, weakness of dorsi- and plantar flexion, together with eversion and extensor hallucis longus. Tickle sensation was altered over the dorsum and lateral sole of the foot and the anterolateral border of the calf. The left ankle jerk was absent.

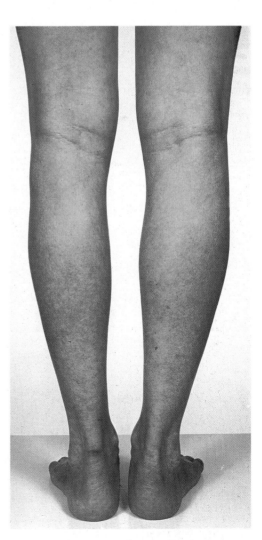

Fig. 2.36. Sciatic palsy. Wasting of the left calf (same patient as in figure 2.35).

Neuralgic Amyotrophy

This condition presents with pain, usually in the region of the shoulder, followed by weakness and wasting of muscles, most commonly of the shoulder girdle group. It may arise spontaneously, or may follow an illness, a vaccination procedure, or injury.

The distribution of muscle weakness is very variable. Sometimes a single peripheral nerve is affected, for example the long thoracic nerve, leading to winging of the scapula when the arm is raised forwards or sideways (Fig. 2.37). On other occasions, the distribution of muscle wasting and weakness suggests a more complex neuropathy, sometimes bilateral (Fig. 38). Sensory changes are rather less conspicuous.

The consequences of mechanical trauma to a peripheral nerve are largely determined by the presence or absence of axonal degeneration. Following complete nerve section, nerve regeneration takes place, in some instances leading to a neuroma which may be markedly tender (Fig. 2.39).

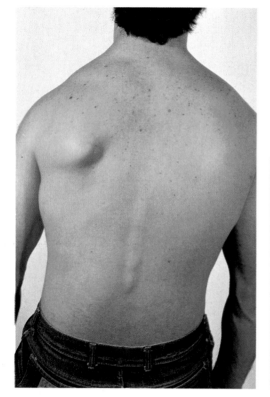

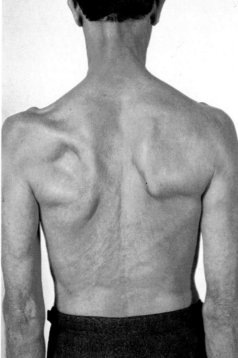

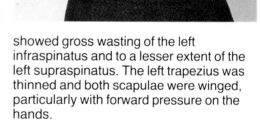

Fig. 2.37. Neuralgic amyotrophy: winging of the left scapula.

The patient, a 22 year old male, had had an episode of pain in the left shoulder one year previously followed by winging of the left scapula.

Fig. 2.38. Neuralgic amyotrophy: wasting of the left spinati and winging of the right scapula.

This 55 year old man had had severe pain in the chest wall on the right 6 months previously for several weeks. Examination showed gross wasting of the left infraspinatus and to a lesser extent of the left supraspinatus. The left trapezius was thinned and both scapulae were winged, particularly with forward pressure on the hands.

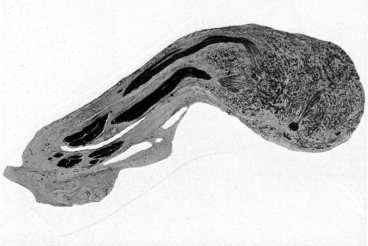

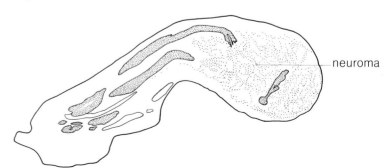

Fig. 2.39. Histology of a digital neuroma. Longitudinal section showing a neuroma composed of interwoven, thin, myelinated nerve fibres, connective tissue and Schwann cells. x 85.

The patient had had a digital nerve divided six months previously. A tender 'neuroma' was subsequently removed at the site of nerve regeneration.

3. Motor Neurone Disease, Primary Muscle Disease and Disorders of the Neuromuscular Junction

Motor neurone disease is a condition of later life, occurring predominantly in the sixth and seventh decades, and slightly more common in men. The pathological changes affect the motor cortex, the pyramidal pathways, the cranial nerve motor nuclei (other than those supplying the eye muscles) and the anterior horn cells (Figs. 3.1 & 3.2). Secondary degenerative changes occur in peripheral nerve and skeletal muscle. Although the signs of the disease are confined to the motor system, subtle pathological changes are detectable in other pathways, for example the posterior columns. The clinical features reflect the distribution of pathological changes, and a number of syndromes have been designated in the past to reflect this. Eventually the picture is fairly uniform

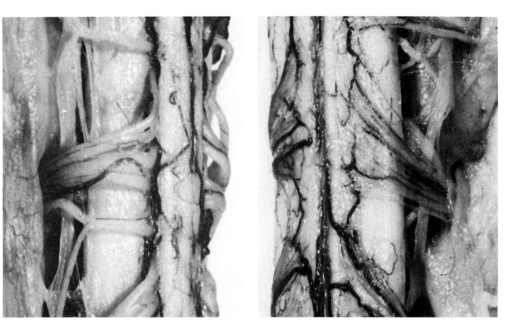

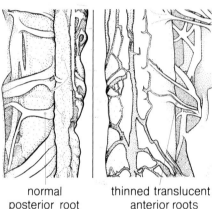

Fig. 3.1 Anterior and posterior nerve roots from the cervical cord of a patient with motor neurone disease. There is a marked discrepancy in size between the normal, posterior roots (left) and the atrophic anterior roots (right).

normal posterior root | thinned translucent anterior roots

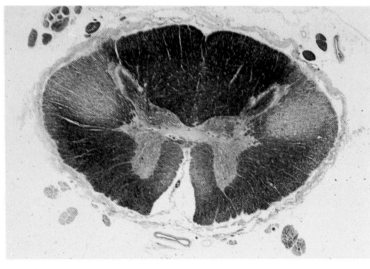

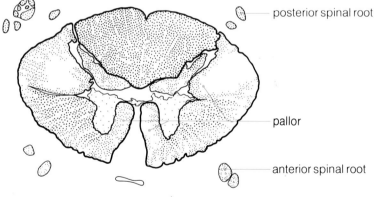

Fig. 3.2 Thoracic cord: myelin preparation showing marked pallor of lateral and anterior corticospinal tracts. Klüver-Barrera stain.

posterior spinal root

pallor

anterior spinal root

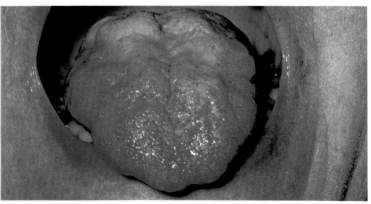

Fig. 3.3 Wasting of the tongue.

The patient, aged 63, had a 9 month history of progressive limb weakness, with more recent dysphagia and dysarthria. Examination revealed a weak palate, a wasted, fasciculating tongue and a combination of lower and upper motor neurone signs in the limbs.

embracing bulbar involvement, with wasting of the tongue, wasting of the limbs, particularly the hands, and evidence of pyramidal involvement with brisk reflexes and extensor plantar responses (Figs. 3.3 & 3.4). Mentation is usually spared, as is sphincter function.

The diagnosis may be difficult when weakness and wasting are initially confined to one limb, suggesting spondylotic disease or even a mononeuropathy (Figs. 3.5 & 3.6).

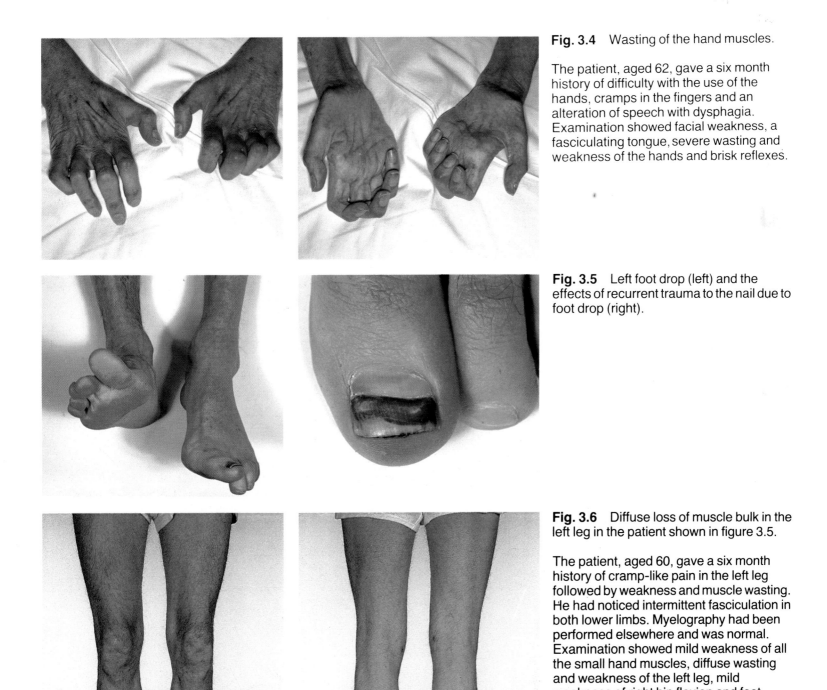

Fig. 3.4 Wasting of the hand muscles.

The patient, aged 62, gave a six month history of difficulty with the use of the hands, cramps in the fingers and an alteration of speech with dysphagia. Examination showed facial weakness, a fasciculating tongue, severe wasting and weakness of the hands and brisk reflexes.

Fig. 3.5 Left foot drop (left) and the effects of recurrent trauma to the nail due to foot drop (right).

Fig. 3.6 Diffuse loss of muscle bulk in the left leg in the patient shown in figure 3.5.

The patient, aged 60, gave a six month history of cramp-like pain in the left leg followed by weakness and muscle wasting. He had noticed intermittent fasciculation in both lower limbs. Myelography had been performed elsewhere and was normal. Examination showed mild weakness of all the small hand muscles, diffuse wasting and weakness of the left leg, mild weakness of right hip flexion and foot dorsiflexion, a brisk left knee jerk, but depressed ankle jerks and fasciculation in both thighs. Sensation was normal. EMG showed normal motor and sensory conduction, but fasciculation potentials in all four limbs.

Electrophysiological investigation shows normal sensory conduction and little abnormality of motor conduction save for a mild slowing of velocity in some cases. Muscle sampling shows fibrillation and fasciculation potentials, (Fig. 3.7) together with prolonged units of increased amplitude. Muscle biopsy shows the changes associated with neurogenic atrophy, namely grouped atrophic fibres, sometimes interspersed with fibre hypertrophy (Fig. 3.8).

Other diseases of the anterior horn cell include spinal muscular atrophy and poliomyelitis. The latter condition is now rare in the United Kingdom. Late sequelae include muscle atrophy, joint deformity and various alterations of limb posture (Figs. 3.9 & 3.10).

PRIMARY MUSCLE DISORDERS

Amongst this group of disorders are those genetically determined, that is, the muscular dystrophies, and a number of acquired conditions which affect muscle directly rather than by involvement of its nerve supply. Primary muscle disease tends to produce a proximal, symmetrical weakness, though this is by no means inevitable. Proximal weakness causes difficulty in walking, in climbing stairs, and in standing from a sitting or lying posture, though a very similar picture may also be encountered in the chronic spinal muscular atrophies (Fig. 3.11).

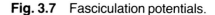

Fig. 3.7 Fasciculation potentials.

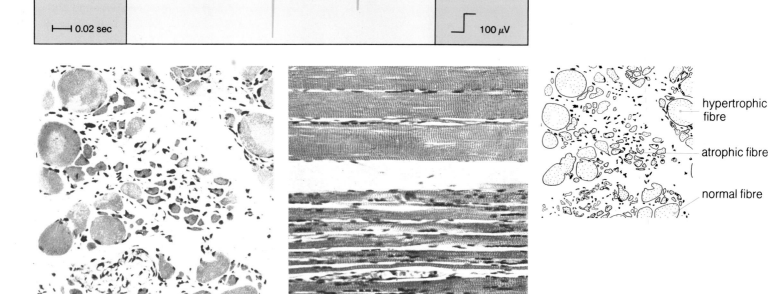

Fig. 3.8 Muscle histology in disseminated neurogenic atrophy. This transverse section shows a mixture of normal, atrophic and hypertrophic fibres (left, haematoxylin and eosin, × 380). Focal neurogenic atrophy: longitudinal section (right) showing normal muscle fibres (above) with atrophic fibres (below). H&E stain, × 140.

Fig. 3.10 Atrophy of the calf and anterior tibial compartment in poliomyelitis (same patient as shown in figure 3.9).

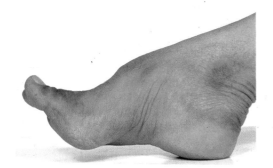

Fig. 3.9 Pes cavus deformity in poliomyelitis.

The patient, aged 48, had had a deformity of the right foot for as long as he could remember, together with wasting of the right calf. Further enquiry revealed a history of an acute febrile illness at the age of three compatible with poliomyelitis.

The Muscular Dystrophies

PSEUDOHYPERTROPHIC MUSCULAR DYSTROPHY (DUCHENNE DYSTROPHY)

This condition, inherited as an X-linked recessive, becomes apparent in early childhood associated with difficulty in walking and climbing stairs. Pseudohypertrophy of muscle occurs, most commonly in the calves, and an associated cardiomyopathy is usual.

BECKER MUSCULAR DYSTROPHY

Though also inherited as an X-linked recessive, this condition progresses far more slowly than Duchenne dystrophy. The distribution of weakness is similar and pseudohypertrophy of the calves is again seen (Fig. 3.12).

LIMB GIRDLE MUSCULAR DYSTROPHY

This condition is usually inherited as an autosomal recessive, although sporadic cases occur. It most commonly presents in early adult life, shows a rather slow progression, and is less often associated with pseudohypertrophy. Cardiomyopathy does not occur. As the title implies, proximal muscles, particularly of the pelvic girdle, are most severely affected (Fig. 3.13). The overlap of the clinical picture with that produced by some of the spinal muscular atrophies is very considerable.

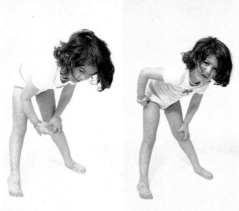

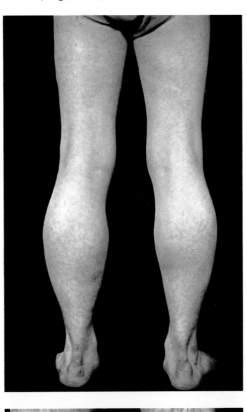

Fig. 3.12 Pseudohypertrophy of the calves in Becker muscular dystrophy.

This 19 year old man had a five year history of difficulty with walking. No upper limb symptoms were apparent. Examination showed mild weakness of triceps with bulky deltoids. There was pseudohypertrophy of the calves, and lower limb weakness maximal in hip extension, plantar flexion and extensor hallucis longus.

Fig. 3.11 Gowers manoeuvre. This is a procedure in which the upper limbs are used to compensate for weakness of the hip and knee extensors.

This 4 year old child had a history of an abnormal gait, but no upper limb symptoms. The creatine phosphokinase (CPK) level was normal. Muscle biopsy suggested neurogenic changes compatible with spinal muscular atrophy.

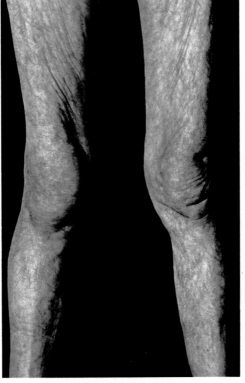

Fig. 3.13 Muscle wasting in limb girdle muscular dystrophy.

The patient gave a one year history of difficulty with walking and climbing stairs. Examination showed mild facial weakness, weakness of neck flexion, proximal upper limb weakness and severe proximal lower limb weakness, maximal in the quadriceps.

FACIOSCAPULOHUMERAL DYSTROPHY

This variant is inherited as an autosomal dominant. Initial involvement predominates in the face and shoulder girdle with later spread to the lower limbs. Weakness of tibialis anterior is prominent. Lack of scapular fixation may produce a typical deformity of the shoulder outline, and gross winging on forward pressure on the hands (Figs. 3.14 & 3.15)

OCULAR MYOPATHY

In some instances, this myopathic disorder is confined to the extra-ocular muscles, in others it is combined with pharyngeal weakness, and sometimes associated with muscle involvement elsewhere, neuropathic disorders, retinal pigmentation and many other syndromes.

Ptosis is followed by a progressive ophthalmoplegia, usually without diplopia (Fig. 3.16). In the oculo-pharyngeal form, extension to the facial muscles occurs, sometimes with later limb involvement.

Other myopathic disorders include scapuloperoneal dystrophy and the rare distal myopathy.

Though differences in the appearance of muscle biopsy specimens occur in the various muscular dystrophies, certain features are characteristic. An increased variation

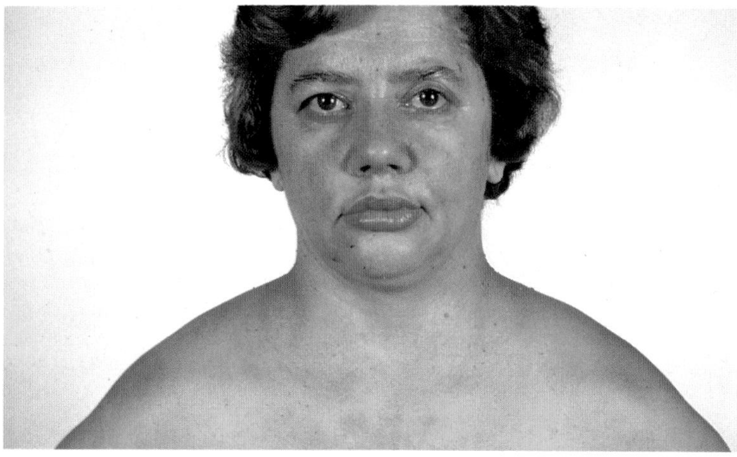

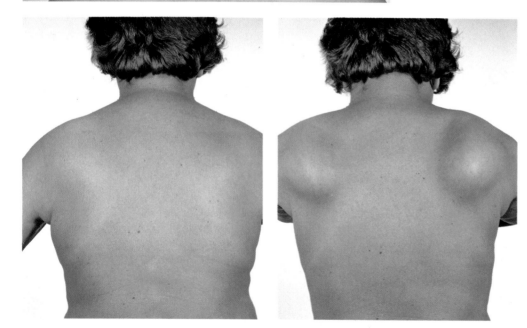

Fig. 3.14 Facioscapulohumeral dystrophy: deformity of shoulder outline due to elevation of the scapulae.

This is a 42 year old female with an 8 year history of weakness, principally of the upper limbs. Examination showed facial weakness and marked proximal upper limb weakness, maximal in biceps and brachioradialis. In the lower limbs, the weakness was both proximal and distal, maximally affecting the dorsiflexors of the feet.

Fig. 3.15 Facioscapulohumeral dystrophy: winging and elevation of the scapulae during forward pressure on the hands (same patient as shown in figure 3.14).

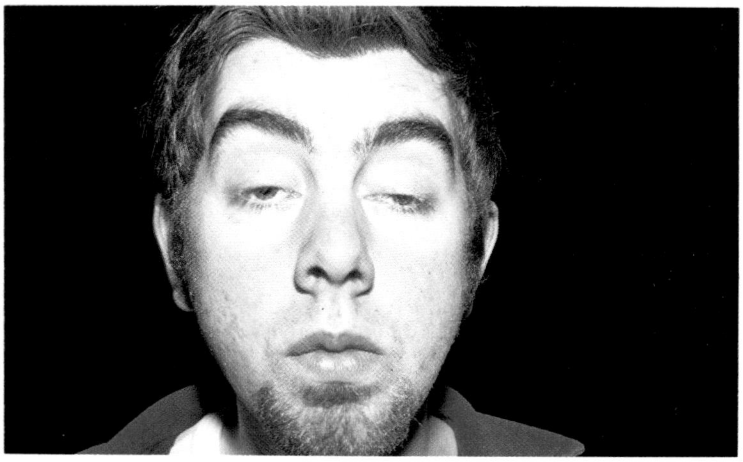

Fig. 3.16 Ocular myopathy: severe bilateral ptosis with considerable facial weakness.

This 20 year old male had ocular myopathy, facial involvement, retinal pigmentation and a cardiac conduction defect.

in fibre size, a tendency for Type I fibre predominance, and an increase in central nuclei and necrotic fibres may occur (Fig. 3.17). Electromyography may show positive sharp waves and fibrillation potentials, particularly in Duchenne dystrophy, with an interference pattern comprising polyphasic low amplitude units of short duration (Fig. 3.18).

Dystrophia Myotonica

This is the most common condition in which myotonia is seen, and the most frequently encountered muscular dystrophy commencing in adult life. It is inherited as an autosomal dominant, with onset usually occurring early in adult life. The presenting symptom may be myotonia, muscle weakness or a reflection of one of the conditions associated with this disorder, for example cataract. Forme fruste variants are encountered which have remained largely asymptomatic at the time of diagnosis. The facial appearance is typical with frontal baldness in men, ptosis and facial weakness (Fig. 3.19). Atrophy of the sternomastoid muscles is striking. Limb involvement is predominantly distal, with wasting of the leg muscles below the knees and the forearms (Fig. 3.20).

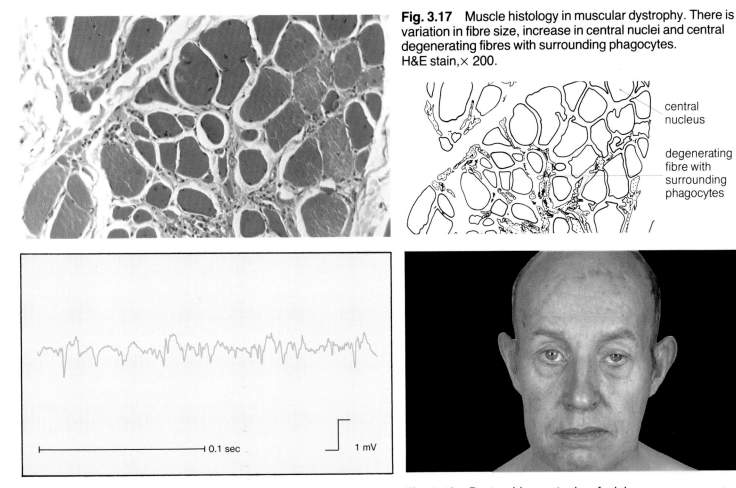

Fig. 3.17 Muscle histology in muscular dystrophy. There is variation in fibre size, increase in central nuclei and central degenerating fibres with surrounding phagocytes. H&E stain,× 200.

central nucleus

degenerating fibre with surrounding phagocytes

Fig. 3.18 EMG recorded from the left deltoid in limb girdle muscular dystrophy showing polyphasic units of low amplitude.

Fig. 3.19 Dystrophia myotonica: facial appearance.

The patient, aged 54, gave a history of myotonia of grip and premature baldness. Examination showed frontal baldness, left ptosis, failure of adduction on lateral gaze, and weakness of the facial muscles and sternomastoid. There was distal wasting and weakness of the upper limbs.

Fig. 3.20 Dystrophia myotonica: limb wasting in the same patient as shown in figure 3.19.

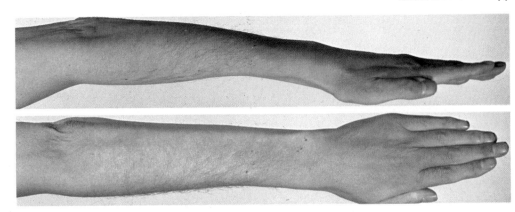

An ophthalmoplegia is sometimes encountered, reflecting either myopathic involvement, or a selective myotonia of certain extra-ocular muscles (Fig. 3.21). Myotonia is most conspicuous in the hands, sometimes presenting as a failure of relaxation of grip, particularly in the cold. The disease affects a number of other systems causing, for example, cardiomyopathy, abnormalities of oesophageal and colonic motility and endocrinological disorders.

EMG analysis reveals high frequency myotonic discharges which tend to decline spontaneously in both amplitude and firing rate (Fig. 3.22). Muscle biopsy shows an abnormal variation in fibre size with an increased proportion of central nuclei.

Myotonia is also a feature of paramyotonia congenita and Thomsen's disease (congenital myotonia) (Fig. 3.23).

Polymyositis

This condition is either confined to muscle or involves the skin in addition (dermatomyositis). The latter condition, when arising in the elderly, is commonly associated with malignancy.

Polymyositis presents as proximal muscle weakness, sometimes fulminating in quality, and associated with tenderness in florid cases. Dysphagia is prominent, facial involvement not infrequent but an ophthalmoplegia rare. In some patients there are signs of joint or other organ disease, particularly where the condition is a reflection of an underlying collagen vascular disease.

Muscle enzyme levels, for example CPK, are usually elevated. EMG analysis reveals high frequency discharges (pseudomyotonia), fibrillation potentials and

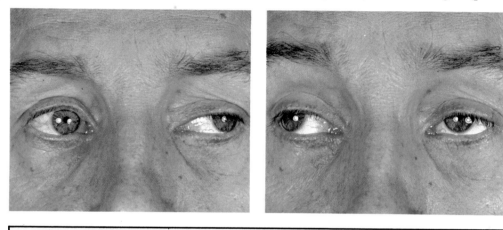

Fig. 3.21 Incomplete adduction on right and left lateral gaze in the same patient as shown in figure 3.19.

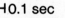

Fig. 3.22 Dystrophia myotonica: myotonic discharge showing rapid decline in amplitude and firing rate.

The patient, aged 35, had had difficulty running for several years, with lesser problems of articulation and swallowing. He was aware of myotonia of grip. Examination revealed frontal baldness, ptosis, facial weakness and severe weakness of neck flexion. There was distal upper and lower limb weakness with myotonia of grip.

┤0.1 sec

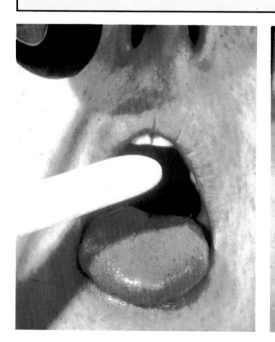

Fig 3.23 Tongue myotonia in myotonia congenita.

motor units of short duration and low amplitude. Abnormalities on muscle biopsy depend on the chronicity of the disorder. There may be variations in fibre size but, more typically, areas of muscle fibre necrosis with infiltration by lymphocytes or polymorphs (Fig. 3.24). More chronic forms of the disease may be difficult to distinguish, at least clinically, from limb-girdle muscular dystrophy. Some patients respond to treatment with either corticosteriods or immunosuppressants.

Other Inflammatory Myopathies
Infiltration of skeletal muscle by inflammatory cells, sometimes with granuloma formation, may occur in sarcoidosis, even in the absence of muscle symptoms or signs (Fig. 3.25). Symptomatic muscle disease in sarcoidosis is less common, presenting as either an acute or subacute myopathy.

Endocrine Myopathies
Thyrotoxic myopathy is said to be common, with up to 50 per cent of thyrotoxic patients giving a history of muscle weakness. Proximal limb involvement is the rule, principally affecting the spinati and deltoids (Fig. 3.26). Periodically bulbar and extra-ocular muscles are affected.

Other endocrine disorders sometimes associated with muscle disease include myxoedema and Cushing's disease. A similar condition can be induced by corticosteroid therapy.

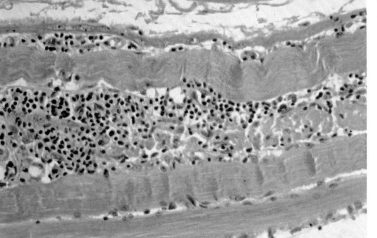

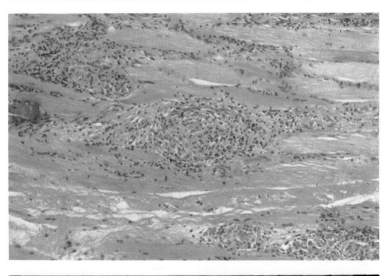

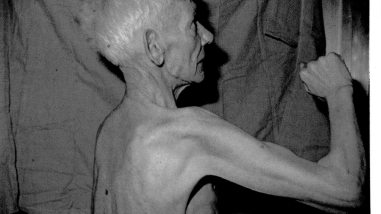

Fig. 3.24 Muscle biopsy in polymyositis showing a disintegrating fibre, inflammatory cell infiltration and a slender regenerating fibre with large subsarcolemmal nuclei. H&E stain, × 450.

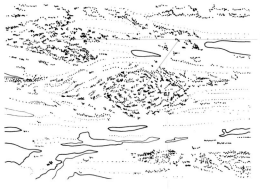

Fig. 3.25 Multiple sarcoid granuloma in skeletal muscle. Haematoxylin and van Gieson stain, × 450.

Fig. 3.26 Thyrotoxic myopathy with evidence of proximal upper limb wasting.

MYASTHENIA GRAVIS AND MYASTHENIC SYNDROME

Myasthenia Gravis

This condition presents with muscle fatiguability, sometimes generalised, at other times confined to the extra-ocular muscles. Many patients present with either diplopia or ptosis, with a characteristic response to intravenous edrophonium (Fig 3.27).

Complex ophthalmoplegias may occur, sometimes mimicking a neuronal disturbance such as internuclear ophthalmoplegia (Fig. 3.28). A triple furrowing of the tongue is said to be a pathognomonic feature but is present in only a small proportion of cases (Fig. 3.29). Remissions occur in some patients, particularly when the disease is confined to the extra-ocular muscles, and may be permanent. In longstanding cases persistent weakness is likely, sometimes with wasting.

Myasthenia gravis is associated with a number of other conditions, including thyroid disease, various auto-immune disorders and polymyositis. A post-synaptic defect exists at the neuromuscular junction, where the number of acetylcholine receptor sites is reduced. A circulating antibody to acetylcholine (ACh) is detected in some 90% of cases. Deposits of immune complexes containing the antibody are found on the post-synaptic membrane. The antibody probably originates from thymic B cells, the numbers of which are increased in patients with this condition. Some patients have an increased number of germinal centres in the thymus (Fig. 3.30).

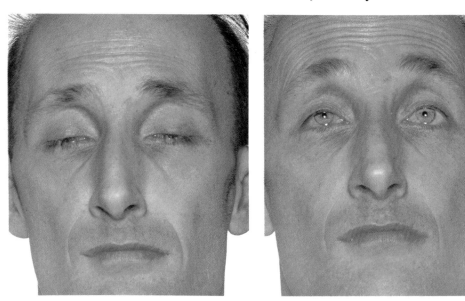

Fig. 3.27 Myasthenia gravis: facial appearance before (left) and after (right) injection of edrophonium.

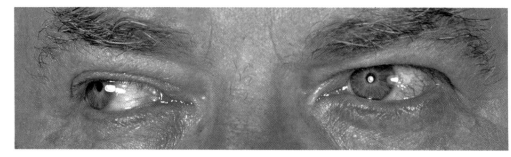

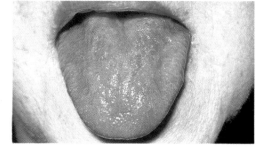

Fig. 3.28 Myasthenia gravis: pseudo-internuclear ophthalmoplegia.

This patient, a 49 year old male, had had unilateral ptosis for several months 30 years previously. He presented with a year's history of intermittent diplopia. Examination showed a failure of left adduction responding within 30 seconds to intravenous edrophonium.

Fig. 3.29 Myasthenia gravis: triple furrowing of the tongue.

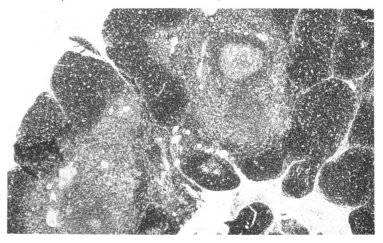

Fig. 3.30 Myasthenia gravis: thymic pathology. H&E stain, × 60.

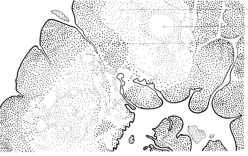

— medulla
— germinal centre
— cortex

Pharmacological tests are of considerable value in diagnosis. Most commonly edrophonium, in a dose of 10 mg, is injected intravenously after a trial dose of 2 mg. Response occurs within a minute and is complete within three to four minutes.

Electrophysiological investigation is also helpful. Repetitive stimulation at less than 3Hz produces a decrement in the amplitude of the evoked response in many patients, sometimes with a paradoxical increment at higher frequencies. Single fibre EMG analysis demonstrates intermittent blocking of action potentials when two or more from the same motor unit can be studied simultaneously (Fig. 3.31). Even when the disease is clinically confined to the extra-ocular muscles,

single fibre analysis of limb muscles may reveal abnormalities.

Some 10% of myasthenic patients are found to have a thymoma on radiological investigation (Figs. 3.32 & 3.33). In approximately 65% of the remainder, pathological changes occur in the thymus, including an increased number of germinal centres. There is some negative correlation between thymic hyperplasia and germinal centres, and a good response to thymectomy. Alternative treatments include anti-cholinesterase therapy, to which response is very variable, and some form of immunosuppression. Long-term corticosteroid therapy, best given as an alternate day regime, is of great value in resistant cases.

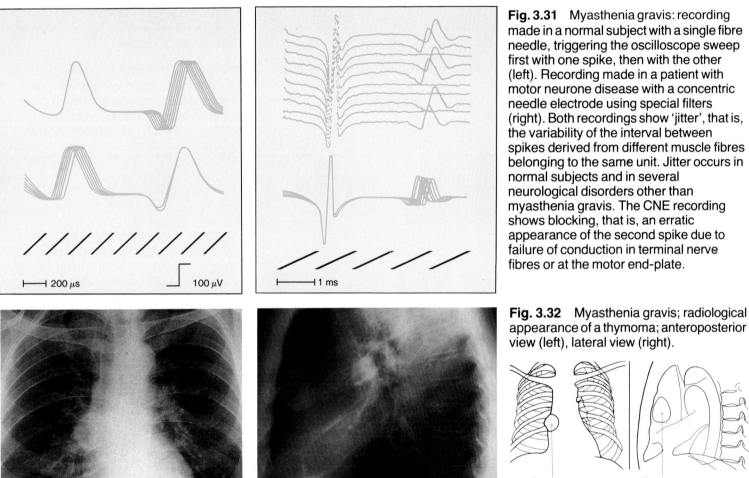

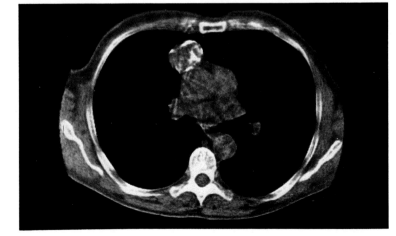

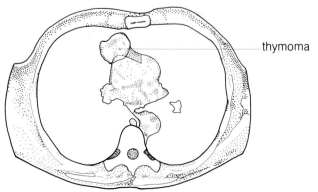

Fig. 3.31 Myasthenia gravis: recording made in a normal subject with a single fibre needle, triggering the oscilloscope sweep first with one spike, then with the other (left). Recording made in a patient with motor neurone disease with a concentric needle electrode using special filters (right). Both recordings show 'jitter', that is, the variability of the interval between spikes derived from different muscle fibres belonging to the same unit. Jitter occurs in normal subjects and in several neurological disorders other than myasthenia gravis. The CNE recording shows blocking, that is, an erratic appearance of the second spike due to failure of conduction in terminal nerve fibres or at the motor end-plate.

Fig. 3.32 Myasthenia gravis; radiological appearance of a thymoma; anteroposterior view (left), lateral view (right).

Fig. 3.33 Myasthenia gravis: CT scan of the mediastinum demonstrating a thymoma.

EATON-LAMBERT SYNDROME

This condition typically occurs in association with oat-cell carcinoma of the bronchus, but sometimes arises *de novo*. The clinical features may mimic a myopathy, with proximal muscle weakness and sometimes pain. Oculomotor involvement is rare and fatiguability not a feature. Deep tendon reflexes are usually depressed, but often augment after a period of sustained muscle contraction. Electrophysiological investigation reveals evoked muscle action potentials of low amplitude which increase dramatically after a period of repetitive contraction (Fig. 3.34). With repetitive nerve stimulation at high frequency, the size of the evoked potential is again augmented (Fig. 3.35).

In this condition, the quanta of ACh released from the nerve ending are reduced in number, though of normal size. Clinical improvement sometimes results from the use of guanidine, which enhances ACh release, or corticosteroids.

VOLKMANN'S ISCHAEMIC CONTRACTURE

In this condition, contractures of forearm muscles occur in association with fractures in the region of the elbow. The contractures are the consequence of muscle necrosis with secondary fibrosis, secondary to ischaemia. There may be associated ischaemic nerve injury, particularly to the median nerve. Figure 3.36 shows an area of muscle necrosis with inflammatory cell infiltration.

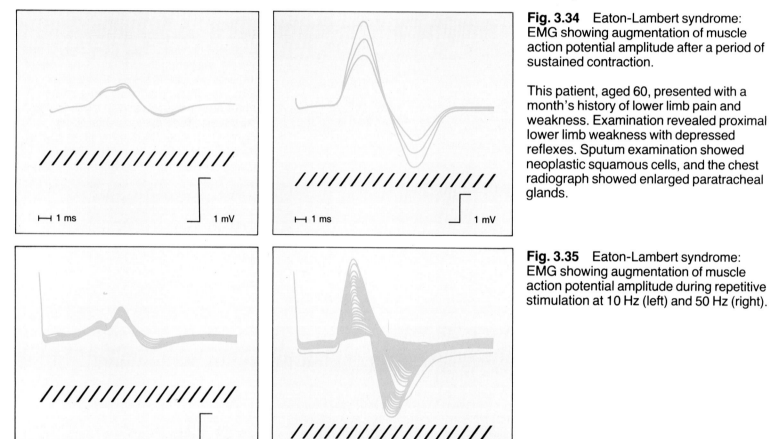

Fig. 3.34 Eaton-Lambert syndrome: EMG showing augmentation of muscle action potential amplitude after a period of sustained contraction.

This patient, aged 60, presented with a month's history of lower limb pain and weakness. Examination revealed proximal lower limb weakness with depressed reflexes. Sputum examination showed neoplastic squamous cells, and the chest radiograph showed enlarged paratracheal glands.

Fig. 3.35 Eaton-Lambert syndrome: EMG showing augmentation of muscle action potential amplitude during repetitive stimulation at 10 Hz (left) and 50 Hz (right).

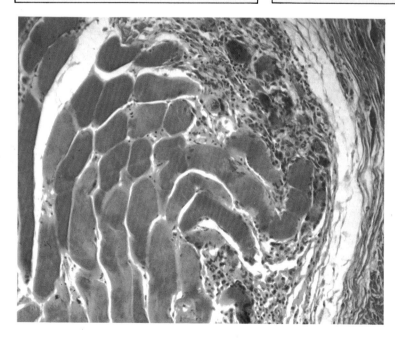

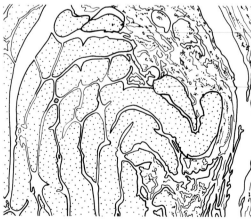

inflammatory cells

necrotic muscle cell

Fig. 3.36 Volkmann's ischaemic contracture: histology showing muscle necrosis and inflammatory cells. H&E stain, × 225.

4. Cerebrovascular Disease I: Cerebral Infarction

The internal carotid artery has no branches in the neck. Within the skull, prior to its termination in the anterior and middle cerebral arteries, its three main branches are the ophthalmic, posterior communicating and anterior choroidal arteries. In some twenty per cent of individuals, the posterior cerebral artery also originates from the internal carotid artery (Fig. 4.1).

The vertebral arteries pass through the transverse foramina of the upper six cervical vertebrae, turn posteriorly over the posterior arch of the atlas and, having entered the cranial cavity, unite to form the basilar artery at the level of the junction of pons with medulla. The posterior inferior cerebellar artery arises from the vertebral artery, whilst the main branches of the basilar artery, visible angiographically, are the paired anterior and superior cerebellar arteries. At its termination, the basilar artery bifurcates into the posterior cerebral arteries (Fig. 4.2).

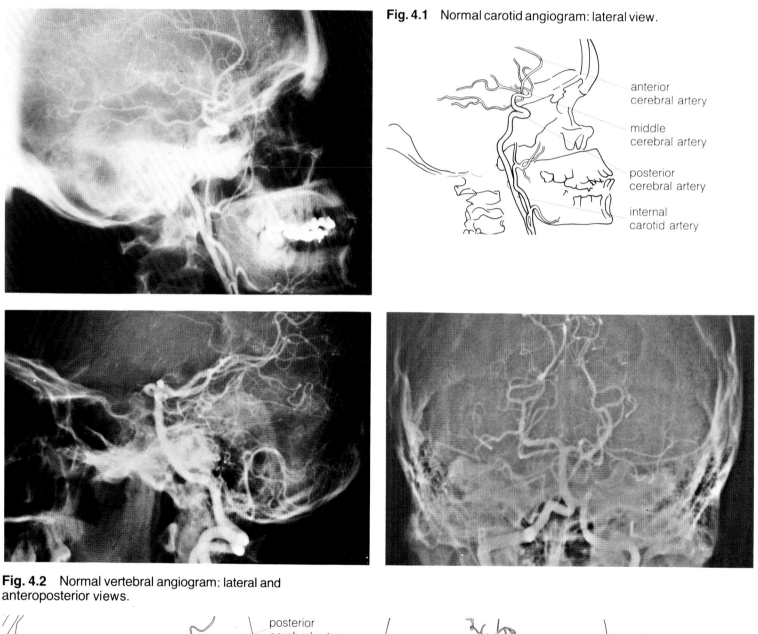

Fig. 4.1 Normal carotid angiogram: lateral view.

anterior cerebral artery

middle cerebral artery

posterior cerebral artery

internal carotid artery

Fig. 4.2 Normal vertebral angiogram: lateral and anteroposterior views.

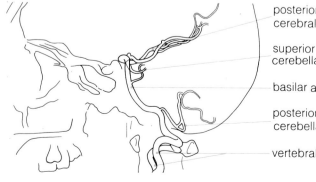

posterior cerebral artery

superior cerebellar artery

basilar artery

posterior inferior cerebellar artery

vertebral arteries

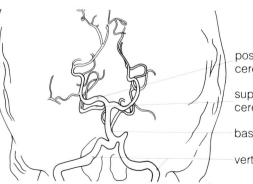

posterior cerebral artery

superior cerebellar artery

basilar artery

vertebral arteries

The anterior cerebral artery supplies the medial portion of the inferior frontal lobe and the medial surface of the frontal and parietal lobes. On the lateral surface of the hemisphere it supplies a narrow parasagittal zone in the frontal and parietal lobes (Fig. 4.3; red). From the proximal segment of the anterior artery arise the medial lenticulostriate arteries, the largest of which is the recurrent artery of Heubner. Together, they supply the anteromedial part of the basal ganglia (Fig. 4.4; red).

The middle cerebral artery supplies a large part of the lateral surface of the frontal, temporal and parietal lobes (Fig. 4.3; blue). Lenticulostriate arteries arise from the first part of the middle cerebral artery and supply much of the corpus striatum and internal capsule (Fig. 4.4; blue).

The posterior cerebral artery, via its cortical branches, supplies the inferior and medial surfaces of the temporal and occipital lobes together with a small area on the lateral surface of the hemisphere (Figs. 4.3 & 4.4; green).

Fig. 4.3 Arterial supply of the lateral surface of the cerebral hemisphere: anterior cerebral artery (red), middle cerebral artery (blue), posterior cerebral artery (green).

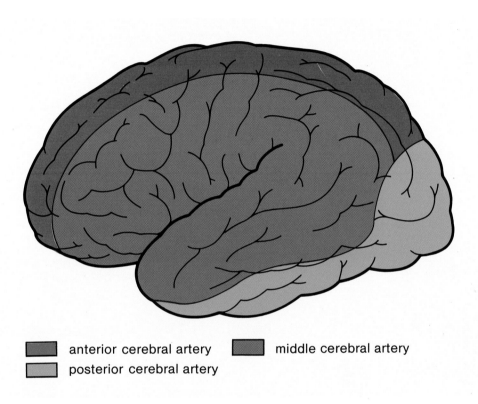

anterior cerebral artery   middle cerebral artery
posterior cerebral artery

Fig. 4.4 Arterial supply of a coronal section of the cerebral hemisphere.

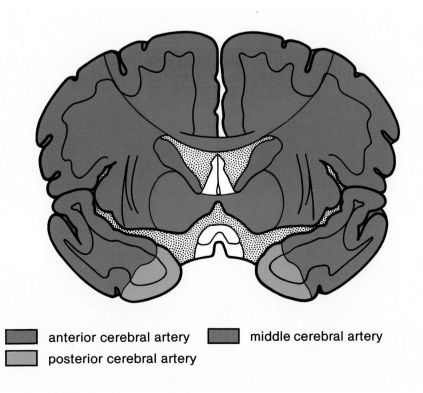

anterior cerebral artery   middle cerebral artery
posterior cerebral artery

Variation in the size and distribution of individual cerebral vessels is considerable. The vertebral artery may originate from the aortic arch or even the carotid system. An asymmetry of size of the vertebral arteries is common, and is prominent in some ten per cent of individuals, the hypoplastic vessel being more usually on the right (Fig. 4.5). Similarly, variations of the circle of Willis from the classical configuration have been demonstrated in as many as 50 per cent of post-mortem specimens, consisting either of differing calibres of component vessels or reduplication of one of the communicating arteries (Fig. 4.6).

Where occlusion or critical stenosis of an internal carotid artery exists, flow through the circle of Willis from the vertebrobasilar circulation may be sufficient to maintain middle cerebral filling (Fig. 4.7).

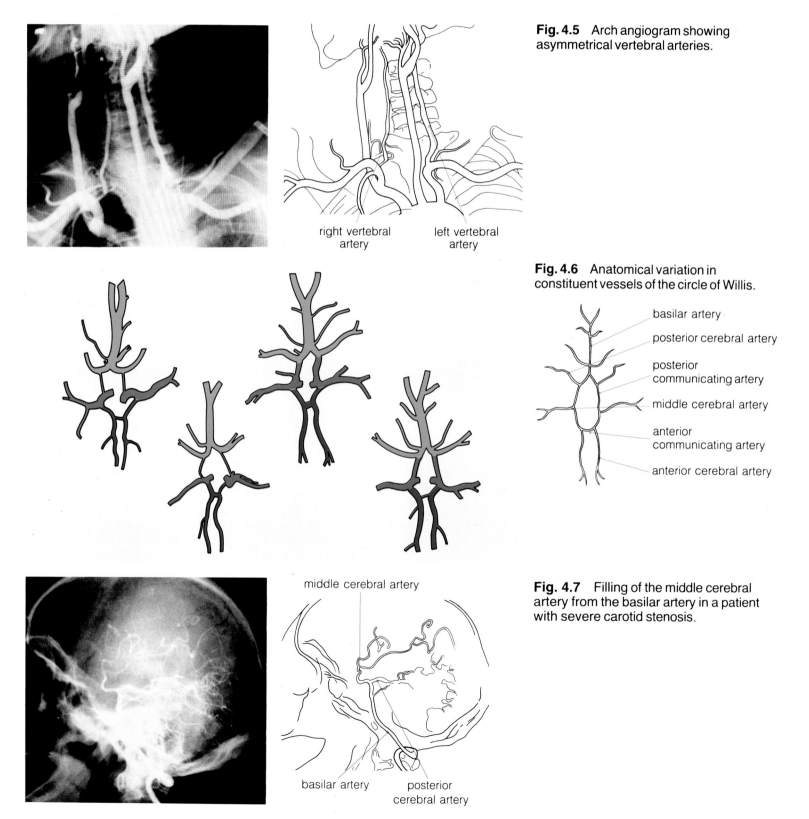

Fig. 4.5 Arch angiogram showing asymmetrical vertebral arteries.

right vertebral artery

left vertebral artery

Fig. 4.6 Anatomical variation in constituent vessels of the circle of Willis.

basilar artery

posterior cerebral artery

posterior communicating artery

middle cerebral artery

anterior communicating artery

anterior cerebral artery

Fig. 4.7 Filling of the middle cerebral artery from the basilar artery in a patient with severe carotid stenosis.

middle cerebral artery

basilar artery

posterior cerebral artery

The Pathological and Physiological Consequences of Cerebral Infarction

Soon after the onset of an extensive cerebral infarction, swelling of both grey and white matter appears with the grey matter sometimes showing petechial haemorrhages. Later, small infarcts evolve into scar tissue containing necrotic neurones with proliferation of capillaries and macroglia. Larger infarcts show cystic degeneration with shrinkage of the affected hemisphere and dilatation of the ipsilateral lateral ventricle (Fig. 4.8). Destruction of pyramidal fibres or the parent Betz cell causes degeneration of the distal pyramidal pathways. Consequently, in the spinal cord, demyelination appears in the uncrossed anterior and crossed lateral corticospinal tracts (Fig. 4.9).

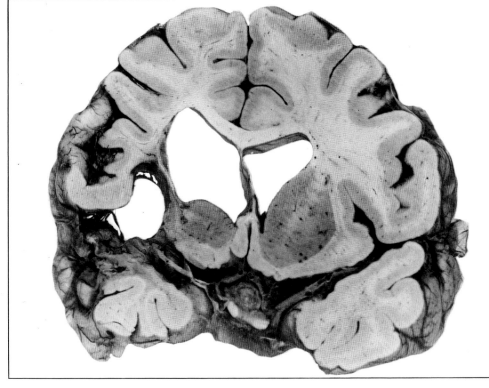

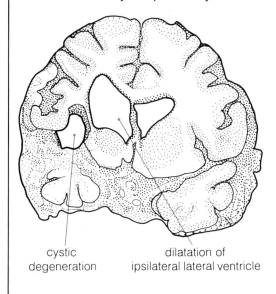

Fig. 4.8 Cystic degeneration of central white matter and internal capsule consequent to middle cerebral artery occlusion several years previously.

cystic degeneration   dilatation of ipsilateral lateral ventricle

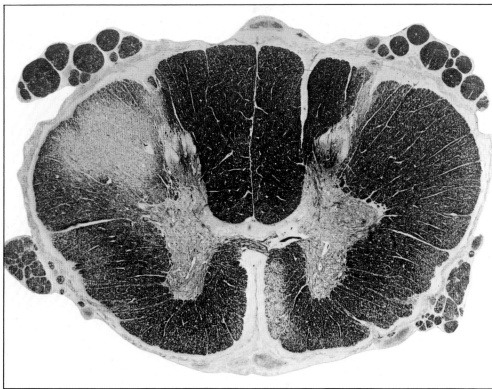

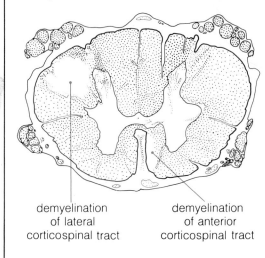

Fig. 4.9 Degeneration of lateral and anterior corticospinal tracts in the cervical cord consequent to the pathological changes described in the previous figure.

demyelination of lateral corticospinal tract   demyelination of anterior corticospinal tract

Computerised axial tomography has allowed the *in vivo* demonstration of cerebral infarction and haemorrhage in a way previously available only at post-mortem examination (Fig. 4.10).

Assessment of cerebral blood flow in healthy individuals and those with cerebrovascular disease depended initially on the surface counting over the cerebral hemisphere of radioactive xenon injected directly into the internal carotid artery. Autoregulation of cerebral blood flow suffices to maintain that flow despite wide variations in perfusion pressure. The arterial tension of carbon dioxide is of particular importance in the regulation of cerebrovascular resistance, retention of carbon dioxide being associated with cerebral vasodilatation.

Mean cerebral blood flow tends to fall in areas of acute cerebral infarction, but more meaningful information has come from the analysis of regional blood flow in such cases. A syndrome of luxury perfusion in association with cerebral infarction has been described, referring to areas adjacent to the infarct in which inappropriately high blood flow exists for the metabolic requirements of that region. Such areas are liable to lose their autoregulatory capacity, with a failure to respond to alteration in carbon dioxide tension.

As an alternative to intracarotid injection, techniques have been developed for the analysis of cerebral blood flow using either intravenous or inhaled xenon. The combination of xenon inhalation and the technique of

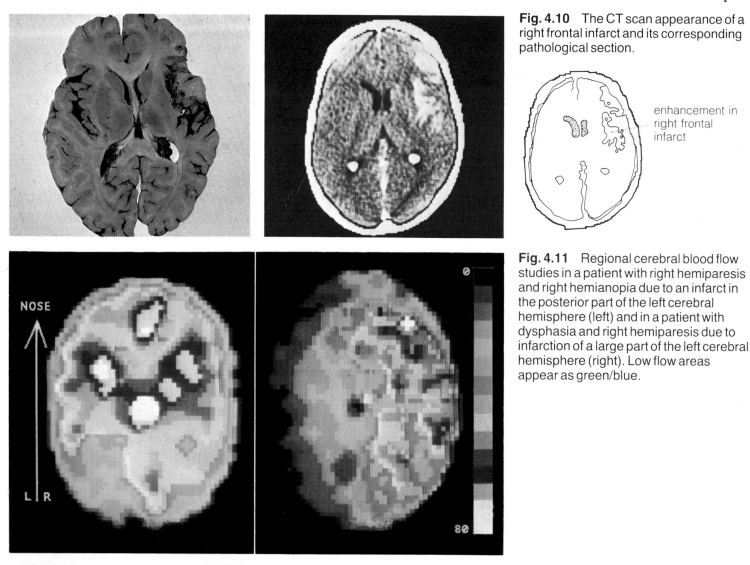

Fig. 4.10 The CT scan appearance of a right frontal infarct and its corresponding pathological section.

enhancement in right frontal infarct

Fig. 4.11 Regional cerebral blood flow studies in a patient with right hemiparesis and right hemianopia due to an infarct in the posterior part of the left cerebral hemisphere (left) and in a patient with dysphasia and right hemiparesis due to infarction of a large part of the left cerebral hemisphere (right). Low flow areas appear as green/blue.

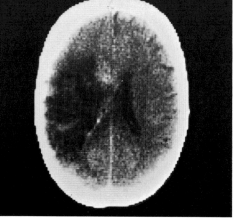

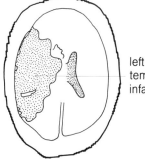

left temporoparietal infarct

Fig. 4.12 CT scan appearance of an infarct in the left temporoparietal region.

emission tomography enables an assessment of flow in horizontal brain slices analogous to those represented by computerised axial tomography (Fig. 4.11).

The procedure has been further developed by combining the findings from intravenous xenon with the simultaneous measurement of gamma ray emission from radioactive isotopes of oxygen and carbon dioxide. The oxygen extraction can be correlated with regional metabolic activity and the carbon dioxide emission with regional blood flow. These changes can be analysed using a gamma camera or by computerised tomography producing a picture of the metabolic activity and blood flow in selected brain sections. An area showing a relatively greater reduction of metabolic activity, as expressed by

oxygen extraction compared to flow, as measured by emission from labelled carbon dioxide, is by definition, an area of luxury perfusion. But where metabolic activity exceeds flow, an area of critical perfusion can be defined, improvement of flow through which can theoretically aid neurological recovery. Figure 4.12 shows a left hemisphere infarct on CT scan and the corresponding emission CT scans demonstrate the evolution of the affected area from a critical perfusion state at 8 hours to an area of luxury perfusion at 4 days (Fig. 4.13).

Following the intravenous injection of Conray, some fifty per cent of cerebral infarcts show enhancement on computerised axial tomography, most prominently between one and three weeks after onset (Fig. 4.14).

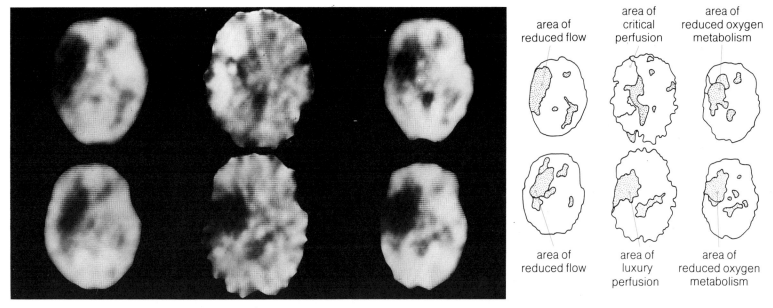

Fig. 4.13 Emission CT scans showing an infarct in the left temporoparietal region: at 8 hours (upper) and 4 days (lower). The scans on the left indicate cerebral blood flow as expressed by emission from labelled CO$_2$; those on the right show metabolic activity as expressed by oxygen extraction, and the middle scans indicate the oxygen extraction ratio.

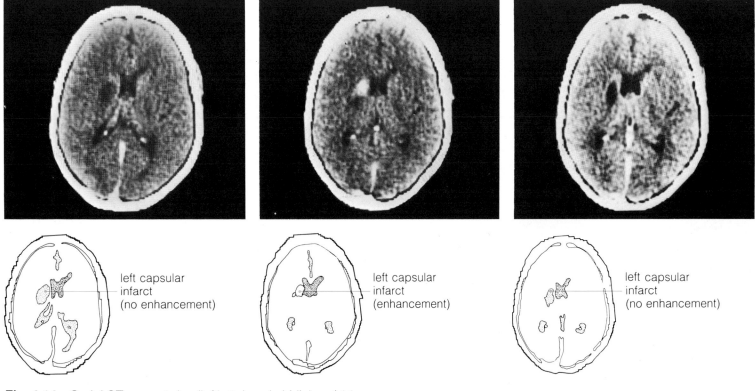

Fig. 4.14 Serial CT scans 1 day (left), 8 days (middle) and 14 weeks (right) after the onset of a right hemiparesis demonstrating transient contrast enhancement in a capsular infarct.

The enhancement predominates in grey matter, is often patchy and generally correlates, in its temporal relationship, with the presence of an abnormal isotope scan. Enhancement may partly reflect luxury perfusion adjacent to the infarct and partly the consequences of vascular proliferation in the early stages after onset.

Serial scanning has enabled the time course of cerebral oedema in relationship to infarction to be assessed in detail. The series of CT scans in figure 4.15 shows the development and resolution of cerebral oedema after the onset of a left hemiparesis due to a right cerebral infarct. Oedema reaches a maximum after four to five days, tending to obscure the cortical gyral pattern and causing a mass effect in a minority of cases. The same evolution

had been previously studied from post-mortem specimens. Figure 4.16 shows the time course for the development of midline shift measured at post-mortem in cases of proven infarction due to middle cerebral artery occlusion. The sequence matches that observed from serial scanning. This swelling of the affected hemisphere is also responsible for transtentorial herniation and is an important contributory factor to the mortality of cerebral infarction in the first week after onset.

CEREBRAL INFARCTION

The CT scanner has enabled the pathological basis of stroke syndromes to be established more accurately. Accordingly, cerebral haemorrhage can be distinguished

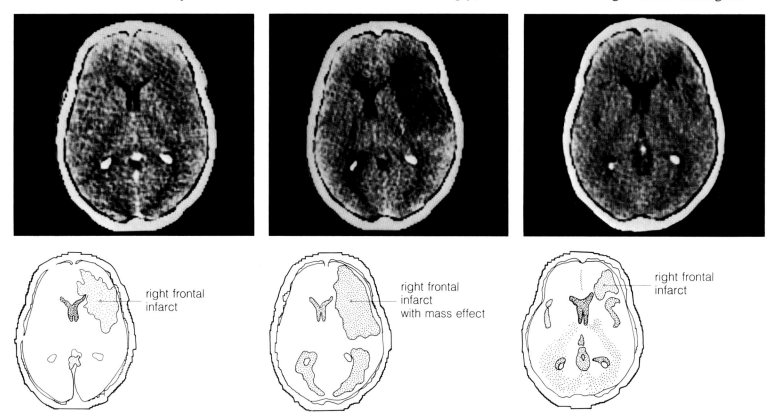

Fig. 4.15 Serial CT scans showing development and resolution of cerebral oedema: ill-defined low density area in right frontal lobe after 6 hours (left); extensive right frontal infarct with shift of lateral ventricles to the left after 8 days (middle); right frontal infarct with resolution of oedema after 16 days (right).

Fig. 4.16 The degree of midline shift according to elapse of time from the onset of ischaemic infarction in middle cerebral artery territory.

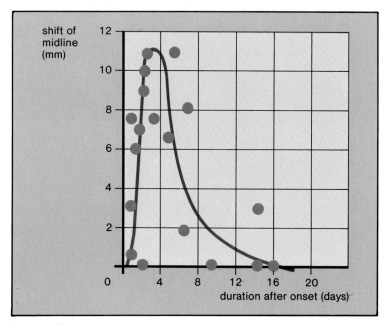

from infarction, and a haemorrhagic element of the latter identified with some certainty. Abnormal scans in patients with cerebral infarction were initially recorded in only fifty per cent of cases, but with the use of more sophisticated scanners, the positive yield has increased dramatically.

As a consequence of arterial occlusion, a number of specific infarction syndromes, many eponymous, have been described. However, incomplete forms of these classical syndromes frequently occur, and moreover, in many patients multiple territory infarcts further complicate the clinical picture.

Infarction in anterior cerebral territory results in a deficit, the severity of which is partly influenced by whether the recurrent artery of Heubner is occluded. When it is,

infarction of the anterior inferior striatum coincides with the cortical and subcortical lesions, and the resulting hemiparesis is often nearly complete (Fig. 4.17). Sparing of the recurrent artery leads to a hemiparesis in which the lower limb is much more severely affected. Disturbances of mood and sphincter control are commonly encountered. The CT scan in such cases shows a low density area in the frontal region alongside the midline (Fig. 4.18). Angiographic confirmation of an anterior cerebral occlusion demands bilateral studies since in many normal individuals both anterior cerebral vessels are supplied by one carotid artery, with cross-flow through the anterior communicating artery (Fig. 4.19).

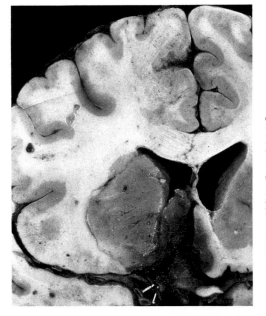

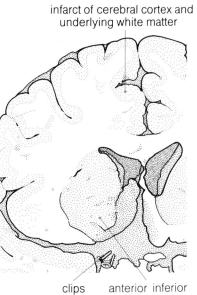

infarct of cerebral cortex and underlying white matter

clips   anterior inferior striatum

Fig. 4.17 Infarction of the cerebral cortex and underlying white matter, and anterior inferior striatum following clipping of the anterior cerebral artery in a case of subarachnoid haemorrhage.

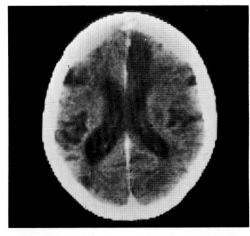

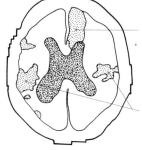

right anterior cerebral territory infarct

additional infarcts

Fig. 4.18 Infarct in the right anterior cerebral territory. There are additional infarcts in both the left and right cerebral hemispheres.

The patient, aged 68, presented with left-sided weakness and incontinence. There was a history of hypertension, a previous episode of right-sided weakness, and evidence of deteriorating mental function.

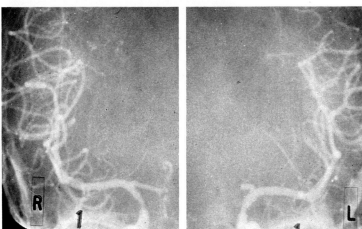

Fig. 4.19 Right (left) and left (right) carotid angiograms showing bilateral anterior cerebral artery occlusions.

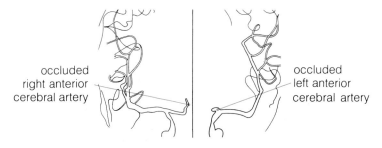

occluded right anterior cerebral artery

occluded left anterior cerebral artery

The patient, aged 70, presented with a year's difficulty in walking. Examination revealed a severe dementia and bilateral pyramidal signs including extensor plantar responses.

4·9

Infarction due to occlusion of the middle cerebral artery usually, but not inevitably, produces a profound neurological deficit with hemiparesis, hemianaesthesia and homonymous hemianopia. Dysphasia occurs when the dominant hemisphere is affected. The infarct appears on the CT scan as an extensive low density area occupying much of the hemisphere, sometimes with mass effect, and can occur with either occlusion of the internal carotid artery or the middle cerebral branch (Figs. 4.20 & 4.21).

Posterior cerebral artery occlusion may produce occipital infarction alone, with a consequent congruous homonymous hemianopia, or a more conspicuous deficit if parietal cortex and, or, deeper stuctures are affected. These may include the posterior part of the internal capsule, part of

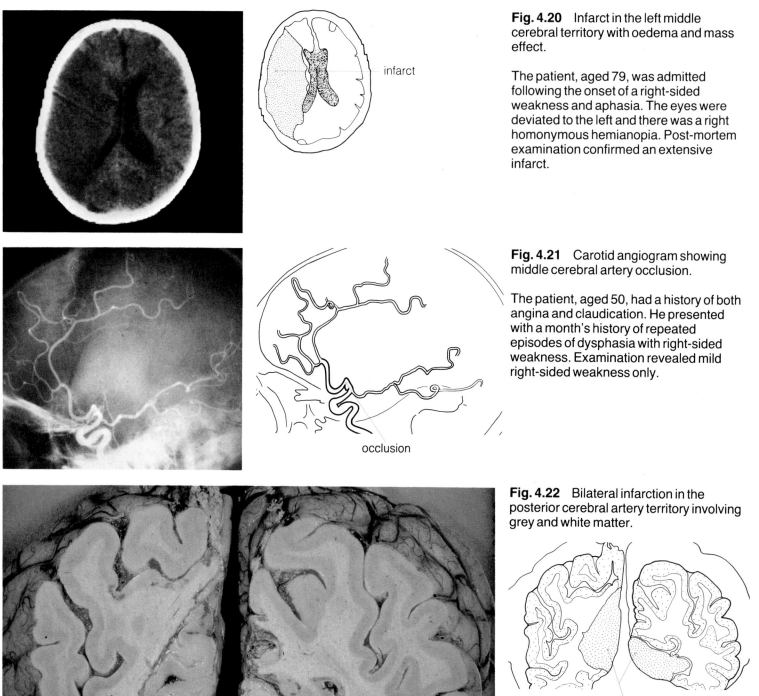

Fig. 4.20 Infarct in the left middle cerebral territory with oedema and mass effect.

The patient, aged 79, was admitted following the onset of a right-sided weakness and aphasia. The eyes were deviated to the left and there was a right homonymous hemianopia. Post-mortem examination confirmed an extensive infarct.

infarct

Fig. 4.21 Carotid angiogram showing middle cerebral artery occlusion.

The patient, aged 50, had a history of both angina and claudication. He presented with a month's history of repeated episodes of dysphasia with right-sided weakness. Examination revealed mild right-sided weakness only.

occlusion

Fig. 4.22 Bilateral infarction in the posterior cerebral artery territory involving grey and white matter.

infarcts

the visual radiation, and the thalamus. A thalamic syndrome can result in association with a hemianopia and a hemisensory disturbance. Simultaneous bilateral occipital infarction usually implies occlusion of the terminal basilar artery, unilateral infarction occlusion of the appropriate posterior cerebral vessel (Figs. 4.22–4.24).

Patients with hypertension and a history of multiple stroke-like episodes may present with arteriosclerotic dementia, comprising dementia with signs of diffuse hemispheric damage. The CT scan in such cases demonstrates multiple low density zones scattered throughout both cerebral hemispheres (Fig. 4.25).

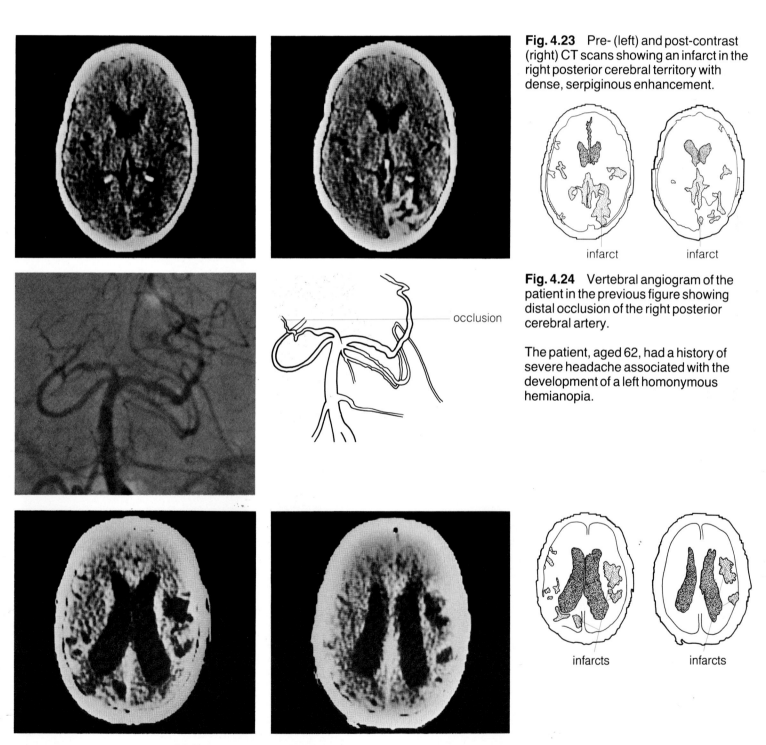

Fig. 4.23 Pre- (left) and post-contrast (right) CT scans showing an infarct in the right posterior cerebral territory with dense, serpiginous enhancement.

infarct   infarct

Fig. 4.24 Vertebral angiogram of the patient in the previous figure showing distal occlusion of the right posterior cerebral artery.

The patient, aged 62, had a history of severe headache associated with the development of a left homonymous hemianopia.

occlusion

infarcts   infarcts

Fig. 4.25 CT scans in two planes showing multiple areas of diminished density in both cerebral hemispheres with ventricular dilatation due to ischaemic atrophy.

The patient, aged 73, was admitted following the development of dysphasia, right-sided visual and sensory inattention and bilateral extensor plantar responses.

Watershed or boundary zone infarction describes ischaemic zones at the junction of the territories of the major cerebral vessels. They may result from occlusion of a major supplying vessel, such as the internal carotid, or from a period of profound hypotension. The watershed infarctions in figure 4.26 occurred in the early childhood of a patient with epilepsy, rheumatic heart disease and the sickle cell trait, and may have resulted from intracerebral sickling during status epilepticus.

The various eponymous brain stem vascular syndromes, beloved of writers of medical texts, are in practice, relatively uncommon. Benedikt's syndrome results from unilateral infarction of the medial mid-brain. An ipsilateral, and frequently incomplete third nerve paresis results. Figure 4.27 shows such a paresis with sparing of the pupil, but typical downward and outward deviation of the globe due to the unopposed action of the superior oblique and lateral rectus muscles. There was an associated

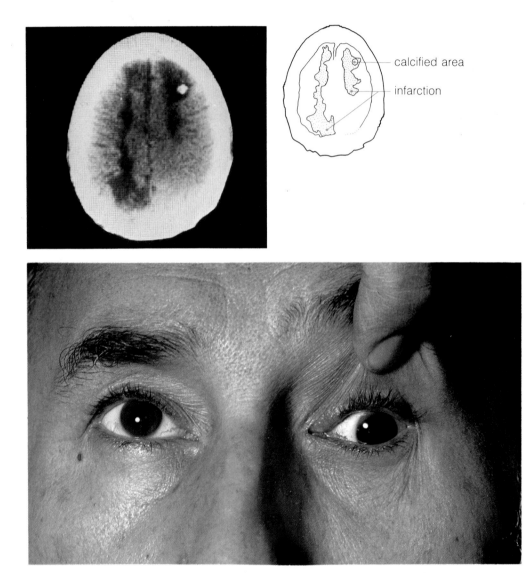

Fig. 4.26 CT scan showing an infarct in the left hemisphere in the peripheral distribution of the anterior cerebral artery and in the right hemisphere, in the watershed between anterior and middle cerebral territory. This infarct contains a calcified area.

The patient, aged 22, had been admitted following a generalised convulsion. Examination showed a right hemi-atrophy and evidence of mitral regurgitation. He was sickle cell positive. In the past he had suffered prolonged convulsions at the age of 10 months and rheumatic fever at 3 years.

Fig. 4.27 Benedikt's syndrome. The left eyelid is being retracted to show the left eye deviated downwards and laterally. The pupil is not dilated.

The patient, aged 56, had developed a left ptosis, diplopia, dysarthria and right-sided clumsiness four weeks before admission. Examination showed dysarthria, a pupil-sparing left third nerve paresis and right-sided cerebellar signs.

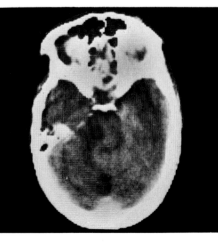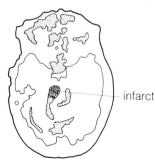

Fig. 4.28 CT scan showing an infarct in the left side of pons.

contralateral limb ataxia. If such infarcts are of sufficient size they appear as low density areas on the CT scan (Fig. 4.28). The most commonly quoted brain stem ischaemic syndrome is that of lateral medullary infarction (Fig. 4.29). The syndrome is often identified with posterior inferior cerebellar artery occlusion, but more often results from occlusion of the parent vertebral artery. The clinical picture is predictable from the area of the medulla affected, with ipsilateral Horner's syndrome, facial spinothalamic loss, palatal palsy and limb cerebellar signs, together with contralateral limb spinothalamic loss.

Cerebellar infarction, previously often identified only at post-mortem examination can be readily detected by CT scanning (Figs. 4.30 & 4.31). The patients tend to have a depressed level of consciousness with nystagmus, horizontal ocular deviation, cranial nerve palsies and an ipsilateral limb cerebellar disturbance.

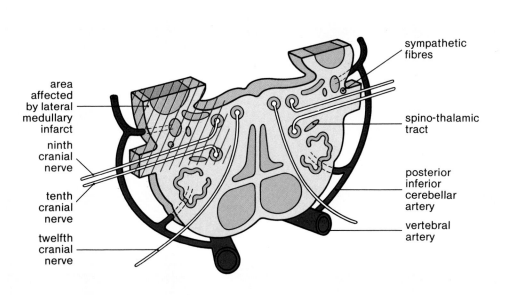

Fig. 4.29 Diagrammatic cross-section of the medulla indicating the structures affected by a lateral medullary infarct.

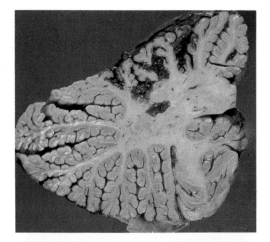

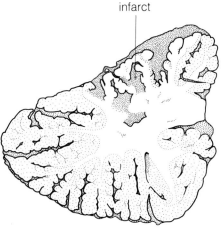

Fig. 4.30 An old cystic haemorrhagic infarct in the cerebellar hemisphere.

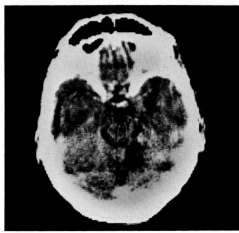

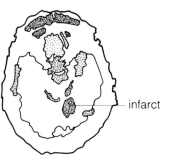

Fig. 4.31 CT scan appearance of a cerebellar infarct in the territory of the superior cerebellar artery.

The patient, aged 70, was admitted with a history of collapse and vomiting. Examination showed dysarthria, bilateral cerebellar signs, more marked on the right, and a gait ataxia.

The Pathogenesis of Cerebral Infarction

Post-mortem analysis of cases of cerebral infarction, particularly of the haemorrhagic type, indicates that a high proportion have a potential embolic source in either the heart or the major neck vessels (Fig. 4.32 & 4.33). Primary atherosclerotic thrombosis causing occlusion of intracranial vessels is unusual except in the case of the basilar artery.

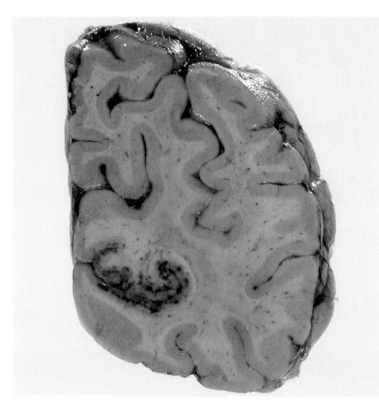

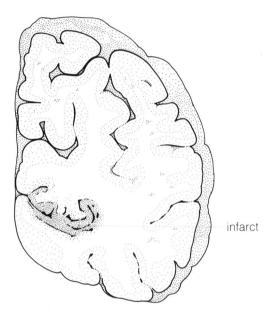

Fig. 4.32 Haemorrhagic infarct. The visual cortex has been infarcted due to compression of the posterior cerebral artery following parahippocampal herniation through the notch in the tentorium cerebelli.

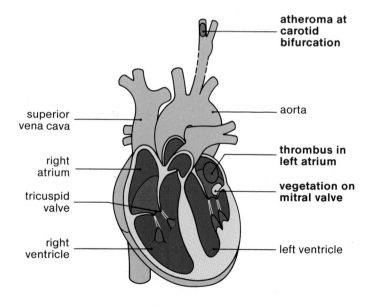

Fig. 4.33 Diagram showing potential sources for emboli reaching the cerebral circulation.

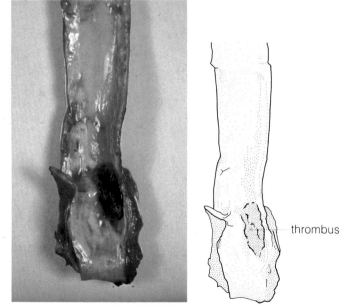

Fig. 4.34 Thrombus adherent to the wall of the carotid artery at, and above, the carotid bifurcation.

The patient had died five days after the onset of a hemiplegia.

Atherosclerosis at the carotid bifurcation, frequently with overlying thrombus (Fig. 4.34), is common and can often be accurately defined by angiography. In some patients with a history of cerebral ischaemic episodes, post-mortem studies establish the presence of cerebral vessels occluded by material containing cholesterol crystals, presumably embolic in origin (Fig. 4.35). *In vivo* demonstration of such emboli can be achieved by finding cholesterol emboli in retinal vessels, sometimes leading to areas of retinal infarction (Figs. 4.36 & 4.37).

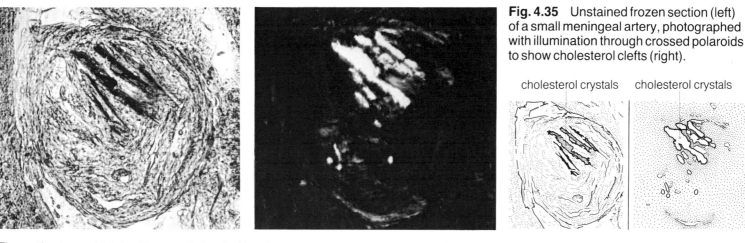

Fig. 4.35 Unstained frozen section (left) of a small meningeal artery, photographed with illumination through crossed polaroids to show cholesterol clefts (right).

cholesterol crystals   cholesterol crystals

The patient, aged 69, had been admitted with a three week history of increasing confusion. There was a past history of hypertension. Examination showed a confused, disorientated individual with limb rigidity and pyramidal signs. At post-mortem examination there was extensive atheroma in the aorta, numerous areas of ischaemic necrosis in the cerebral white and grey matter and multiple occlusions of small cerebral arteries by material containing needle-like clefts of cholesterol.

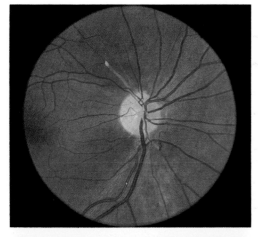
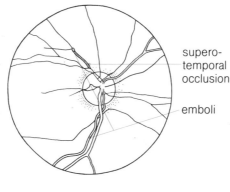

supero-
temporal
occlusion

emboli

Fig. 4.36 Multiple cholesterol emboli with occlusion of the superotemporal branch of the central retinal artery.

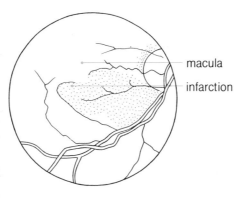

macula

infarction

Fig. 4.37 Branch retinal artery occlusion causing an area of retinal infarction below the macula.

To delineate an embolic source from the major neck arteries angiography is essential. Atheroma at the carotid bifurcation may appear as plaques, with or without ulceration, or as a critical area of stenosis (Figs. 4.38-4.40). Only when stenotic lesions exceed ninety per cent of the lumen does impaired flow become relevant as a cause of symptoms, as opposed to distal embolisation. The development of carotid occlusion may result in a completed stroke, or in the

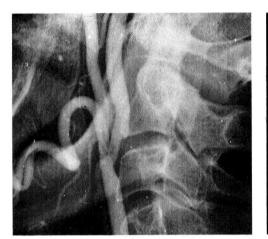

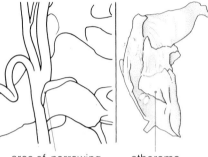

area of narrowing   atheroma

Fig. 4.38 Irregularity and slight narrowing at the origin of the internal carotid artery: angiogram (left) and endarterectomy specimen (right).

The patient, aged 66, had had a brief episode of heaviness and altered feeling in the left arm and leg.

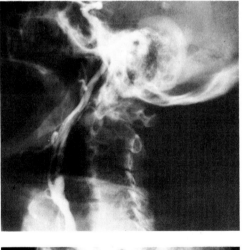

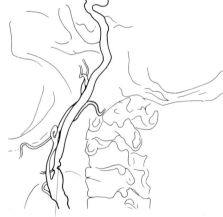

marked irregularity

Fig. 4.39 Irregularity and narrowing of the proximal internal carotid artery with additional irregularity at the carotid bifurcation and narrowing of the external carotid artery.

The patient, aged 71, gave a history of mild right hemiparesis two years previously, and a more recent attack of weakness of the left leg with recovery. There was a right carotid bruit.

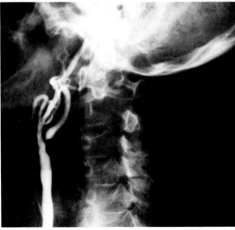

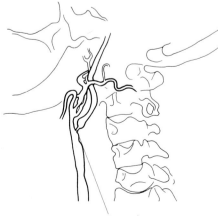

severe stenosis

Fig. 4.40 Severe stenosis at the origin of the left internal carotid artery.

The patient, aged 69, had had numerous vertebrobasilar ischaemic attacks, with deafness, vertigo and ill-defined visual blurring.

cessation of transient ischaemic attacks (Fig. 4.41). Demonstration of an external carotid stenosis serves as a reminder that not all carotid bifurcation bruits are of clinical significance (Fig. 4.42).

Atherosclerotic disease is not confined to the carotid bifurcation. Disease less accessible to surgical intervention may be demonstrated in the carotid siphon or in the intracranial arteries (Fig. 4.43).

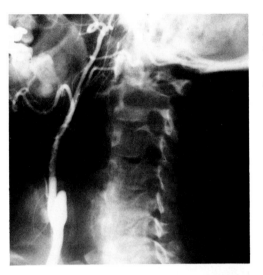

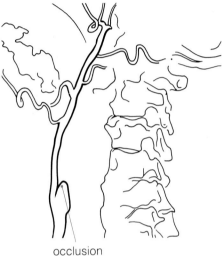

occlusion

Fig. 4.41 Occlusion of the internal carotid artery.

The patient, aged 48, gave a history of sudden onset of dyslexia, followed three months later by recurrent episodes of right-sided weakness, culminating in a right hemiparesis with aphasia.

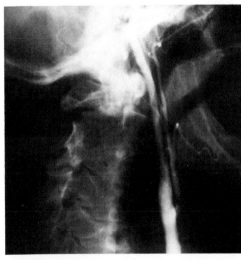

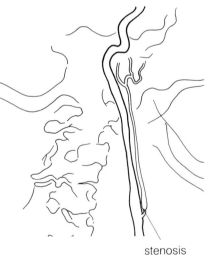

stenosis

Fig. 4.42 Stenosis at the origin of the external carotid artery with some irregularity below the carotid bifurcation.

The patient, aged 72, presented with a history of recurrent attacks of dysphasia, unsteadiness and visual disturbance. There was a left carotid bruit.

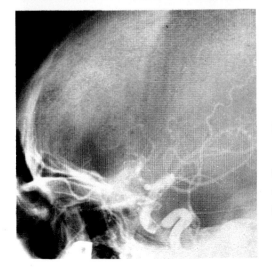

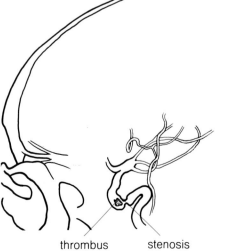

thrombus   stenosis

Fig. 4.43 Stenosis of the right carotid siphon with a probable clot distally.

The patient, aged 54, had had frequent attacks of left-sided paraesthesiae, one episode of right amaurosis fugax and a two day history of persistent weakness of the left hand. Examination showed a severe weakness of the left hand and left-sided hyper-reflexia.

Middle cerebral artery stenosis is not amenable to direct surgical intervention, but its effects may possibly be mitigated by extracranial to intracranial bypass surgery (Fig. 4.44). Basilar artery occlusion, usually thrombotic, is not inevitably fatal but is likely to produce profound neurological deficit (Fig. 4.45).

The subclavian steal syndrome arises when occlusion of a subclavian artery occurs proximal to the origin of the vertebral artery. Flow through the distal subclavian artery, particularly during use of the limb, may then be maintained by reverse flow down the ipsilateral vertebral artery (Fig. 4.46). Stenotic lesions of the subclavian or

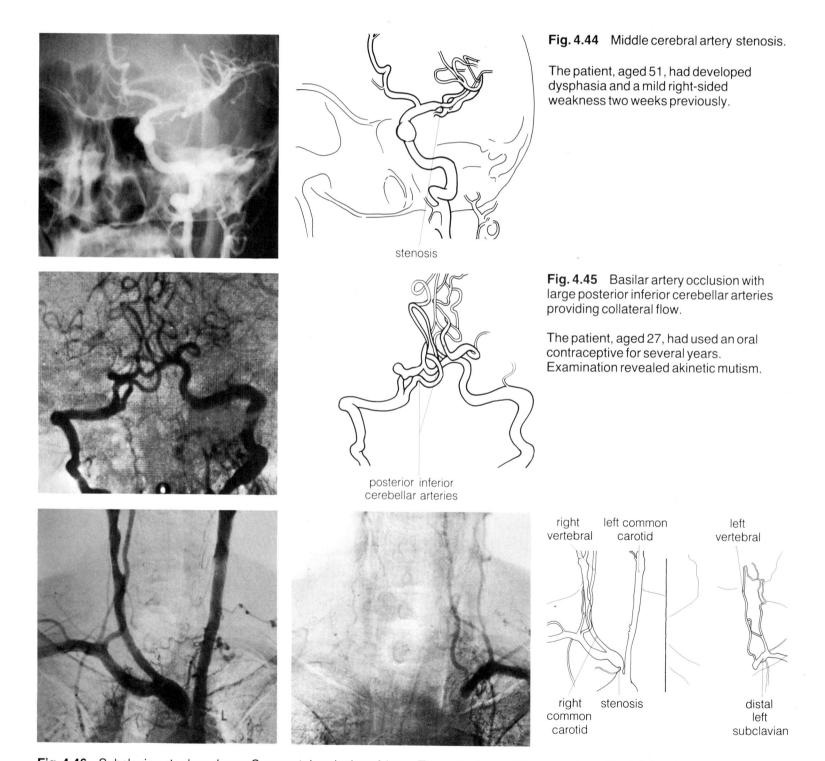

stenosis

Fig. 4.44 Middle cerebral artery stenosis.

The patient, aged 51, had developed dysphasia and a mild right-sided weakness two weeks previously.

Fig. 4.45 Basilar artery occlusion with large posterior inferior cerebellar arteries providing collateral flow.

The patient, aged 27, had used an oral contraceptive for several years. Examination revealed akinetic mutism.

posterior inferior cerebellar arteries

right vertebral   left common carotid   left vertebral

right common carotid   stenosis   distal left subclavian

Fig. 4.46 Subclavian steal syndrome. Segmental occlusion of the first part of the left subclavian artery and stenosis at the origin of the innominate artery (left) with delayed distal collateral filling via the left vertebral artery (right).

The patient, aged 59, presented with a left hemiparesis, had bilateral neck bruits, and radiological evidence of diffuse arterial disease.

vertebral arteries may act as a source of emboli to the vertebrobasilar circulation.

The heart is an important source of emboli, not only to the smaller intracranial vessels but, with large emboli, to the major neck vessels themselves. Patients with mitral stenosis and atrial fibrillation are liable to peripheral and cranial embolisation from left atrial thrombi (Fig. 4.47). Mitral valve prolapse may be relatively innocuous in haemodynamic terms, but is probably capable of acting as a source of micro-emboli to the brain (Fig. 4.48).

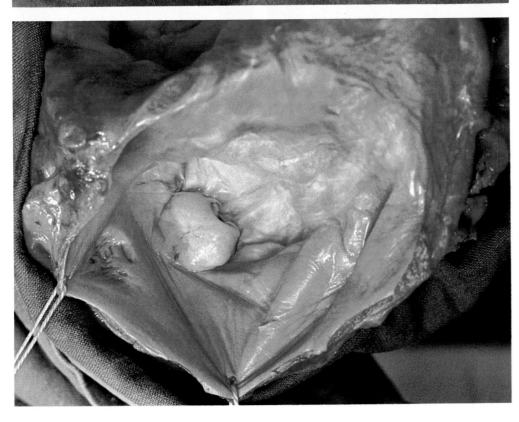

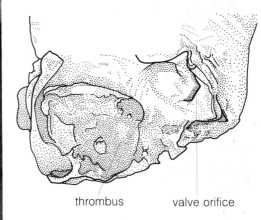

Fig. 4.47 Mitral valve stenosis with a large thrombus almost filling the atrium.

thrombus   valve orifice

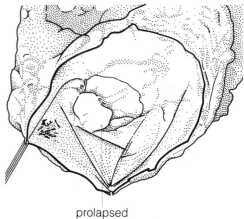

Fig. 4.48 Prolapsed mitral valve viewed from the left atrium.

prolapsed mitral valve

Subacute bacterial endocarditis, most commonly arising in mitral or aortic valves, may present with a cerebral embolus (Fig. 4.49). The pattern of this disease has changed, with fewer young patients with histories of rheumatic heart disease, and an increasing proportion of older patients, many without clinical or pathological evidence of rheumatic valvular lesions. At the bacteraemic stage, emboli are formed from vegetations separating from the valvular lesion. Subsequently, immune complexes may develop in such patients, sometimes

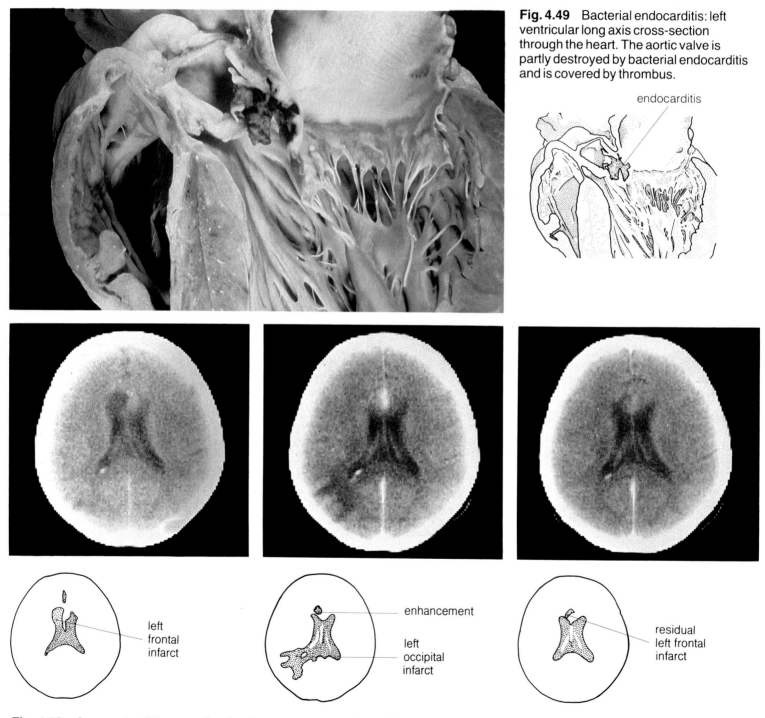

Fig. 4.49 Bacterial endocarditis: left ventricular long axis cross-section through the heart. The aortic valve is partly destroyed by bacterial endocarditis and is covered by thrombus.

endocarditis

left frontal infarct

enhancement

left occipital infarct

residual left frontal infarct

Fig. 4.50 Successive CT scans showing the appearance and resolution of low density areas with variable enhancement in the left frontal and occipital lobes.

The patient, aged 40, developed a staphylococcal septicaemia. There was a history of a ventricular septal defect diagnosed in childhood. Following recovery, the development of proteinuria and haematuria was found to be associated with the deposition of immune complexes of IgA, IgG and C3 in the kidneys.

manifesting as haematuria or proteinuria due to renal deposition, and sometimes as single or multiple areas of cerebral infarction (Fig. 4.50).

Marantic, or non-bacterial thrombotic endocarditis tends to occur in association with carcinoma, and hence in older subjects, but at times it may present in young individuals without evidence of an underlying condition (Figs. 4.51 & 4.52). In either case, systematic embolisation is often the first manifestation of the cardiac lesion.

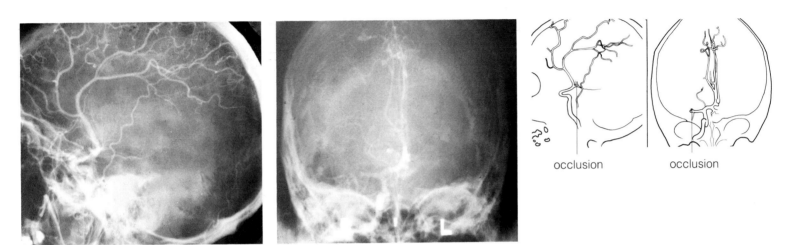

Fig. 4.51 Distal 'calyceal' embolic occlusion of the right middle cerebral artery: lateral view (left) and anteroposterior view (right).

The patient, aged 26, presented with headache, left homonymous hemianopia and left-sided motor and sensory deficit. Post-mortem examination revealed a middle cerebral embolus composed of white gelatinous material, vegetations of which were also found on the aortic valve.

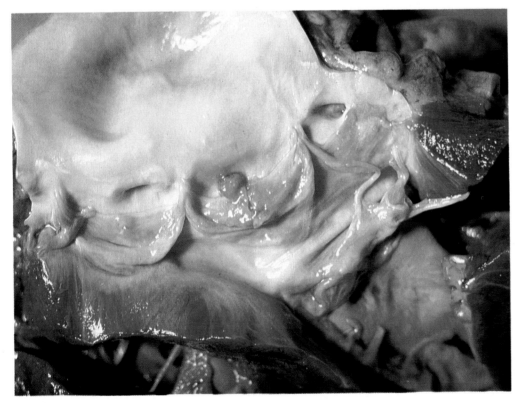

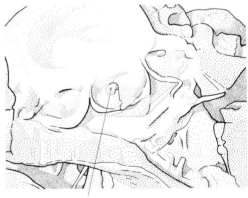

Fig. 4.52 Aortic valve with vegetations from the patient described in the previous figure.

A patent foramen ovale, of the size seen in figure 4.53 is likely to present with haemodynamic problems. Smaller defects, of at least 7mm, have been reported in some six per cent of autopsies and may allow paradoxical embolisation of material from the leg or pelvic veins in the presence of pulmonary hypertension due to concomitant pulmonary emboli.

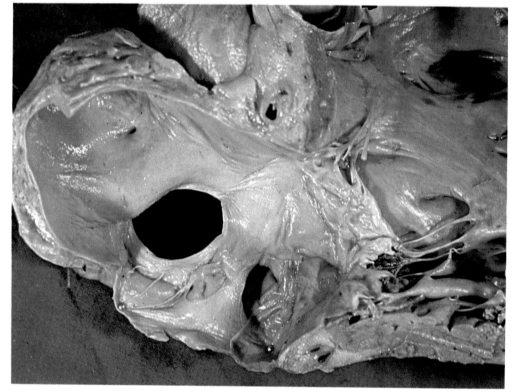

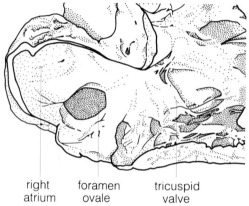

Fig. 4.53   Patent foramen ovale.

right   foramen   tricuspid
atrium   ovale   valve

5. Cerebrovascular Disease II: Cerebral Haemorrhage and Other Disorders

The effects of hypertension on the cerebral circulation are numerous. Hypertensive encephalopathy typically results from an acute rise in blood pressure in an individual without a previous history of hypertension. CT scanning in such patients shows diffuse areas of low attenuation which resolve once the blood pressure is satisfactorily controlled (Fig. 5.1).

Closely correlated with the presence of hypertension are lacunes, cystic cavities around 1cm in diameter in the basal ganglia and centrum semiovale in senile atherosclerotic brains (Fig. 5.2). The lesions, rather than being small infarcts, which are often found in the pons, centrum semiovale and basal ganglia, may represent expanded perivascular spaces, or even the sequelae of previous haemorrhage. It has been suggested that lacunes in particular sites can be correlated with specific neurological syndromes.

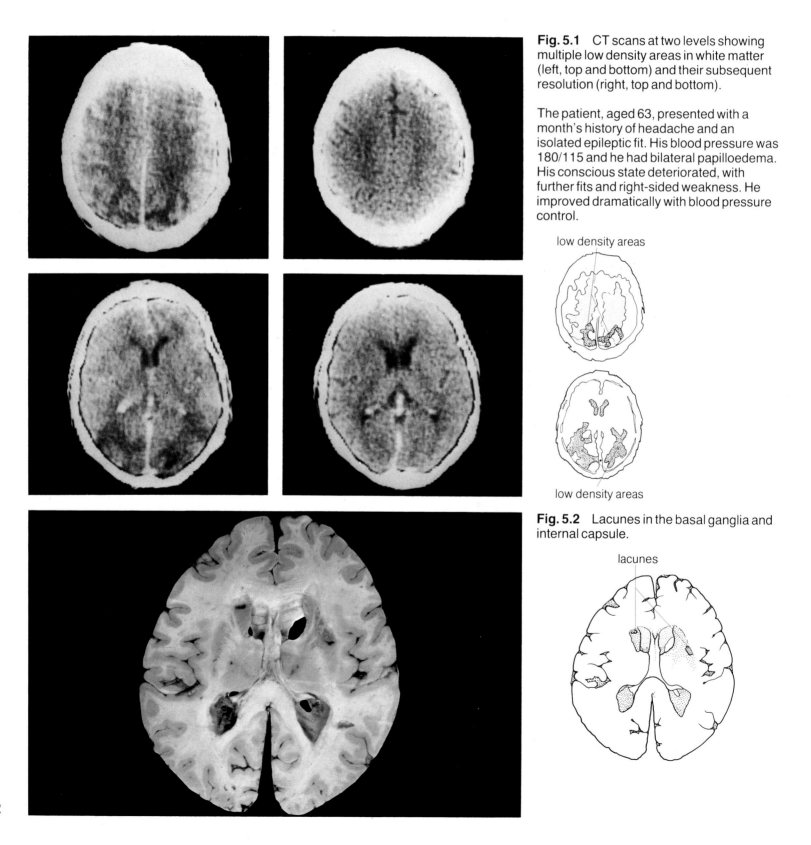

Fig. 5.1 CT scans at two levels showing multiple low density areas in white matter (left, top and bottom) and their subsequent resolution (right, top and bottom).

The patient, aged 63, presented with a month's history of headache and an isolated epileptic fit. His blood pressure was 180/115 and he had bilateral papilloedema. His conscious state deteriorated, with further fits and right-sided weakness. He improved dramatically with blood pressure control.

low density areas

low density areas

Fig. 5.2 Lacunes in the basal ganglia and internal capsule.

lacunes

The importance of hypertension in the genesis of intracerebral haemorrhage, particularly in the pons and cerebellum, has long been recognised. Charcot and Bouchard described aneurysms in small cerebral arteries in patients with cerebral haemorrhage, and suggested that the phenomena were associated. Analysis of the distribution of these aneurysms, ranging up to 2mm in diameter, has been performed on the brains of hypertensive and normotensive individuals. Their distribution, mainly in the internal capsule, corpus striatum, pons and cerebellum mirrors the sites of spontaneous intracerebral haemorrhage (Fig. 5.3). Injection studies at post-mortem examination outline the aneurysms and sometimes demonstrate leakage of contrast material through the wall (Fig. 5.4).

Hypertensive cerebral haemorrhage most commonly occurs in the cerebral hemisphere, particularly in the region of the striatum and internal capsule (Fig. 5.5).

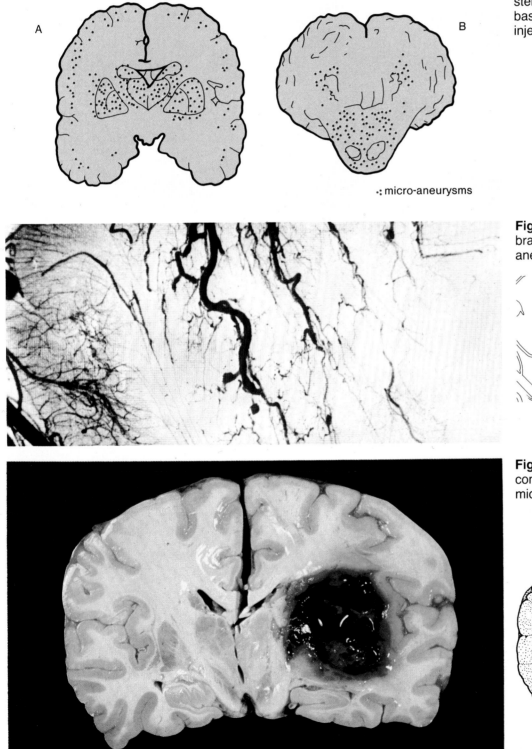

•: micro-aneurysms

Fig. 5.3 Sites of hemispheric (A) and brain stem (B) micro-aneurysms in 53 subjects, based on post-mortem analysis using an injection technique.

Fig. 5.4 Two aneurysms on the lateral branches of a main striate artery. Other aneurysms are also visible.

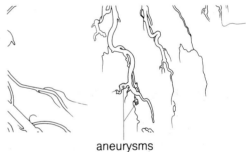

aneurysms

Fig. 5.5 Recent capsular haematoma with compression of the lateral ventricle and midline shift.

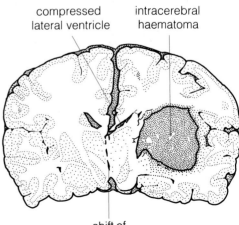

compressed lateral ventricle

intracerebral haematoma

shift of midline structures

Initially the affected hemisphere is swollen, and the haematoma may extend into the lateral ventricle. Clinical differentiation between cerebral haemorrhage and infarction is notoriously inaccurate, but the CT scanner allows the identification of cerebral haemorrhages with almost complete accuracy (Fig. 5.6). It is now appreciated that severe headache can be a manifestation of infarction, that seizures occur with both conditions and that hypertension is not uncommon in those presenting with a cerebral infarct. Alteration of the conscious level is by no means inevitable in the presence of haemorrhage; some haemor-

rhages may present subacutely rather than abruptly.

Cerebellar haematoma is an important condition to recognise, since, in contradistinction to haemorrhage at other sites, surgical intervention may improve prognosis. The clinical features include headache, vomiting, clouding of consciousness, brain stem and ipsilateral cerebellar signs. It usually occurs in the region of the dentate nucleus with occupation of the medial part of the cerebellar hemisphere sometimes extending into the fourth ventricle (Fig. 5.7). Multiple cerebral haematomata are usually consequent to a blood dyscrasia, though they may arise spontaneously.

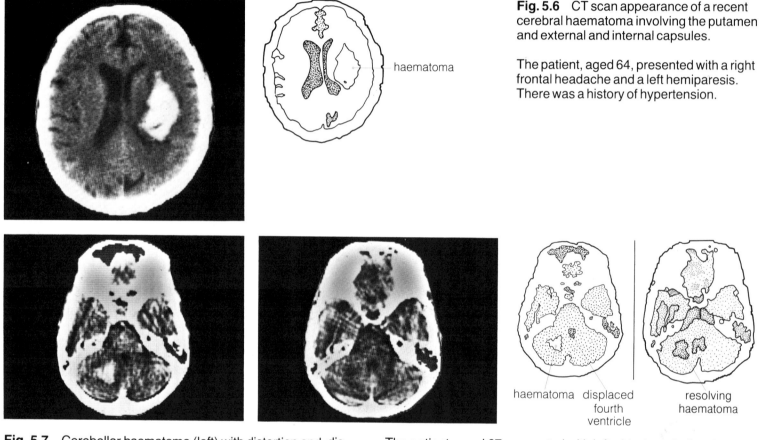

Fig. 5.6 CT scan appearance of a recent cerebral haematoma involving the putamen and external and internal capsules.

The patient, aged 64, presented with a right frontal headache and a left hemiparesis. There was a history of hypertension.

Fig. 5.7 Cerebellar haematoma (left) with distortion and displacement of the fourth ventricle and subsequent resolution (right). The patient, aged 67, presented with left-sided cerebellar signs.

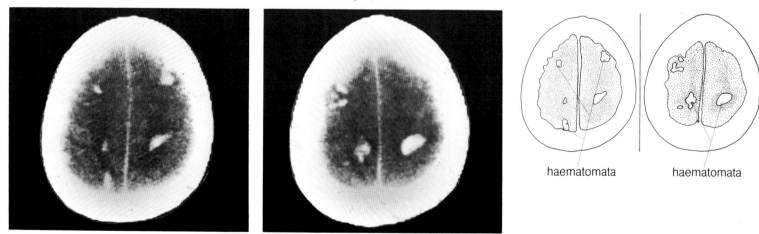

Fig. 5.8 CT scan at two levels showing multiple cerebral haematomata in both hemispheres.

The patient, aged 32, was admitted following an overdose of an unidentified substance. He was found to have multiple areas of small bowel necrosis and developed disseminated intravascular coagulation with a low platelet count and increased concentration of fibrin degradation products. At post-mortem, numerous areas of fresh haemorrhage were found throughout both cerebral hemispheres.

Those shown in figure 5.8 occurred in a patient with disseminated intravascular coagulation induced by self-poisoning.

Subarachnoid haemorrhage may arise from extension of an intracerebral haematoma, but more usually results from rupture of a berry aneurysm. Typically, patients present with sudden, severe headache often with vomiting, and are found to have some degree of clouding of consciousness, neck stiffness and a positive Kernig's sign. The sudden increase in intracranial pressure may cause retinal haemorrhages which extrude into the pre-retinal or subhyaloid space often displaying a horizontal upper margin due to the effects of gravity (Fig. 5.9). Berry aneurysms tend to occur at particular sites, for example at the origin of the posterior communicating artery, and their position may produce focal neurological signs as well as those of subarachnoid bleeding (Fig. 5.10). An expanding posterior communicating aneurysm may compress the adjacent third cranial nerve, producing an oculomotor paresis with pupillary dilatation (Fig. 5.11).

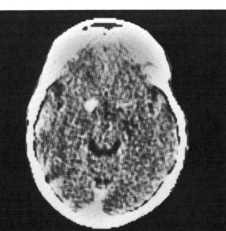

haemorrhage

Fig. 5.9 A subhyaloid haemorrhage.

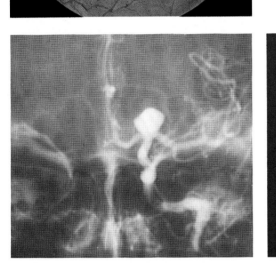

Fig. 5.10 Aneurysm arising from the termination of the left internal carotid artery: angiogram (left) and CT scan (right).

aneurysm   aneurysm

The patient, aged 39, with a long history of migraine, presented with a two-week history of severe left-sided headache associated with vomiting.

Fig. 5.11 Left eyelid elevated to show third nerve paresis (eye deviated down and out) with a dilated pupil.

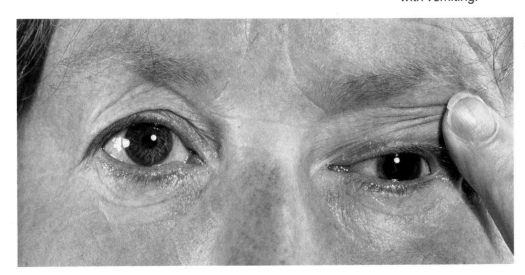

Large intracranial aneurysms are uncommon and usually present with symptoms due to space occupation. Cavernous aneurysms compress the oculomotor nerves, some or rarely all the divisions of the trigeminal nerve and, when placed anteriorly, the optic nerve (Fig. 5.12). Such aneurysms may fill with laminated thrombi often with strands of calcification (Fig. 5.13). The CT scan of such aneurysms may show a calcified rim, with peripheral and

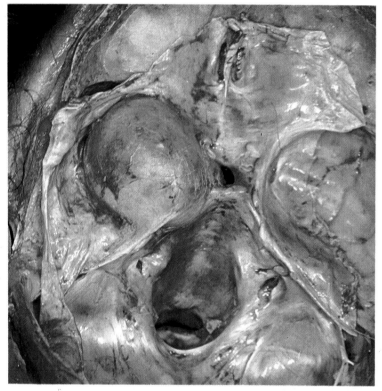

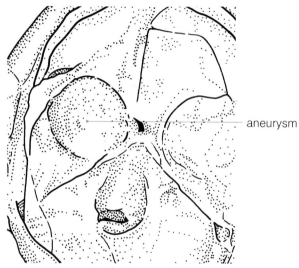

Fig. 5.12 A giant aneurysm arising from the intracavernous carotid artery.

Fig. 5.13 A giant 6 cm aneurysm arising from the anterior communicating artery and causing frontal lobe compression. There was extensive central and peripheral calcification.

The patient, aged 64 at his death, had had subarachnoid haemorrhages at the age of 24 and 46. His final illness with severe gait ataxia as the most prominent symptom, was due to a glioblastoma of the cerebellar vermis.

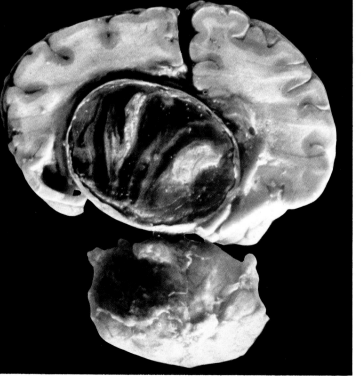

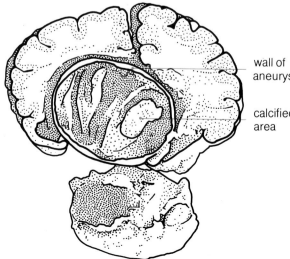

central or more uniform enhancement (Figs. 5.14 & 5.15).

Aneurysms of the posterior circulation are uncommon in comparison to those of the carotid group, but may arise from the vertebral or basilar arteries or from their branches such as the posterior inferior cerebellar artery (Fig. 5.16).

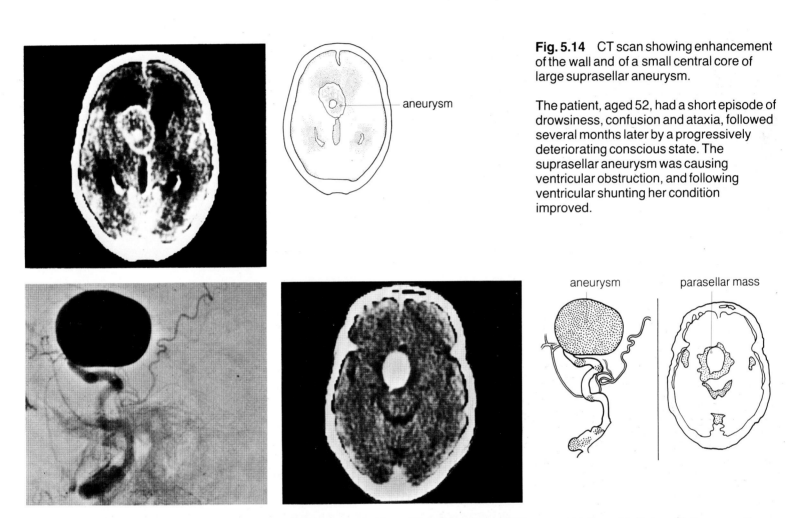

Fig. 5.14 CT scan showing enhancement of the wall and of a small central core of large suprasellar aneurysm.

The patient, aged 52, had a short episode of drowsiness, confusion and ataxia, followed several months later by a progressively deteriorating conscious state. The suprasellar aneurysm was causing ventricular obstruction, and following ventricular shunting her condition improved.

Fig. 5.15 A giant aneurysm arising from the left internal carotid artery (left) appearing on an enhanced CT scan (right) as a uniformly dense parasellar mass.

The patient, aged 62, gave a history of left visual failure over three years. Examination revealed a fixed dilated pupil, a blind left eye with optic atrophy and temporal constriction of the right visual field.

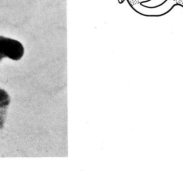

Fig. 5.16 Aneurysm at the origin of the left posterior inferior cerebellar artery.

The patient, aged 37, gave a week's history of severe headache of sudden onset with vomiting and neck stiffness. A further episode occurred two days prior to admission. The cerebrospinal fluid was uniformly blood-stained.

Other Conditions

Capillary, venous and arteriovenous angiomata have been described, but the last is the one most likely to be encountered clinically. Arteriovenous angiomata comprise both arterial and venous components with the former showing degenerative changes. Despite this, the source of bleeding from such malformations is usually venous, with accordingly less severe consequences than from haemorrhages arising from an arterial source.

These malformations may also present with epilepsy, recurrent headache, focal neurological deficit or rarely with a progressive dementia. On CT scan the malformation appears as an area of mixed density with a pattern on enhancement tending to outline the serpiginous vessels which comprise the lesion (Fig. 5.17). In addition, angiography or CT scanning may indicate the presence of recent intracerebral haemorrhage (Fig. 5.18).

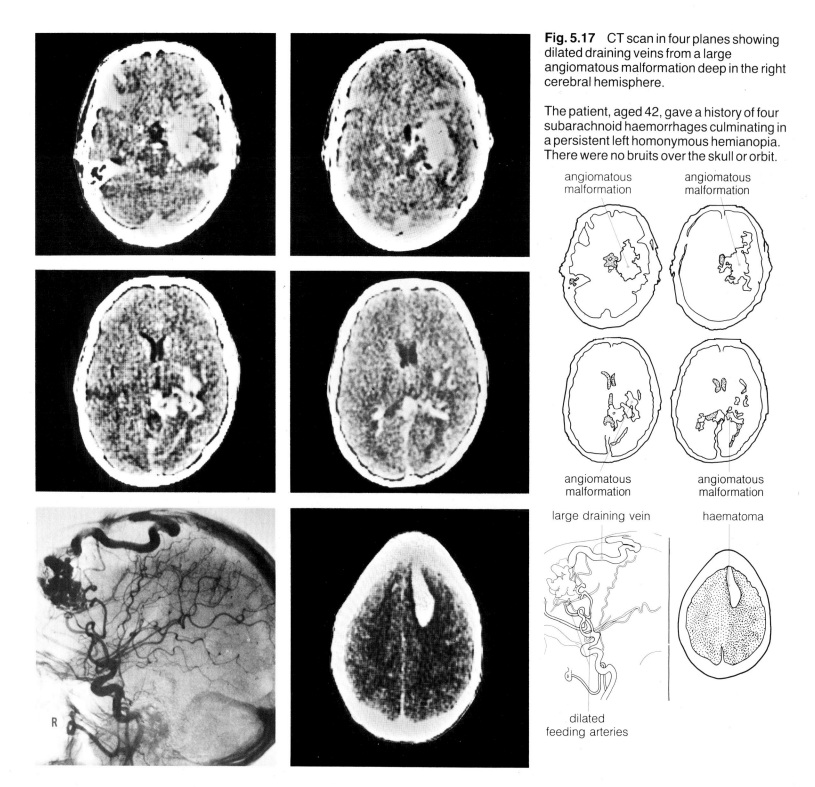

Fig. 5.17 CT scan in four planes showing dilated draining veins from a large angiomatous malformation deep in the right cerebral hemisphere.

The patient, aged 42, gave a history of four subarachnoid haemorrhages culminating in a persistent left homonymous hemianopia. There were no bruits over the skull or orbit.

angiomatous malformation

angiomatous malformation

angiomatous malformation

angiomatous malformation

large draining vein

haematoma

dilated feeding arteries

Fig. 5.18 Carotid angiogram (left) showing dilated feeding arteries of a frontal angiomatous malformation with a large vein draining into the superior sagittal sinus. The CT scan (right) of the same patient shows a right frontal haematoma.

In the Sturge-Weber syndrome, angiomata involving the meninges in the posterior part of the hemisphere, which are demonstrable as calcification corresponding to the cortical gyral pattern, are associated with facial naevi (Fig. 5.19).

The syndrome of moya moya presents in childhood or young adults. Severe narrowing or occlusion of the distal internal carotid arteries and of the circle of Willis leads to the development of anastomotic channels from perforat-ing and pial vessels and, in some cases, from branches of the external carotid artery (Fig. 5.20). In children the presentation is usually with episodes of cerebral ischaemia, in young adults with recurrent subarachnoid or intracerebral bleeding. Post-mortem examination reveals numerous anastomotic channels in conjunction with large vessel occlusion and cerebral atrophy (Fig. 5.21).

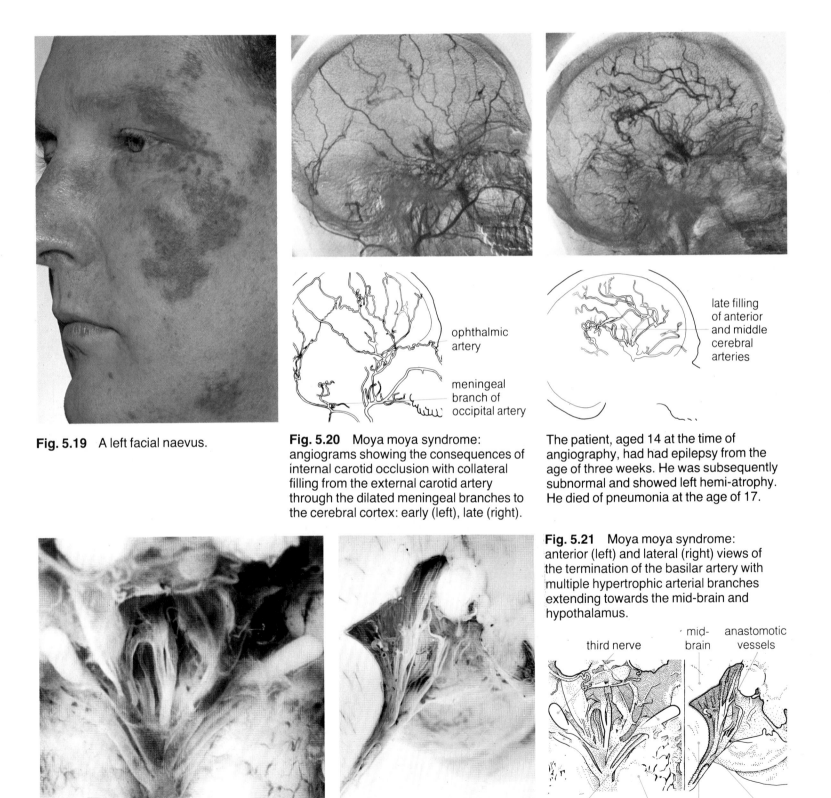

Fig. 5.19 A left facial naevus.

ophthalmic artery

meningeal branch of occipital artery

Fig. 5.20 Moya moya syndrome: angiograms showing the consequences of internal carotid occlusion with collateral filling from the external carotid artery through the dilated meningeal branches to the cerebral cortex: early (left), late (right).

late filling of anterior and middle cerebral arteries

The patient, aged 14 at the time of angiography, had had epilepsy from the age of three weeks. He was subsequently subnormal and showed left hemi-atrophy. He died of pneumonia at the age of 17.

Fig. 5.21 Moya moya syndrome: anterior (left) and lateral (right) views of the termination of the basilar artery with multiple hypertrophic arterial branches extending towards the mid-brain and hypothalamus.

third nerve

mid-brain

anastomotic vessels

basilar artery   pons   pons   basilar artery

Venous thrombosis may occur secondary to infection of the ear or paranasal sinuses but can also develop spontaneously. Superior sagittal sinus thrombosis results in acute brain swelling associated with a clinical picture which includes headache, alteration of consciousness, epilepsy and papilloedema (Fig. 5.22).

Subdural haematomata may arise in the supra- or infratentorial space and may be bilateral or unilateral. The sources of the haemorrhage are veins lying on the surface of the brain which are susceptible to relatively minor degrees of trauma, particularly in the elderly. They may develop acutely, subacutely or chronically. Prior to CT scanning being introduced, the diagnosis rested on the use of conventional isotope scanning together with cerebral angiography. Technetium scanning shows a superficial rim of increased activity whilst angiography reveals an avascular area between the surface of the brain

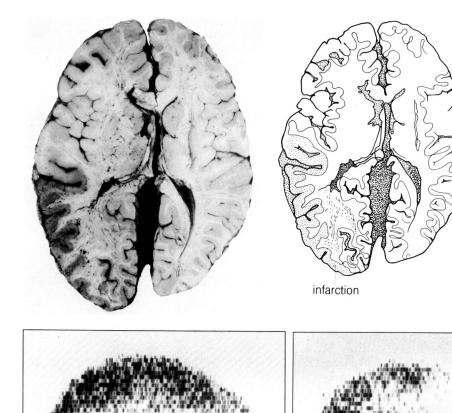

infarction

Fig. 5.22 Horizontal brain slice showing venous infarction of the cortex maximal in the occipital region.

The patient, a child, had suffered vomiting and diarrhoea. Post-mortem examination revealed a superior sagittal sinus thrombosis.

Fig. 5.23 Technetium scan showing a superficial rim of abnormal uptake due to a subdural haematoma: lateral view (left) and anteroposterior view (right).

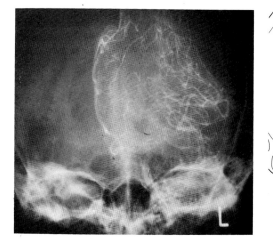

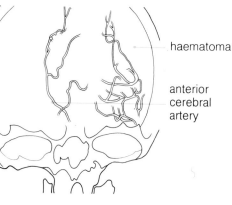

haematoma

anterior
cerebral
artery

Fig. 5.24 Carotid angiogram showing a large lenticular area of diminished density between the inner table of the skull and the underlying compressed brain, with marked shift of the midline structures and herniation of the anterior cerebral artery beneath the falx.

The patient, aged 40, gave a history of increasingly severe, generalised headaches for two months. Examination revealed bilateral papilloedema and slightly increased reflexes on the right. In retrospect, he recalled a fall downstairs three months previously.

and the table of the skull together with a shift of midline structures (Figs. 5.23 & 5.24).

CT scanning detects subdural haematomata with a high degree of accuracy and can to some extent, by the characteristics of the uptake, indicate the pathological state of the effusion and its possible duration. Acute lesions present within a few days of injury and appear as high density crescentic areas, adjacent to the skull table, often with associated midline shift (Fig. 5.25). With a longer history, lysis of the haematoma results in a low density area sometimes with a medially placed enhancing membrane (Fig. 5.26). Occasionally the haematoma is isodense with respect to cerebral tissue and its detection, by CT scanning, depends on the demonstration of ipsilateral ventricular compression and midline shift (Fig. 5.27).

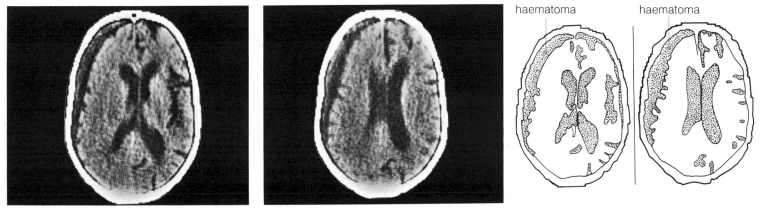

Fig. 5.25 CT scan in two planes showing an extensive peripheral haematoma (area of increased density) in the frontoparietal region causing cerebral compression and displacement of the midline structures.

The patient, aged 82, had fallen four hours previously. He was unconscious, responding only to painful stimuli, and had a left hemiparesis.

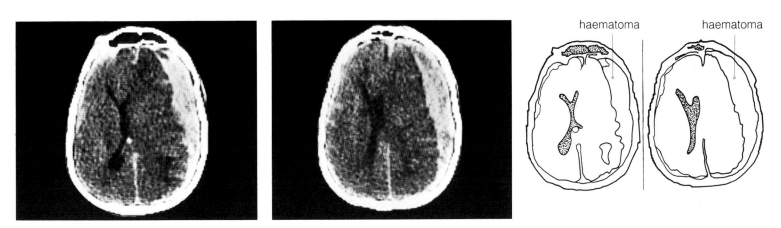

Fig. 5.26 A large chronic subdural haematoma in a patient with cerebral atrophy.

The patient, aged 81, was admitted with a history of drowsiness and confusion. He recovered spontaneously and surgical intervention was not required.

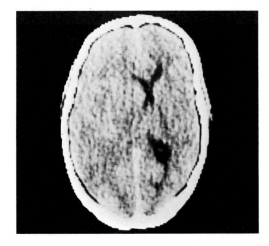 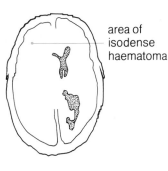

area of isodense haematoma

Fig. 5.27 A large isodense subdural haematoma compressing the left lateral ventricle and causing midline shift.

The patient, aged 24, had received a head injury one week previously, and complained of weakness in the right arm.

Extradural haematoma usually results from trauma to the middle meningeal artery secondary to skull fracture (Fig. 5.28). Classically, following injury, there is a lucid interval before the development of impaired consciousness with focal neurological signs. The CT scan shows a high density localised mass with ventricular compression and displacement (Fig. 5.29). There may be associated cerebral oedema.

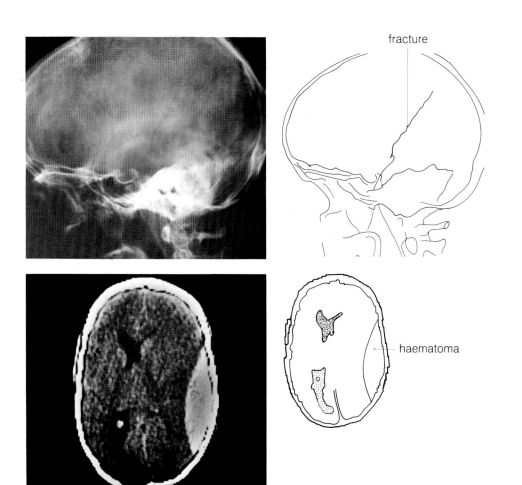

fracture

haematoma

Fig. 5.28 A lateral skull radiograph showing a right temporoparietal fissure fracture crossing the posterior branch of the middle meningeal artery.

The patient, aged 27, had been found unconscious. No focal neurological signs were recorded.

Fig. 5.29 A large peripheral haematoma in the right temporoparietal region adjacent to the inner table, causing cerebral compression and shift of midline structures. This is the same patient as in the previous figure.

6. Cerebral Degeneration and Movement Disorders

The aetiological basis of most of the conditions to be described here has yet to be established. The discovery of severely depleted brain dopamine levels in Parkinson's disease, secondary to relatively selective degeneration of dopaminergic neurones, raised expectations that dopa replacement therapy would control the clinical manifestations of the disease. This view neglected the progressive degeneration of dopaminergic neurones underlying the disorder, a progression which determines the waning response to drug therapy with the passage of time. Subsequently, the finding of substantial loss of gaba-containing neurones in Huntington's chorea, and cholinergic neurones in Alzheimer's disease has been interpreted with greater caution. Indeed, GABA therapy has no effect on the clinical features of Huntington's chorea whilst choline, the precursor of acetyl choline, produces little response in patients with Alzheimer's disease.

Recognition of the role of dopamine and other neurotransmitters in the genesis of movement disorders has led to the use of dopaminergic blocking agents in controlling, for example, the choreiform movements of Huntington's chorea. Apart from in Parkinson's disease, however, manipulation of brain amine levels in this manner has proved of limited value in the conditions described here.

Although toxic or nutritional factors operate in some cases (for example, in Wilson's disease and in Wernicke's encephalopathy) they are of no relevance in others. Further progress in the management of these disorders is unlikely until the basis of the initiating pathological insult is better understood.

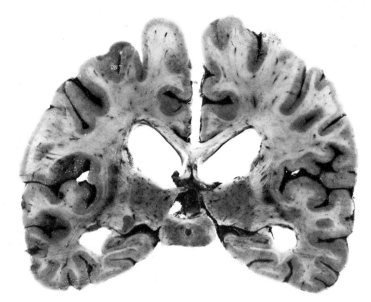

Fig. 6.1 Alzheimer's disease: coronal section through the cerebral hemispheres showing widened cortical sulci and dilated lateral ventricles.

The onset, which occurred around 34 years, was of progressive memory impairment with occasional jerking movements of the limbs. The patient's twin brother and mother were affected by the disease.

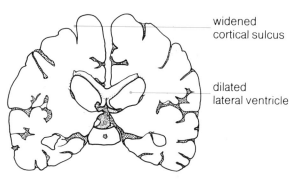

widened cortical sulcus

dilated lateral ventricle

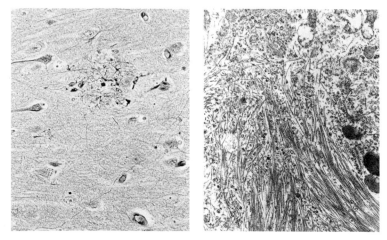

Fig. 6.2 Alzheimer's disease: senile plaque and neurofibrillary tangles in the hippocampus (left, Palmgren stain, ×280) and an electron micrograph showing part of a neurofibrillary tangle in a nerve cell from a right frontal brain biopsy (right, ×3,000).

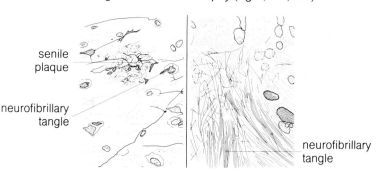

senile plaque

neurofibrillary tangle

neurofibrillary tangle

Fig. 6.3 Alzheimer's disease: frozen section of frontal cortex showing numerous senile plaques and neurofibrillary tangles. Von Braumuhl stain, ×210.

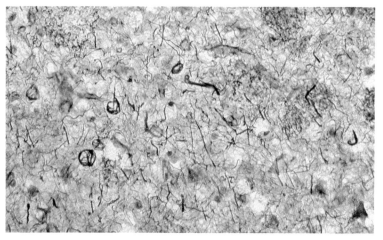

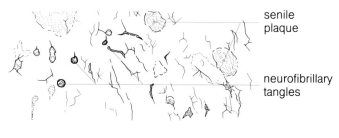

senile plaque

neurofibrillary tangles

Dementia

Senile and pre-senile dementia are distinguished by their age of onset, the former beginning after the age of 65. The commonest form of pre-senile dementia is Alzheimer's disease, which shares many clinical and pathological features with senile dementia. In Alzheimer's disease the cerebral atrophy is diffuse (Fig. 6.1) whilst in the rarer Pick's disease the changes are generally confined to the frontotemporal regions. Histological changes in Alzheimer's disease include a loss of neurones, neurofibrillary tangles in degenerating neurones and the presence of senile plaques (Figs. 6.2 & 6.3).

Most cases of Alzheimer's disease present in the sixth decade. The onset is insidious with deterioration of cognitive function and behavioural disturbance. Speech abnormalities, sometimes amounting to a frank dysphasia, may be prominent. In its early stages the diagnosis and differentiation from a depressive illness can be difficult.

Prior to the introduction of the CT scanner, air encephalography was required to assess the degree of cerebral atrophy. Typically this would show dilatation of the ventricular system with enlargement of the cortical sulci (Fig. 6.4). CT scanning is equally capable of demonstrating these changes, but with negligible morbidity (Fig. 6.5).

On occasions dementia may reflect a primary haematological or biochemical disorder, such as vitamin B_{12} deficiency or myxoedema. These can be readily excluded by the appropriate investigations.

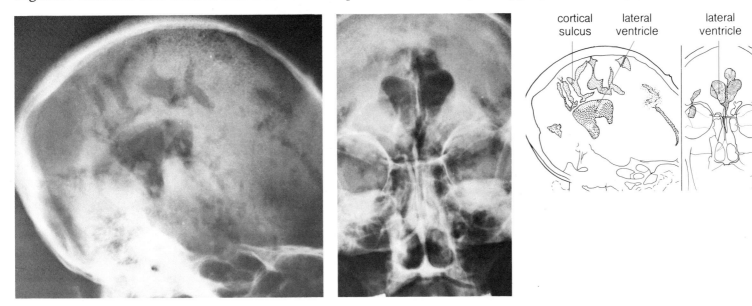

Fig. 6.4   Pre-senile dementia: air encephalogram showing dilated cortical sulci and enlargement of the lateral ventricles.

The patient, aged 53, gave a 4 year history of deteriorating memory. Psychometry indicated a severe, diffuse impairment of cognition, affecting both verbal and non-verbal communication.

Fig. 6.5   Pre-senile dementia: serial CT scans at two levels showing the development of cortical atrophy and ventricular dilatation between 1977 (left) and 1982 (right).

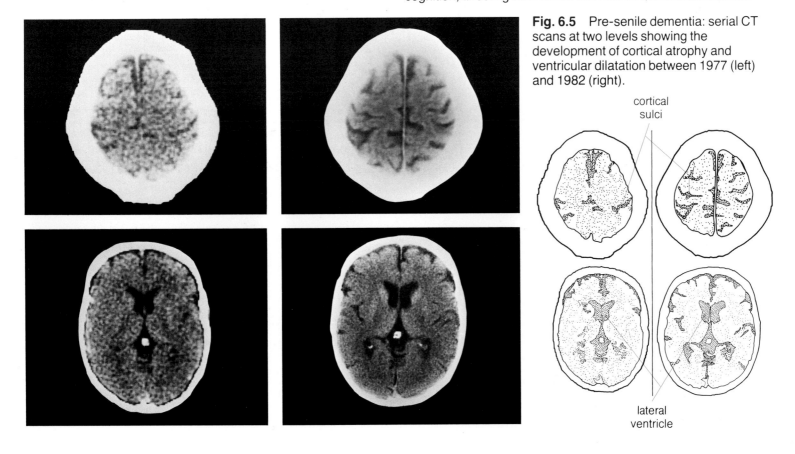

6.3

Parkinson's Disease

The most significant pathological changes in this condition centre on the substantia nigra and locus coeruleus. The substantia nigra shows depletion of melanin-containing nerve cells, maximal in the central part of the zona compacta, producing a characteristic pallor compared to a normal control (Figs. 6.6 & 6.7). A reduction of brain dopamine reflects the fall out of dopaminergic neurons. Cytoplasmic inclusion bodies (Lewy bodies) are found in nerve cells in the substantia nigra and elsewhere (Fig. 6.8). Changes in the cerebral cortex occur, and it is recognised that Parkinsonian patients may show evidence of cognitive dysfunction.

Clinical diagnosis is sometimes difficult in the early stages. A triad of rigidity, tremor and bradykinesia is the hallmark of the condition, but one or two of these components can be initially lacking and rarely the tremor, for example, may never develop. The condition most

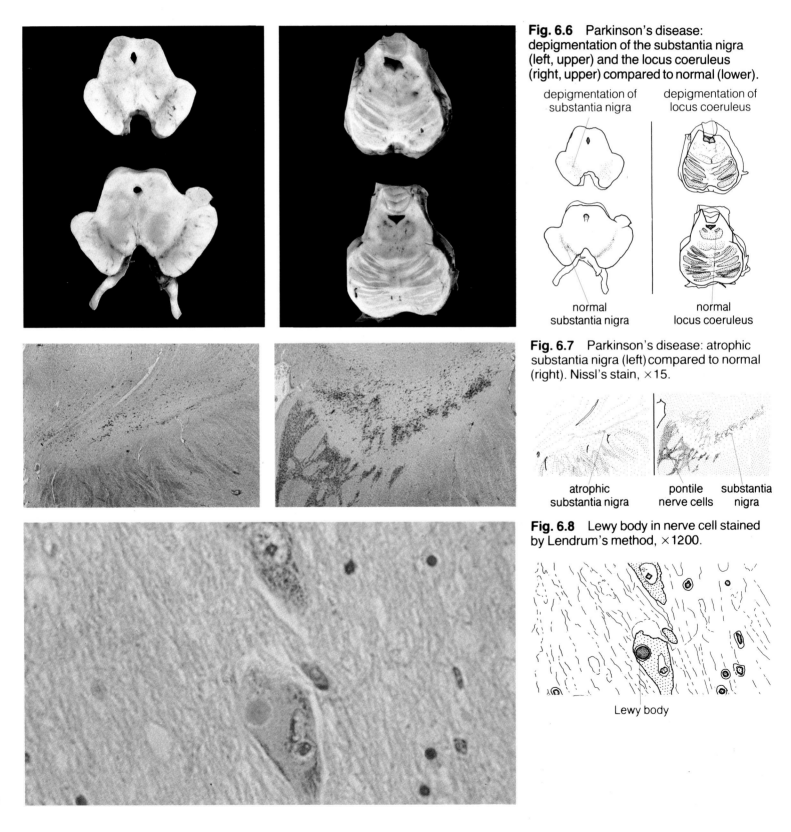

Fig. 6.6 Parkinson's disease: depigmentation of the substantia nigra (left, upper) and the locus coeruleus (right, upper) compared to normal (lower).

depigmentation of substantia nigra

depigmentation of locus coeruleus

normal substantia nigra

normal locus coeruleus

Fig. 6.7 Parkinson's disease: atrophic substantia nigra (left) compared to normal (right). Nissl's stain, ×15.

atrophic substantia nigra

pontile nerve cells

substantia nigra

Fig. 6.8 Lewy body in nerve cell stained by Lendrum's method, ×1200.

Lewy body

commonly begins in the sixth decade and is slightly more common in men.

The patient's facial appearance often declares the diagnosis, with a staring expression, infrequent blinking and impassivity (Fig. 6.9). The patient may complain of excessive salivation, which is more a reflection of impaired tongue movement and a disturbance of swallowing than of increased saliva formation (Fig. 6.10). Postural changes are very characteristic. The stance becomes stooped with flexion of the cervical and lumbar regions (Fig. 6.11), and a tendency to hold the arms flexed across the trunk.

The tremor usually lies between 4–6 Hz and is most often a rest tremor, disappearing briefly during voluntary activity. It is more apparent in the arms than the legs, and is capable of producing an electrical artefact on the ECG (Fig. 6.12).

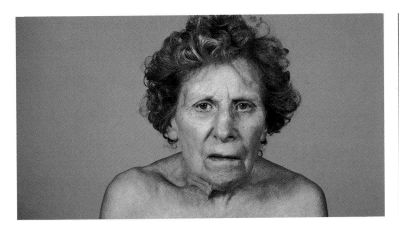

Fig. 6.9 Parkinson's disease: the characteristic facial appearance.

The patient, aged 71, gave a 2 year history of slowness of walking, difficulty in manipulating the fingers and an intermittent tremor of the upper limbs.

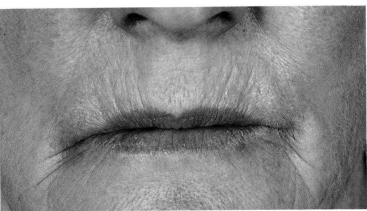

Fig. 6.10 Parkinson's disease: angular stomatitis secondary to dribbling of saliva from the angles of the mouth.

The patient, aged 65, had had a tremor of the right hand for several months. Examination showed mild, predominantly right-sided Parkinsonian signs.

Fig. 6.11 Parkinson's disease: a characteristic posture of the head and neck.

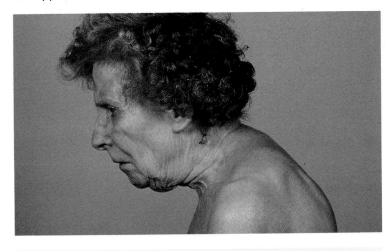

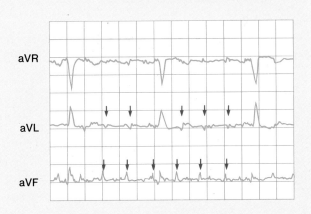

Fig. 6.12 Parkinson's disease: an ECG trace showing an artefact (arrows) produced by a limb tremor.

The patient, aged 77, had a short history of Parkinson's disease in association with a failure of memory. She showed a Parkinsonian tremor, particularly of the right arm.

Although anti-cholinergic drugs, once the mainstay of treatment, still have a useful role, L-dopa, combined with a peripheral dopa decarboxylase inhibitor, is the mainstay of therapy. Alternative approaches include the use of a dopaminergic agonist, such as bromocriptine or an inhibitor of dopamine metabolism, for example deprenyl. The former appears to improve the on-off effect in some patients whilst deprenyl appears capable of reducing end-of-dose akinesia. Response to dopa is often dramatic in the early stages. An analysis of gait or of writing can be used to assess progress (Fig. 6.13). Eventually, however, the response diminishes, no doubt due to progression of the underlying pathological process. In addition, with long-term therapy, a number of side-effects become apparent, including end-of-dose akinesia and the on-off effect, describing a rapid fluctuation in disability. Involuntary, dose dependent, movements may appear at any stage during treatment and include choreiform movements, orofacial dyskinesia, and dystonic postures of the upper or lower limbs (Figs. 6.14 & 6.15). Though the movements

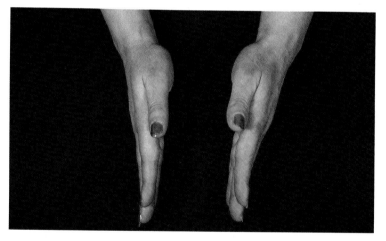

Fig. 6.13 Parkinson's disease: two examples of the patient's writing, showing the improvement related to the introduction of dopa therapy.

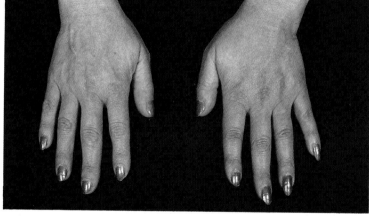

Fig. 6.14 Parkinson's disease: an abnormal posture of the left hand, with hyperextension of the index finger and abduction of the little finger.

The patient, aged 45, had a 3 year history of stiffness and tremor of the left hand. With Sinemet therapy she had noticed a periodic abnormal posture of the left hand.

Fig. 6.15 Parkinson's disease: dystonic posture of the left foot secondary to Sinemet therapy. (Taken from a television picture.)

The patient, aged 65, had had Parkinson's disease for several years. At a critical dose of Sinemet, he was liable to show an orofacial dyskinesia with dystonic posturing of the left foot.

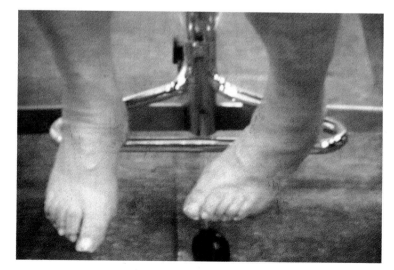

can be partially blocked by various neuroleptic agents, these in turn will partially inhibit the dopa response. In the late stages of the disease, disturbance of mobility may become profound (Fig. 6.16).

Huntington's Chorea

This is an uncommon condition, inherited as an autosomal dominant, and usually commencing in the fourth decade. Pathological changes embrace generalised cerebral atrophy with degeneration of the corpus striatum, particularly the caudate nucleus and putamen, where there is extensive loss of small nerve cells (Fig. 6.17). Post mortem analysis reveals a depletion of brain gamma-amino butyric acid (GABA), suggesting a loss of some 50% of striatal GABA-containing neurones. CT scanning delineates these anatomical changes, including the atrophy of the caudate nucleus (Fig. 6.18).

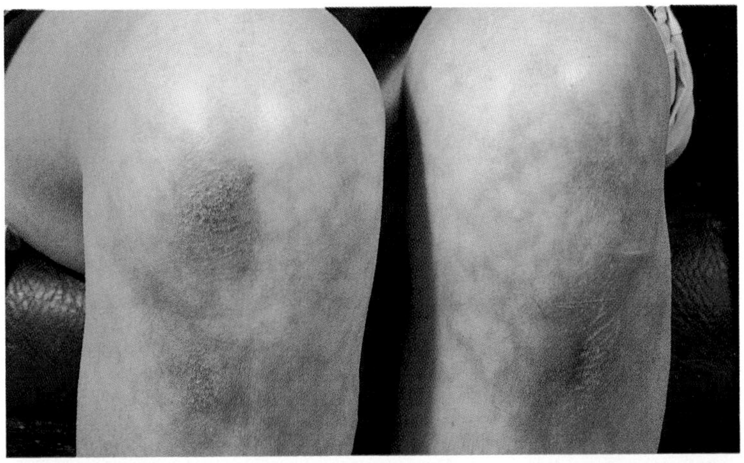

Fig. 6.16 Parkinson's disease: keratotic lesions on both knees. Due to immobility the patient had had to crawl on hands and knees within her home for some time.

The patient, aged 74, had had Parkinson's disease for 12 years Examination showed marked lower limb rigidity.

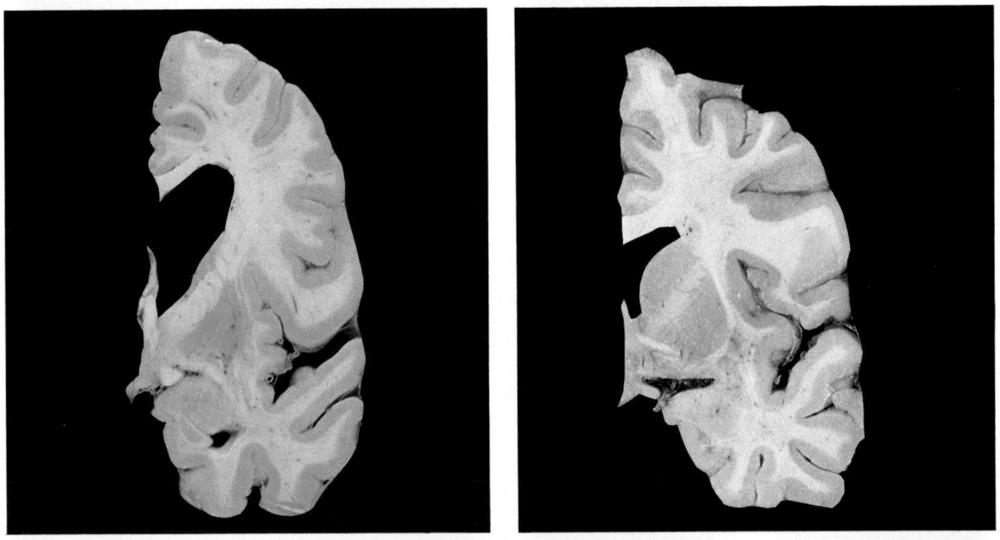

Fig. 6.17 Huntington's chorea: coronal brain section showing a dilated lateral ventricle with atrophy of the caudate and lentiform nuclei (left), and a control section (right).

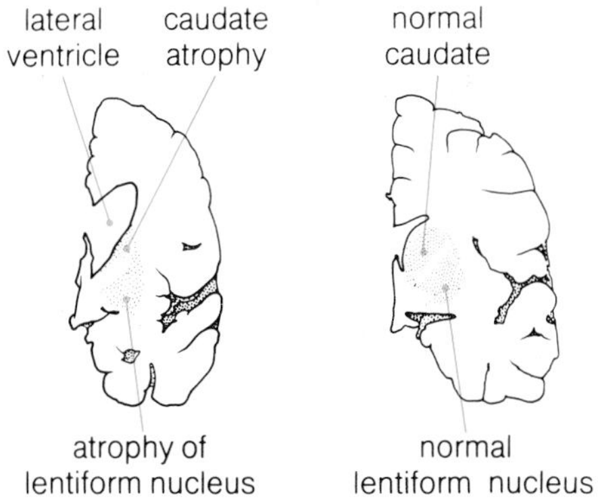

lateral ventricle | caudate atrophy | normal caudate

atrophy of lentiform nucleus | normal lentiform nucleus

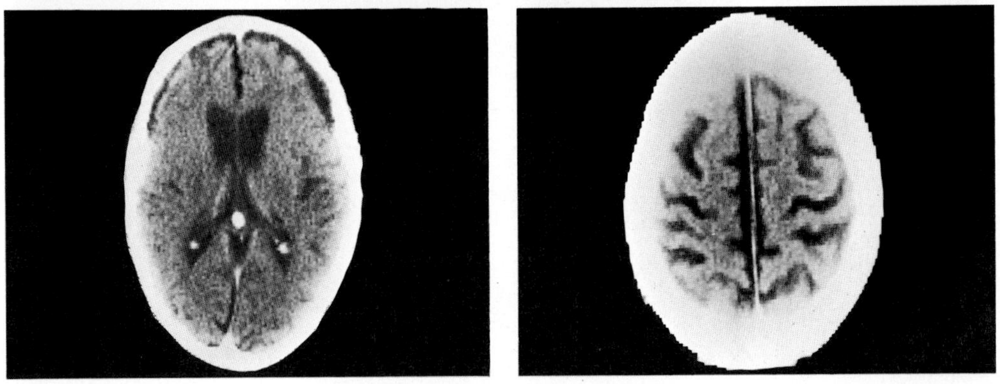

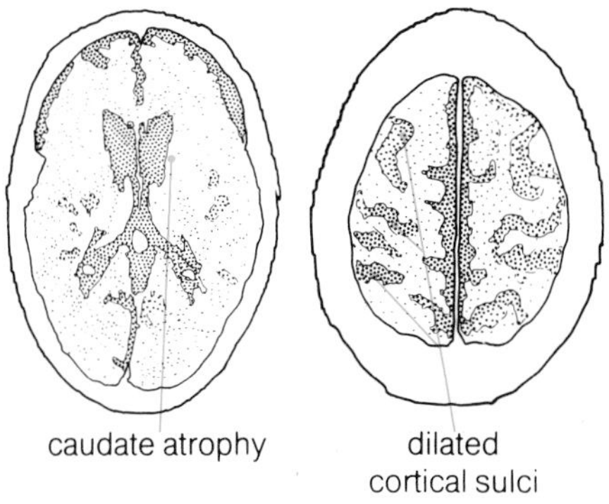

caudate atrophy | dilated cortical sulci

Fig. 6.18 Huntington's chorea: CT scan showing atrophy of the caudate nuclei (left) and cortical atrophy (right).

This man was first seen at the age of 56, when he gave a two to three year history of altered memory, of which he himself was hardly aware. Psychometry indicated a significant impairment of cognitive function. Occasional choreiform movements witnessed then had become florid 4 years later. There was no family history.

In adults the condition begins either with chorea or with behavioural disturbances. The chorea is often very subtle initially and tends to involve the face, head, arms and upper trunk in particular (Fig. 6.19). As well as behavioural disturbances, failure of memory is likely, sometimes leading to a frank dementia. Some patients develop epilepsy.

The condition sometimes presents in childhood (Juvenile Huntington's) when inheritance is usually from an affected father. Rigidity is more conspicuous than chorea, at times suggesting a Parkinsonian syndrome (Fig. 6.20). Dystonic posturing of the limbs may be a prominent feature (Fig. 6.21).

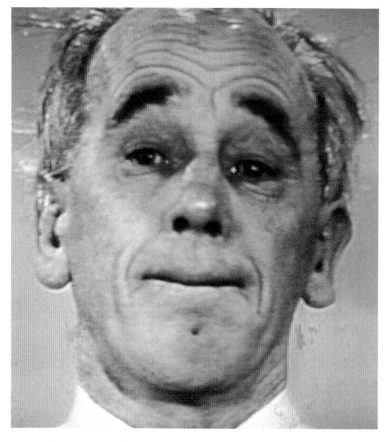

Fig. 6.19 Huntington's chorea: brief choreic contraction of frontalis. (Taken from a television picture.)

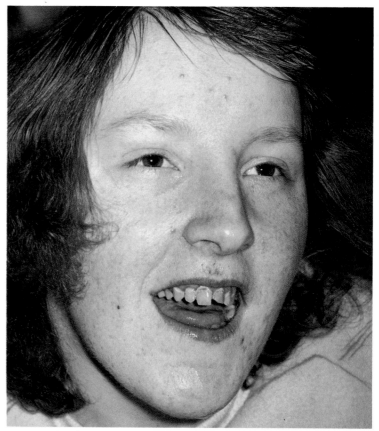

Fig. 6.20 Juvenile Huntington's: a 'Parkinsonian' facial appearance.

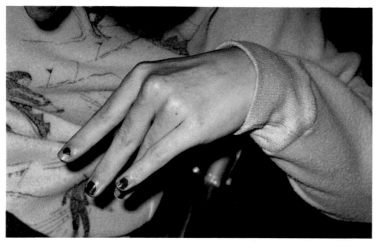

Fig. 6.21 Juvenile Huntington's: abnormal limb posture.

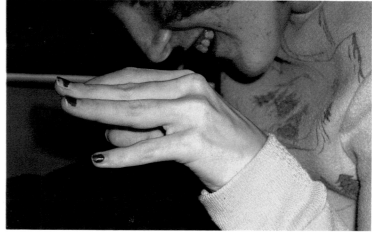

The girl, aged 16, had a three year history of increasing rigidity with alteration of mood and intellectual capacity. Examination showed slowed eye movements, a rigid neck and dystonic posturing of the left hand and right foot. Her father has the disease.

Steele-Richardson-Olszewski Syndrome

Substantia nigra and locus coeruleus are again affected in this condition, but the degenerative changes are widespread involving pons, midbrain, dentate and subthalamic nuclei, globus pallidus and nucleus basalis. In the later stages, brain stem atrophy is considerable (Fig. 6.22). Microscopic changes include neurofibrillary tangles and gliosis (Figs. 6.23 & 6.24).

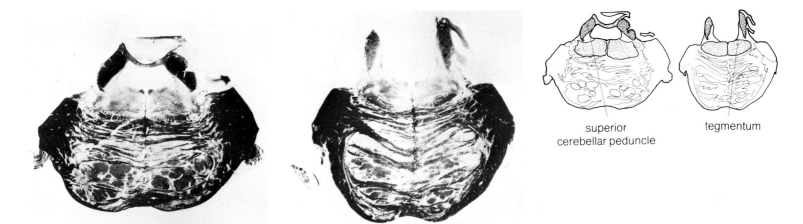

superior
cerebellar peduncle   tegmentum

Fig. 6.22 Steele-Richardson-Olszewski Syndrome. Normal pons (left) and the analagous level from a patient showing pale superior cerebellar peduncles and shrunken tegmentum (right). Myelin stain, ×15.

The woman, at the age of 61, developed falls and unsteadiness when walking. Two years later she became dysarthric, followed by difficulty with eye movement. At the age of 64, she had a vertical gaze paresis with normal doll's-head movements, dysarthria, limb immobility and pyramidal signs. She died at the age of 67.

Fig. 6.23 Steele-Richardson-Olszewski Syndrome: symmetrical gliosis in periaqueductal region and substantia nigra. Holzer preparation, ×5.

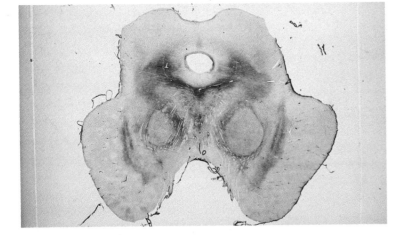

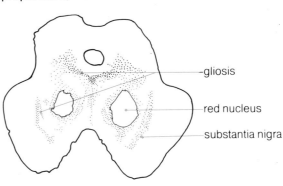

gliosis

red nucleus

substantia nigra

Fig. 6.24 Steele-Richardson-Olszewski Syndrome: neurofibrillary tangle in the mid-brain. Palmgren, ×790.

The patient developed unsteadiness at the age of 58 followed by difficulty in focussing. Examination showed a supranuclear gaze palsy in the vertical plane, dysarthria and dementia. She died at the age of 63.

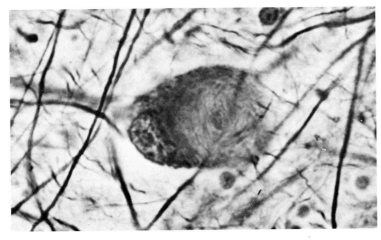

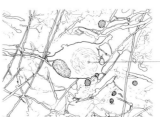

neurofibrillary
tangle

Radiological investigation reveals, in the late stages, widespread atrophic changes affecting both cerebral and cerebellar cortices (Fig. 6.25).

Clinical features of the condition include a supranuclear ophthalmoplegia, limb rigidity, gait disorder and dementia. In some cases, an axial rigidity principally affects neck extensors, causing hyperextension of the neck (Fig. 6.26). The supranuclear gaze palsy produces, at least initially, an impairment particularly of vertical voluntary gaze with preservation of reflex eye movement (Fig. 6.27). Later, failure of horizontal gaze appears, sometimes evolving through a phase suggesting an internuclear ophthalmoplegia (Fig. 6.28). The condition, though sharing some pathological features with Parkinson's disease and often displaying limb rigidity and bradykinesia, seldom responds to dopa therapy.

Shy-Drager Syndrome

Multiple system atrophy, or Shy-Drager syndrome, causes a combination of autonomic failure in association

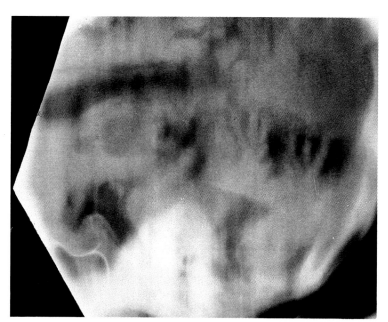

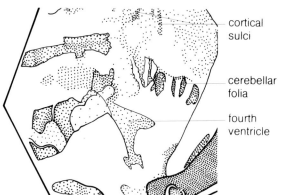

Fig. 6.25 Steele-Richardson-Olszewski Syndrome: air encephalogram showing cerebral and cerebellar atrophy.

At 58, this patient developed clumsiness of the right hand, forgetfulness and experienced frequent falls. Within two years she showed a supranuclear ophthalmoplegia, with limb pyramidal and extra-pyramidal signs.

cortical sulci

cerebellar folia

fourth ventricle

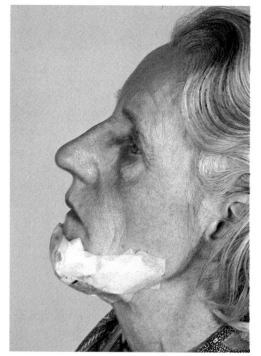

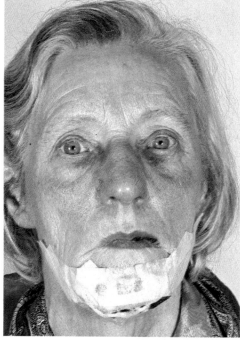

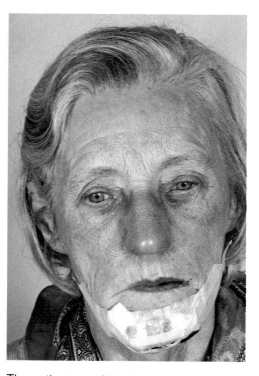

Fig. 6.26 Steele-Richardson-Olszewski Syndrome: head posture with hyperextension of the neck.

Fig. 6.27 Steele-Richardson-Olszewski Syndrome: the patient is attempting to look up (left) and then down (right).

The patient, aged 71, had a year's history of difficulty with walking, associated with frequent falls. There was severe restriction of vertical and, to a lesser extent, of horizontal saccadic eye movements with limb rigidity and a restricted gait.

with cerebellar, pyramidal and extra-pyramidal features. The pathological changes consists of striatonigral degeneration with, or without, olivopontocerebellar degeneration (Fig. 6.29). Autonomic failure is secondary to degeneration of the intermediolateral columns of the spinal cord (Fig. 6.30).

Autonomic failure results in Horner's syndrome in some cases, together with impairment of sphincter control, impotence, anhidrosis and profound postural hypotension. Some patients show a marked hypersensitivity, in terms of blood pressure response, to infusion of tyramine or noradrenaline (Fig. 6.31).

Treatment of the condition is unsatisfactory – a variety of methods to control the blood pressure changes with posture have been suggested, including an anti-gravity suit, fludro-cortisone and tyramine combined with a mono-amine oxidase inhibitor. None has proved particularly successful.

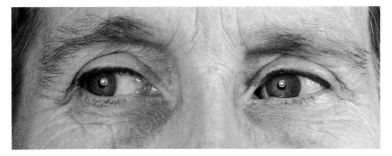

Fig. 6.28 Steele-Richardson-Olszewski Syndrome: the patient has been asked to look to the right. The range of adduction is less than that of abduction.

The patient, aged 58, had a history of depression. For a year she had had difficulty in walking. Her speech had become slurred. Examination showed a severe impairment of vertical saccadic eye movements. Horizontal movements were less severely affected. There was neck and limb rigidity with a gait ataxia.

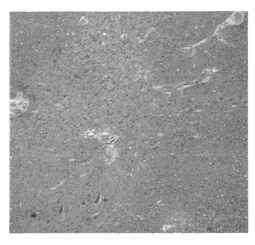

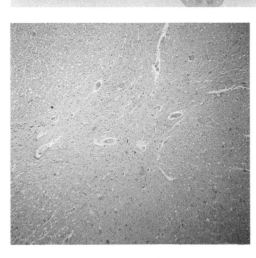

Fig. 6.29 Shy-Drager Syndrome: section of pons and cerebellum showing atrophy of pontine grey matter and middle cerebellar peduncles. Wiegert-Pal stain.

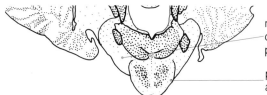

middle cerebellar peduncle

pontine atrophy

Fig. 6.30 Shy-Drager Syndrome: spinal cord section showing loss of intermediolateral column cells (left) compared to normal control (right). H & E stain, ×85.

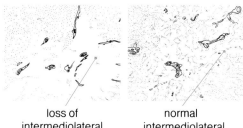

loss of intermediolateral column cells

normal intermediolateral column

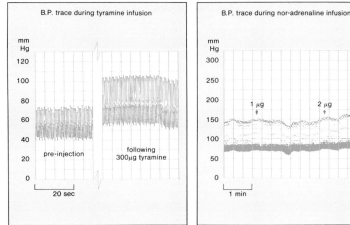

Fig. 6.31 Shy-Drager Syndrome: blood pressure tracings showing hypersensitivity to infusion of tyramine (left) and noradrenaline (right).

The left-hand trace was obtained from a man aged 67, who presented with a 4 year history of impotence, anhidrosis and postural hypotension.
The right-hand trace refers to a man of 64 with a six month history of difficulty walking, together with periodic incontinence of urine. He had been impotent for 3 years and later developed postural hypotension.

Wilson's Disease

This is a rare disorder, inherited as an autosomal recessive. The onset tends to be in the second decade and is rare beyond 40 years of age. As a generalisation, early onset is more likely to occur with manifestations of hepatic disease, and later onset with neurological features.

Pathological abnormalities include cirrhosis of the liver (Fig. 6.32) and degenerative changes of the central nervous system, particularly in the putamen, where cavitation may occur (Fig. 6.33). Changes in the caudate nucleus and globus pallidus are less conspicuous.

Deposition of copper pigment on the undersurface of the cornea in Descemet's membrane produces a brownish-green appearance, the Kayser-Fleischer ring (Fig. 6.34). It is almost invariably found when the disease manifests clinically, particularly if there are neurological signs. These include tremor, dysarthria and dystonia, particularly in children (Fig. 6.35). Psychiatric disturbances and intellectual changes are seen, and some patients develop epilepsy. Abnormal sweating, noted by Wilson to

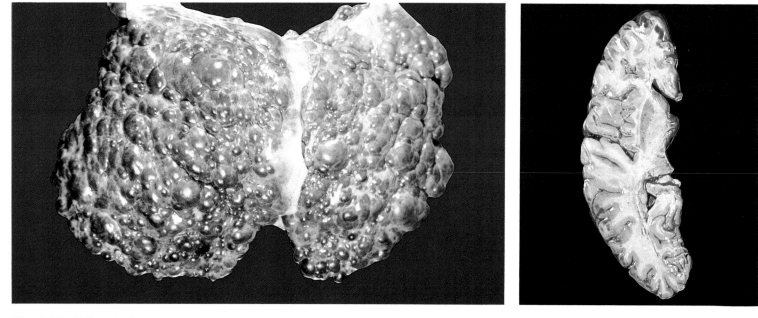

Fig. 6.32 Wilson's disease: liver showing shrinkage with post-necrotic cirrhosis

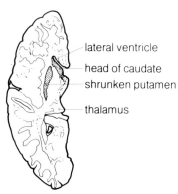

Fig. 6.33 Wilson's disease: horizontal brain slice showing shrunken putamen.

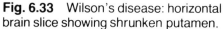

lateral ventricle
head of caudate
shrunken putamen
thalamus

Fig. 6.34 Wilson's disease: the Kayser-Fleischer ring.

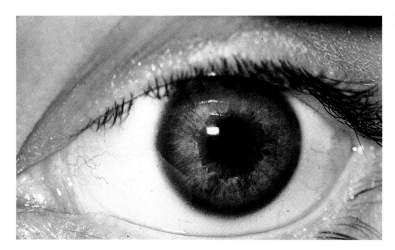

be an occasional feature, was conspicuous in the patient shown in figure 6.35.

Serum copper and coeruloplasmin levels are usually depressed whilst urinary copper excretion is increased. Liver biopsy reveals increased copper stores, the basis also, of the pathological changes in the central nervous system. Treatment is with a combination of a low copper diet plus the chelating agent, penicillamine.

Wernickes Encephalopathy

This condition, precipitated by thiamine deficiency, is usually seen in alcoholics. Its incidence, based on post-mortem studies, is under-reported. The classical triad, described by Wernicke, of mental symptoms, ophthalmoplegia and ataxia, is rather uncommon. Many patients have a related alcoholic neuropathy. A Korsakoff psychosis with memory disturbance and confabulation may coincide with, or follow, the other symptoms. Pathological changes predominate in the mid-brain and hypothalamus, particularly the mamillary bodies (Figs. 6.36 & 6.37).

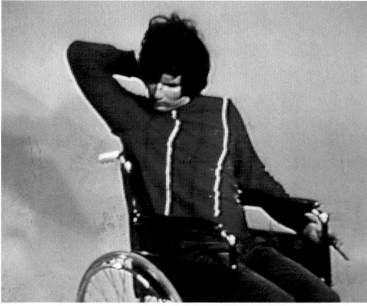

Fig. 6.35 Wilson's disease: dystonic posture of the trunk and limbs. (Taken from a television picture.)

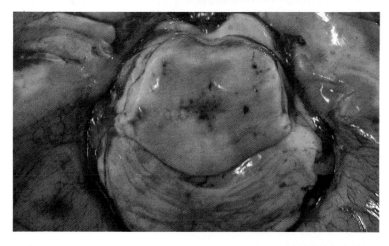

Fig. 6.36 Wernicke's encephalopathy: periaqueductal and inferior collicular haemorrhages.

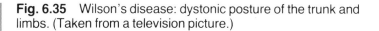
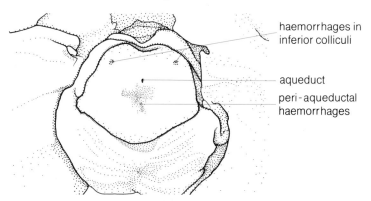

haemorrhages in inferior colliculi

aqueduct

peri-aqueductal haemorrhages

Fig. 6.37 Wernicke's encephalopathy: haemorrhages in floor of fourth ventricle. H & E stain, ×30.

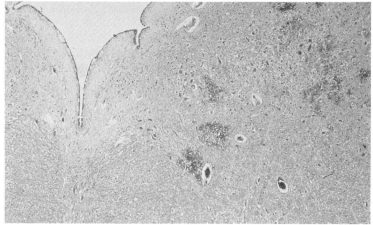
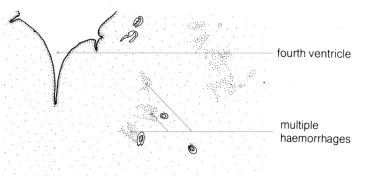

fourth ventricle

multiple haemorrhages

Torsion Dystonia

Dystonia is the description of an abnormal posture of limb, neck or trunk due to a sustained muscle contraction. It may be a manifestation of many disease processes and can be induced by certain drugs. An idiopathic form, torsion dystonia or dystonia musculorum deformans, occurs though as yet the pathological basis for this condition has not been established. Juvenile onset is predominantly in the lower limbs, whilst in the adult the upper limbs or the trunk are more often affected (Fig. 6.38). In adult cases the dystonia tends to remain confined to the site initially involved.

Writer's Cramp

A number of occupational cramps are described, affecting such diverse activities as typing, using scissors and writing. Writer's cramp is by far the commonest form. In most cases the dystonic reaction is confined to a single skilled task but in some patients the condition progresses so that a multiplicity of activities become affected. Abnormal muscle spasm of the fingers and hand develops during writing which tends to become increasingly illegible. A switch to the non-dominant hand may be initially successful (Fig. 6.39) but this hand in turn often then develops the same problem. The condition predominates in males and usually begins in middle life. Treatment is usually unsuccessful.

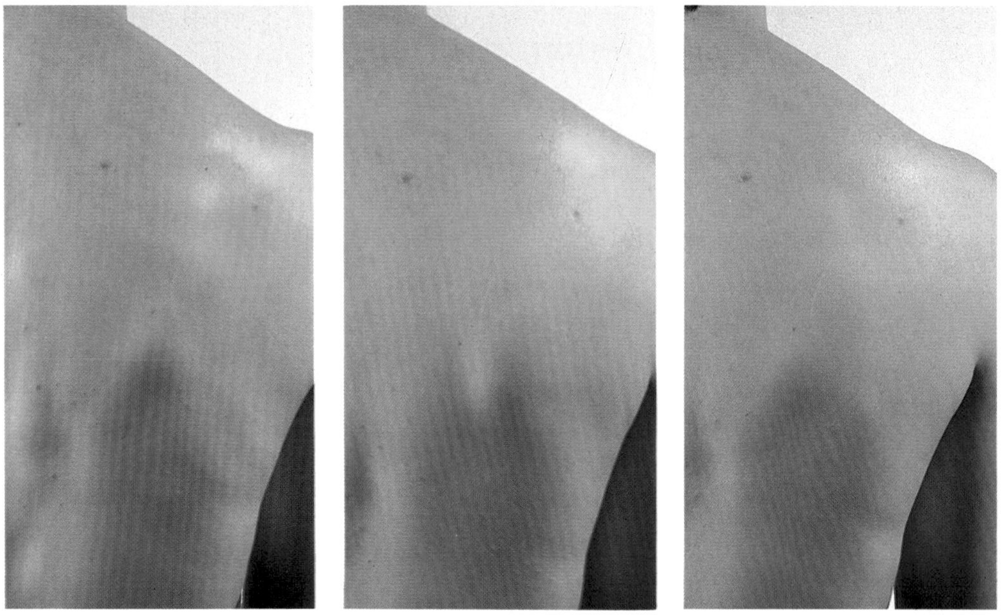

Fig. 6.38 Segmental torsion dystonia: a compendium of still photographs to show the variation in posture of the right shoulder.

The patient, aged 26, had noticed irregular movements of the right shoulder for six weeks. Examination showed variable dystonic posturing of the right shoulder.

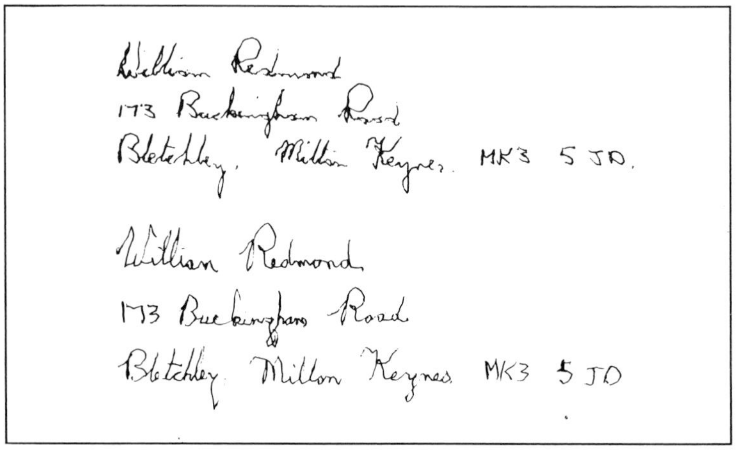

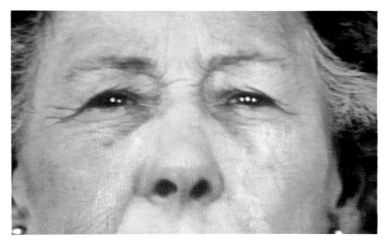

Fig. 6.39 Writer's cramp: an example of the patient's script written with the affected hand (upper) and the unaffected hand (lower) with which the patient had learnt to write.

The patient, aged 64, had had difficulty writing with his left hand for 3 years. Examination showed an excessive use of force when writing with the left hand with a correspondingly cramped script. With his right hand, the script was more open.

Fig. 6.40 Blepharospasm: intermittent contraction of orbicularis oculi. (Taken from a television picture.)

The patient, aged 57, had noticed excessive blinking for 8 years. There was a strong family history of schizophrenia. The abnormalities on examination were confined to blepharospasm.

Blepharospasm

Intermittent contraction of the orbicularis oculi muscles characterises this condition (Fig. 6.40). The movement disorder may remain confined to this area, may spread to the oromandibular muscles – oromandibular dystonia – or become generalised.

Spasmodic Torticollis

Spasmodic contraction of certain muscle groups, particularly the sternomastoid, causes a movement disorder in which the head rotates and flexes towards one shoulder. Involvement of the neck extensors produces a more complex movement (Fig. 6.41). The condition is generally accepted, like writer's cramp and blepharospasm, to be a form of segmental dystonia, and like the others may become more widespread. Some authors have stressed an association with an obsessional personality.

Treatment of the condition is notoriously difficult. Dopaminergic blocking agents, such as tetrabenazine, are of limited value. Thalamotomy has sometimes been used. Tenotomy of the sternomastoid with cervical root section is initially successful (Fig. 6.42) but the condition may later relapse. Sometimes the condition remits or stabilises; in others, derangement of the cervical spine develops.

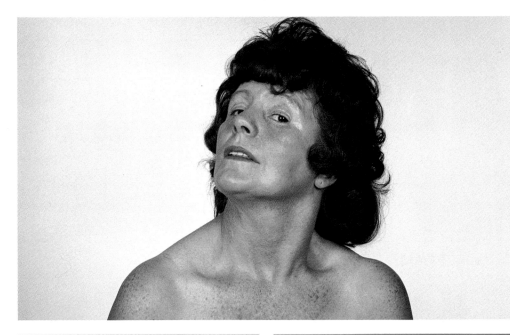

Fig. 6.41 Spasmodic torticollis: a characteristic head posture. Contraction of the left sternomastoid is particularly prominent.

The patient, aged 50, had developed intermittent contraction of the neck muscles seven years previously. Examination showed a tendency for the head to extend and rotate to the right.

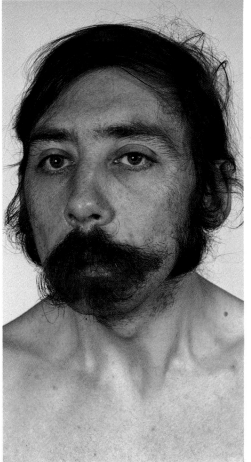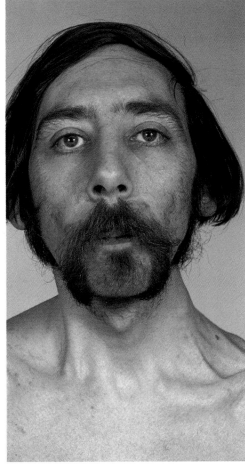

Fig. 6.42 Spasmodic torticollis: neck posture before (left) and after cervical rhizotomy and division of the accessory nerve (right).

The patient, aged 33, gave a two-year history of involuntary rotation of the head to the right. Following division of the left accessory nerve and of the upper three ventral cervical roots there was a considerable improvement in head posture.

Tics

These are stereotyped, repetitive movements which are particularly common in children. The movements may be confined to a single muscle or may involve several groups. The muscles of the head and neck are principally affected (Fig. 6.43).

The syndrome described by Gilles de la Tourette comprises multiple tics in association with vocal utterances. Onset is between the ages of 2 and 15. The condition is chronic though tends to wax and wane. There is a strong familial tendency, possibly on an autosomal dominant basis. Coprolalia occurs in approximately half the cases. The majority respond to haloperidol.

Orofacial Dyskinesia

This clinical syndrome, consisting of involuntary repetitive movements of the mouth and tongue, has multiple causes.

In tardive dyskinesia, associated with long-term ingestion of phenothiazines, tongue protrusion and lip smacking are characteristic features (Fig. 6.44). Paradoxically, the movements may appear for the first time when treatment with such drugs is withdrawn. Dopaminergic blocking agents often reduce the involuntary movements, but at the expense of precipitating Parkinsonian features.

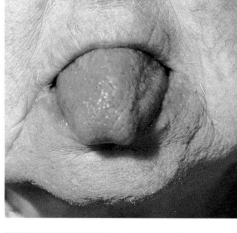

Fig. 6.43 Tic: compulsive head nodding. (Taken from a television picture.)

The patient, aged 75, had noticed repetitive head nodding for several months and had been depressed. There was no history of ingestion of psychotropic drugs. Examination showed repetitive head nodding but no other abnormalities.

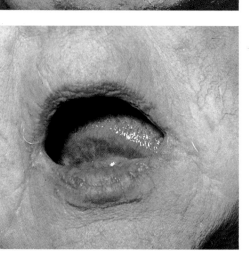
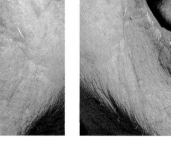

Fig. 6.44 Orofacial dyskinesia: various types of spontaneous tongue movement.

The patient, aged 72, had noticed involuntary movements of the tongue for 3 months. Examination showed frequent lip smacking and pursing with involuntary tongue protrusion.

7. Headache Syndromes and Cerebral Tumours

Although some cerebral tumours will present with headache alone, the majority of patients referred to the neurology clinic with headache suffer from migraine or tension headache. In these cases, the diagnosis is based largely on the patient's history, rather than on the findings on examination or the results of investigations.

Migraine

The headache of migraine tends to be unilateral and is often accompanied by nausea or vomiting (Fig. 7.1). A history of similar headache in first degree relatives is found in over two-thirds of patients. Focal visual, sensory, motor or speech disturbance identifies a minority sub-group of patients with classical, rather than common, migraine. Despite frequent attacks of this nature, persisting neurological deficit is relatively rare (Fig. 7.2).

Certain subgroups of migraine, associated with neurological deficit during the attack, need to be identified with care. Basilar migraine predominates in young females and results in signs of brain stem dysfunction, sometimes with altered awareness, during the course of the attack. Ophthalmoplegic migraine almost always begins in childhood, often with a history of severe headache alone. Subsequently, attacks of headache are associated with an oculomotor paresis which may last for days or weeks, and occasionally is permanent. All the fibres of the oculomotor nerve are affected and, in some cases, the fourth or sixth nerve may be involved. A similar presentation may occur with structural lesions such as an aneurysm, and these require exclusion before the diagnosis is accepted.

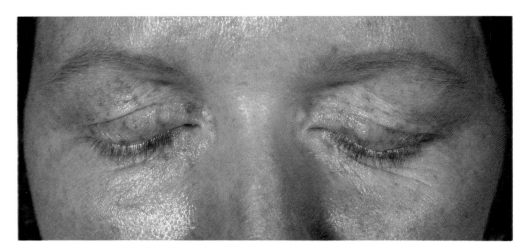

Fig. 7.1 Migraine: petechial haemorrhages on the upper eyelids.

This 40 year old woman gave a 20 year history of migraine. Vomiting occurred in some of the attacks and had been protracted shortly before this photograph was taken.

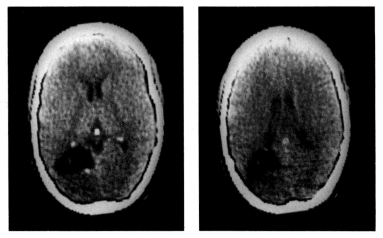

Fig. 7.2 Migraine: CT scan at two levels showing a parieto-occipital infarct.

This 25 year old man had a history of both epilepsy and migraine. Attacks of loss of consciousness were preceded by a right-sided visual aura with bifrontal headache. He had not been aware of a visual defect. Examination showed little limb abnormality but an incomplete right homonymous hemianopia.

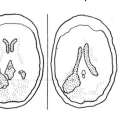

left parieto-occipital infarct

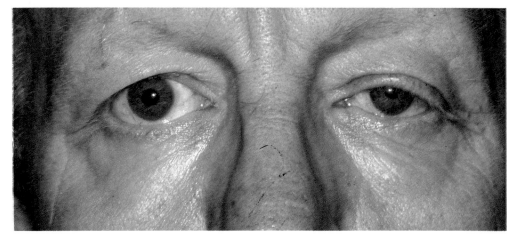

Fig. 7.3 Migrainous neuralgia: acute left Horner's syndrome during an attack of pain.

This 59 year old man had had migrainous neuralgia for many years, with periods of freedom of up to 3 years. Attacks consisted of pain over the left eye, scleral injection, drooping of the eyelid, a constricted pupil and nasal obstruction.

Migrainous Neuralgia (Cluster Headache)

This condition predominates in men, producing attacks of severe pain centred around one eye, lasting a half to two hours and recurring regularly over a period of weeks to be followed by long periods of remission. During attacks the eye ipsilateral to the pain is often congested, with obstruction or discharge from the nostril of that side. The affected eye may develop a Horner's syndrome which usually, though not invariably, remits as the pain subsides (Fig. 7.3).

Cranial Arteritis

In this disorder, an inflammatory reaction, usually with giant cell formation, involves the intima and media of certain vessels. Though typically affecting the superficial temporal artery, the disease is widespread with lesions affecting the aorta, carotid, gut and coronary vessels in some instances. The clinical features of the disease are protean therefore, but most commonly the patient presents with severe headache in association with malaise, low grade fever, sweats and anorexia. There may be associated proximal muscle pains (polymyalgia rheumatica). Examination reveals tender enlarged scalp vessels (Fig. 7.4). Involvement of the posterior ciliary arteries leads to an anterior ischaemic optic neuropathy with severe visual loss. Fundus examination shows a pale, swollen disc with normal retinal vessels (Fig. 7.5).

The ESR is almost always raised, often substantially. The arterial changes are distributed in an uneven fashion so that biopsy may be misleadingly normal. Characteristic changes occur, maximal in the media and internal elastic lamina. The intima is thickened, with inflammatory cells, including giant cells, infiltrating the outer intima (Fig. 7.6). The internal elastic lamina is always affected. Treatment with corticosteroids rapidly eliminates the headache but only rarely reverses established vision loss. It is generally continued for a minimum of twelve months.

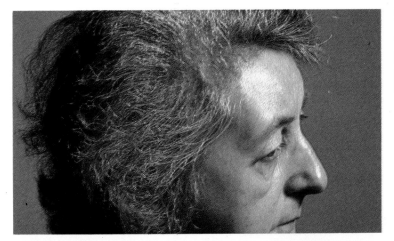

Fig. 7.4 Cranial arteritis: thickened superficial temporal artery.

This patient, aged 70, presented with pain in the forehead followed by the development of a left third nerve palsy. Examination showed gross thickening of the right superficial temporal artery which was tender. Her ESR was 116 mm/hr.

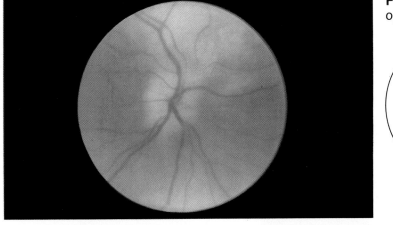

Fig. 7.5 Cranial arteritis: fundus photograph showing ischaemic optic neuropathy.

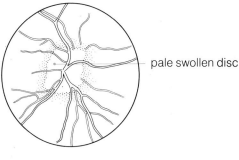

pale swollen disc

irregularity of media   inflammatory cells   multinucleate giant cells

intimal thickening   zone of internal elastic lamina

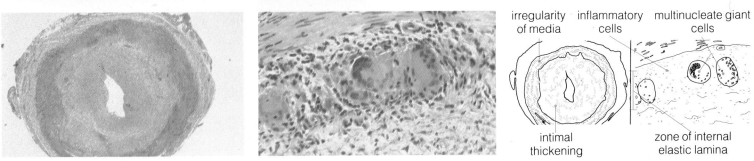

Fig. 7.6 Cranial arteritis: superficial temporal artery biopsy showing intimal thickening and medial damage (left, H&E stain, ×20) and giant cells and inflammatory cell infiltration at the level of the internal elastic lamina (right, H&E stain, ×200).

The patient, a 68 year old woman, had a year's history of shoulder girdle pain and stiffness, and more recent headache.

Cerebral Tumour

The prevalence of intracranial tumour in the population has been reported to be between 3 and 8.4 per 100,000. Gliomas are considered to represent between 31% and 43% of the total. In one series, the frequency in descending order was glioma, metastasis, meningioma, granuloma, pituitary adenoma, sarcoma, haemangioma, haemangioblastoma, craniopharyngioma and neurinoma.

Glioma

A number of classifications of these tumours have been proposed. In that produced by Kernohan and others, astrocytomas, ependymomas and oligodendrogliomas are rated on a four-point scale, according to the degree of malignancy. Grade three and four astrocytomas (glioblastoma multiforme) account for some 50% of the total. Malignant cerebral tumours may spread locally within the

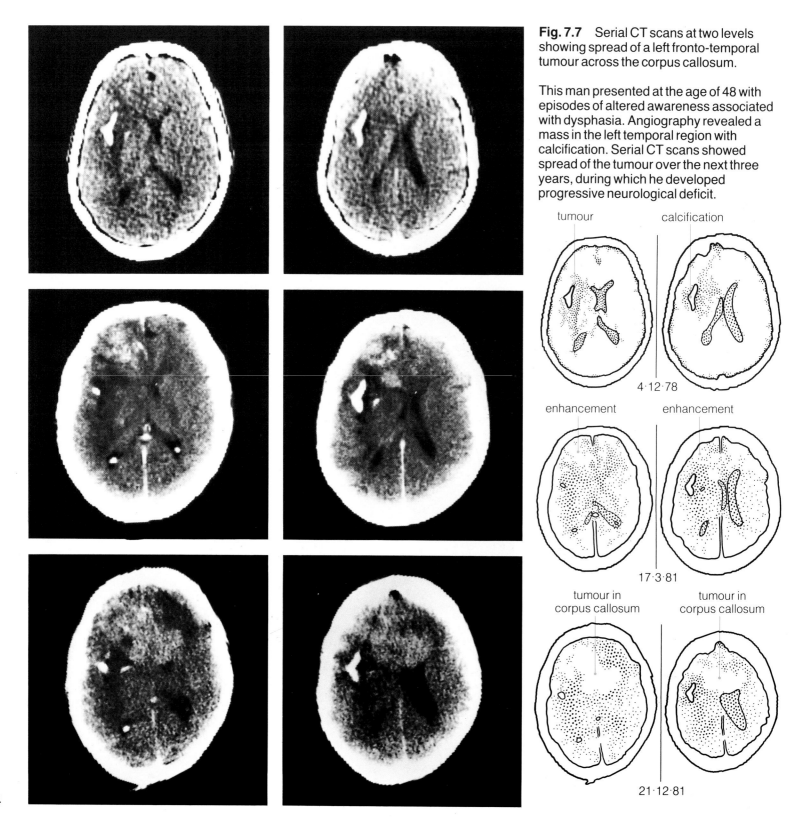

Fig. 7.7 Serial CT scans at two levels showing spread of a left fronto-temporal tumour across the corpus callosum.

This man presented at the age of 48 with episodes of altered awareness associated with dysphasia. Angiography revealed a mass in the left temporal region with calcification. Serial CT scans showed spread of the tumour over the next three years, during which he developed progressive neurological deficit.

tumour   calcification

4·12·78

enhancement   enhancement

17·3·81

tumour in   tumour in
corpus callosum   corpus callosum

21·12·81

brain, either along the ventricular system, under the meningeal surface, along neuronal pathways (Fig. 7.7) and even across the meninges. Spread outside the central nervous system is almost unknown.

The symptomatology of these tumours depends partly on the consequences of raised intracranial pressure, and partly on the site at which the tumour arises. The former, together with the effect of distortion of pain-sensitive structures within the cranium, results in headache, sometimes with vomiting, visual blurring or failure secondary to papilloedema (Fig. 7.8), and on occasions cranial nerve palsies, particularly of the sixth nerve (Fig. 7.9).

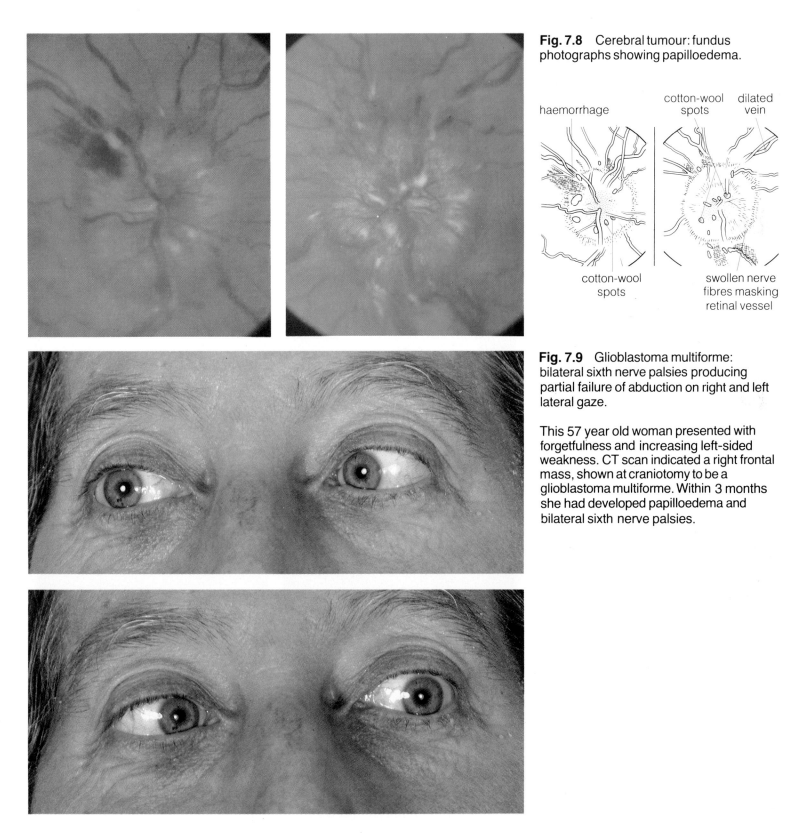

Fig. 7.8 Cerebral tumour: fundus photographs showing papilloedema.

Fig. 7.9 Glioblastoma multiforme: bilateral sixth nerve palsies producing partial failure of abduction on right and left lateral gaze.

This 57 year old woman presented with forgetfulness and increasing left-sided weakness. CT scan indicated a right frontal mass, shown at craniotomy to be a glioblastoma multiforme. Within 3 months she had developed papilloedema and bilateral sixth nerve palsies.

7.5

Tumours arising within the posterior fossa are more likely to produce intracranial hypertension at an early stage, though cerebellar signs are usually prominent in such cases (Fig. 7.10). The focal signs produced by intracranial tumour are understandable on a knowledge of their site of origin, though sometimes these signs are influenced by the local or distant effects of surgical intervention (Fig. 7.11).

Astrocytoma

These tumours have two peak incidences, one in childhood, between the ages of 3 and 8, when they usually arise from the cerebellum, and the other in adults in the fourth decade, usually arising from the cerebral hemispheres. They are slightly more common in men. The less malignant types, grades 1 and 2 show a uniform cell

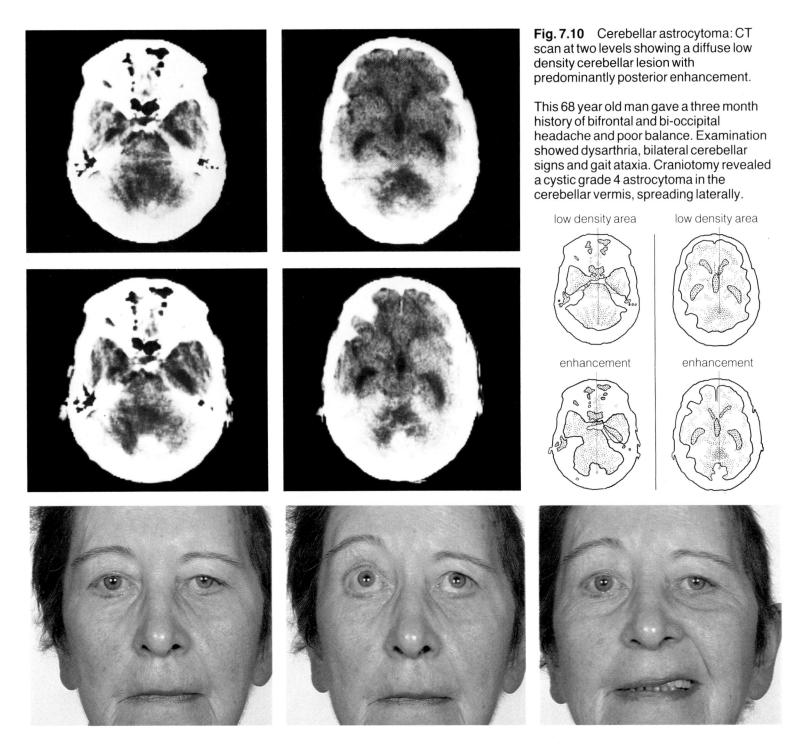

Fig. 7.10 Cerebellar astrocytoma: CT scan at two levels showing a diffuse low density cerebellar lesion with predominantly posterior enhancement.

This 68 year old man gave a three month history of bifrontal and bi-occipital headache and poor balance. Examination showed dysarthria, bilateral cerebellar signs and gait ataxia. Craniotomy revealed a cystic grade 4 astrocytoma in the cerebellar vermis, spreading laterally.

low density area   low density area

enhancement   enhancement

Fig. 7.11 Cerebral tumour: right upper motor neurone facial weakness with paresis of left frontalis due to division of facial nerve fibres to this muscle at the time of surgery. There is depression of the left eyebrow and failure of its elevation (left and middle) together with weakness of the right lower face (right).

This 68 year old woman presented with a short history of dysphasia and right-sided weakness. A large cystic astrocytoma was found in the left frontoparietal area at craniotomy.

pattern with few mitotic figures and poorly defined margins (Fig. 7.12). The most malignant, grades 3 and 4, (glioblastoma multiforme) are rapidly growing, with poorly defined margins, frequent mitotic figures and vascular proliferation (Figs. 7.13 & 7.14).

Post mortem studies suggest that glioblastomas reach a peak incidence in the sixth decade, though clinical series indicate involvement of a rather younger age group. They usually originate in the cerebral hemisphere, particularly the frontal lobe, and carry a poor prognosis.

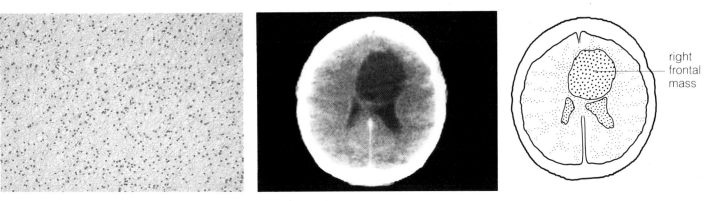

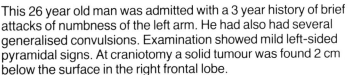

Fig. 7.12 Astrocytoma grade 2 showing increased cellular density with variation in nuclear size and shape (left, H&E stain, × 300), and a CT scan showing a large, apparently cystic, mass in the right frontal lobe (right).

This 26 year old man was admitted with a 3 year history of brief attacks of numbness of the left arm. He had also had several generalised convulsions. Examination showed mild left-sided pyramidal signs. At craniotomy a solid tumour was found 2 cm below the surface in the right frontal lobe.

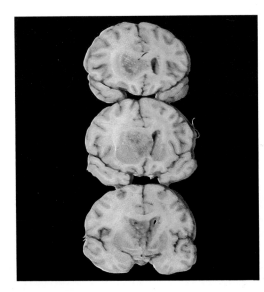

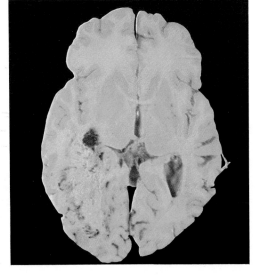

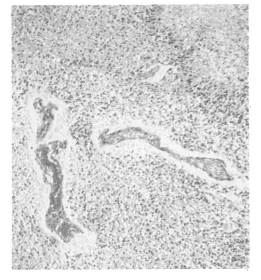

Fig. 7.13 Glioblastoma multiforme infiltrating and expanding the septum pellucidum and corpus callosum.

Fig. 7.14 Astrocytoma grade 3: horizontal brain slice (left) and the microscopic appearance (right, H&E stain, × 120).

This 65 year old woman presented with a short history of dysphasia. Examination showed dysphasia, right homonymous hemianopia, right sensory neglect and mild right pyramidal signs.

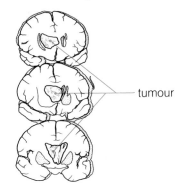

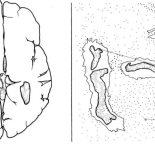

Prior to the introduction of the CT scanner, angiography was the most valuable investigative tool for patients suspected of having a cerebral tumour. With low-grade tumours, angiography simply reveals a mass effect with stretching of vessels or midline shift (Fig. 7.15). With glioblastomas, and certain metastases, the vascularity of the tumour may be revealed as abnormal vessels surrounding the periphery, sometimes with dilated draining veins (Fig. 7.16).

On computerised tomography glioblastomas tend to show more variability in density and enhancement pattern than benign astrocytomas (Fig. 7.17), which are commonly of lower density, with less enhancement and, sometimes, contain areas of calcification.

Ependymoma

The majority of these tumours occur in children and young adults, originating in the posterior fossa in the region of the fourth ventricle (Fig. 7.18) and in the spinal cord.

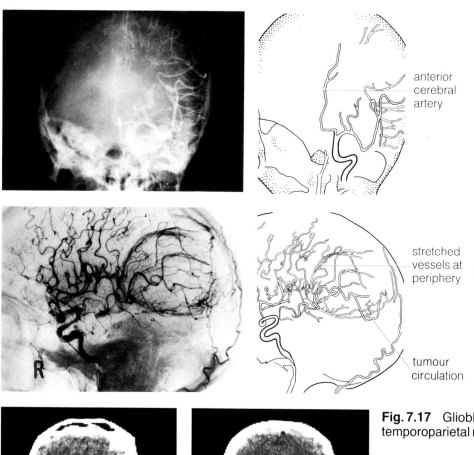

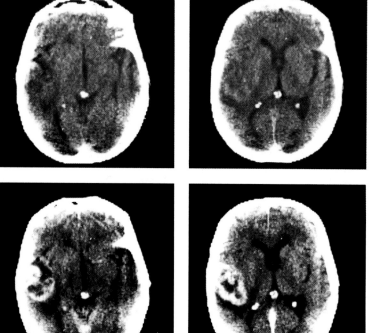

Fig. 7.15 Cerebral tumour: left carotid angiogram showing shift of the anterior cerebral artery to the right.

This 59 year old woman presented with a three month history of fluctuating dysphasia with headache. Examination revealed dysphasia with right-sided visual and sensory neglect. Angiography showed a left temporoparietal mass (a metastasis from a carcinoma of the bronchus) with shift of midline structures.

Fig. 7.16 Glioblastoma multiforme: right carotid angiogram showing a mass in the parieto-occipital region with stretching of vessels and a tumour circulation.

This 66 year old man presented with a short history of left-sided weakness. Examination showed a left homonymous hemianopia and a left hemiparesis. Biopsy of the right parieto-occipital mass showed a glioblastoma multiforme.

Fig. 7.17 Glioblastoma multiforme: CT scan showing a left temporoparietal mass with enhancement.

This man, aged 72, had an unexplained collapse, followed by a slowly progressive dysphasia, which was the major finding on neurological examination. Biopsy of his tumour showed a grade 4 cystic astrocytoma.

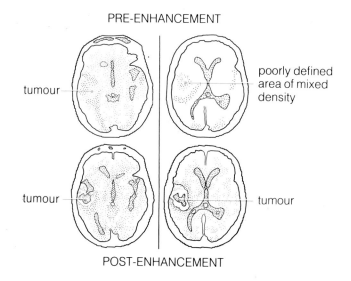

Papilloma of the Choroid Plexus

These are rare tumours, arising within the lateral or fourth ventricle, and causing hydrocephalus or seedling deposits in the spinal subarachnoid space (Fig. 7.19).

Oligodendroglioma

These are estimated to represent between 3% and 5% of all brain tumours. They generally arise in the white matter of the cerebral hemisphere and present in the middle years of life. The tumours often contain calcium, usually within the walls of blood vessels, but sometimes in the parenchyma. They are composed of sheets of uniform cells interspersed with thin-walled vessels (Fig. 7.20). Calcification may be a prominent feature on the skull radiograph or CT scan (Fig. 7.21).

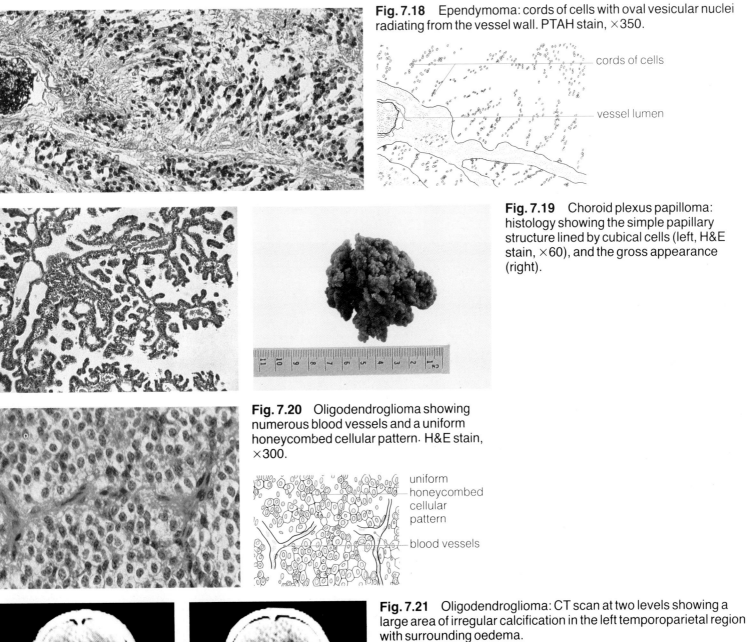

Fig. 7.18 Ependymoma: cords of cells with oval vesicular nuclei radiating from the vessel wall. PTAH stain, ×350.

cords of cells

vessel lumen

Fig. 7.19 Choroid plexus papilloma: histology showing the simple papillary structure lined by cubical cells (left, H&E stain, ×60), and the gross appearance (right).

Fig. 7.20 Oligodendroglioma showing numerous blood vessels and a uniform honeycombed cellular pattern. H&E stain, ×300.

uniform honeycombed cellular pattern

blood vessels

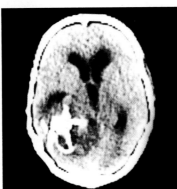

Fig. 7.21 Oligodendroglioma: CT scan at two levels showing a large area of irregular calcification in the left temporoparietal region with surrounding oedema.

This 50 year old woman gave a history of loss of balance and intermittent vomiting. Examination showed papilloedema.

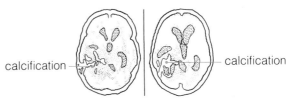

calcification

calcification

Medulloblastoma

Classically these tumours occur in childhood, arising from the vermis of the cerebellum (Fig. 7.22). They seldom arise over the age of 30 and males are more commonly affected. Periodically they originate from the cerebellar hemisphere. The tumours are highly malignant, sometimes spreading via the subarachnoid space (Fig. 7.23).

Cerebral Metastases

It has been suggested that the incidence of metastatic brain tumours at routine autopsy in patients with any form

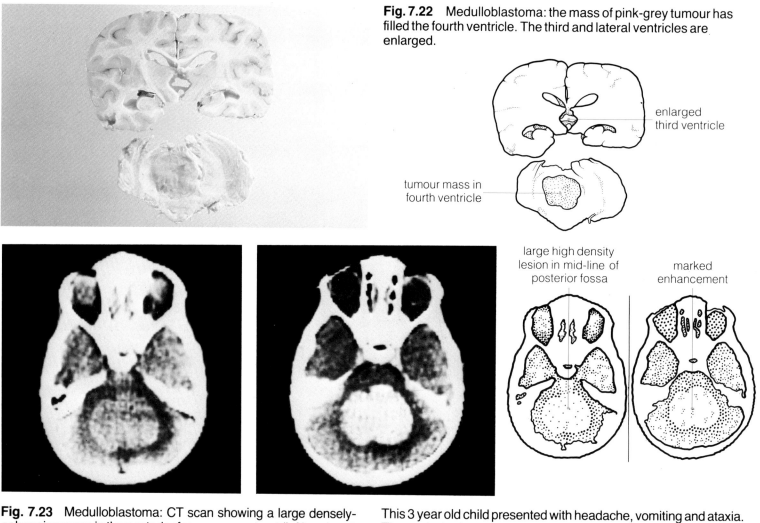

Fig. 7.22 Medulloblastoma: the mass of pink-grey tumour has filled the fourth ventricle. The third and lateral ventricles are enlarged.

enlarged third ventricle

tumour mass in fourth ventricle

large high density lesion in mid-line of posterior fossa

marked enhancement

Fig. 7.23 Medulloblastoma: CT scan showing a large densely-enhancing mass in the posterior fossa: pre-contrast (left) and post-contrast (right).

This 3 year old child presented with headache, vomiting and ataxia. The posterior fossa mass proved to be a medulloblastoma at craniotomy.

Fig. 7.24 Metastases: multiple deposits of malignant melanoma in a Nissl-stained brain section.

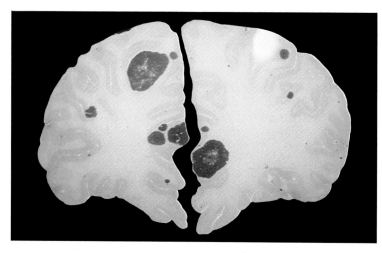

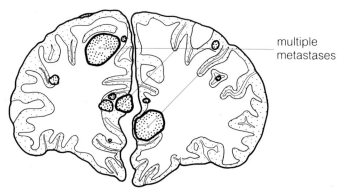

multiple metastases

of malignancy reaches 20%. The percentage of intracranial tumours reported to be metastatic may be as high as 40%. The most frequent primary tumours responsible for cerebral metastases arise from the breast and bronchus. In the majority of cases, the metastases are multiple (Figs. 7.24 & 7.25). They tend to be well demarcated, sometimes with areas of necrosis, cyst formation or haemorrhage (Fig. 7.26). Less frequent primary sources include renal and gut tumours, choriocarcinoma and melanoma. These, with breast and bronchus, account for some 95% of metastases. For bronchial tumours, some 33% of autopsies show cerebral metastases (Fig. 7.27).

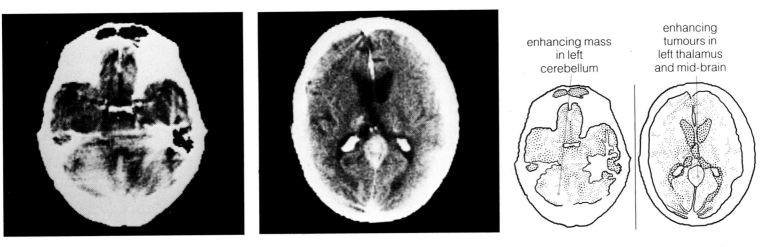

Fig. 7.25 Metastases: CT scan at two levels showing deposits in the left cerebellum (left), and left thalamus and mid-brain (right).

This man, aged 61, presented with loss of feeling in the left leg, left facial numbness and ataxia. There were complex neurological signs including a right sixth and seventh nerve weakness, reduced pain and temperature sensation in the left arm and leg, and ataxia. The CT scan showed multiple metastases and later he developed superior vena caval obstruction due to a carcinoma of the bronchus.

Fig. 7.26 Haemorrhagic metastasis in the cerebellum.

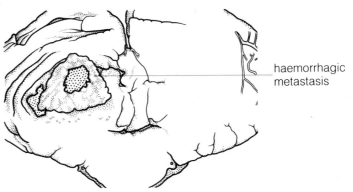

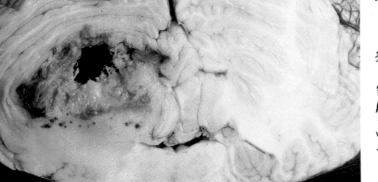

Fig. 7.27 Metastasis from an adenocarcinoma (×30, left), and a metastasis from a squamous cell carcinoma of the bronchus (×120, right). H&E stain.

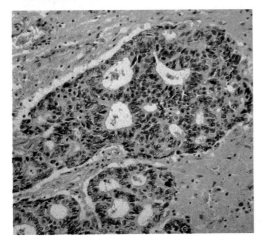

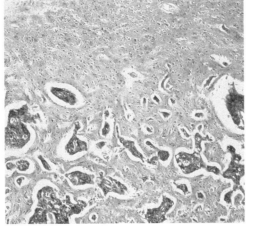

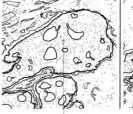

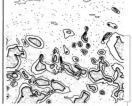

For tumours of the breast around 15% to 20% show cerebral metastases. Other primary tumours metastasize only rarely to the brain (Figs. 7.28 & 7.29).

The cerebrum, cerebellum and brain stem are affected in that order of frequency. The orbit is an uncommon site for metastatic disease (Figs. 7.30 & 7.31). The clinical picture in patients with metastases may well be complex, due to the likelihood of multiple lesions contributing to the clinical findings (Fig. 7.32).

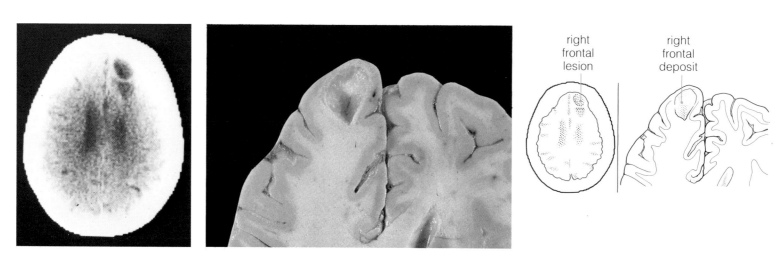

Fig. 7.28 Cystic metastasis from carcinoma of the vulva: CT scan (left) and corresponding brain slice (right, photographed from below).

This 72 year old woman had had a carcinoma of the vulva treated one year previously. She presented with epilepsia partialis continua, consisting of repetitive jerking of the left shoulder and leg. EEG showed periodic complexes with a right central emphasis, and the CT scan an enhancing lesion in the right frontal lobe.

Fig. 7.29 Metastasis from carcinoma of the vulva, H&E stain, ×180. Same patient as in figure 7.28.

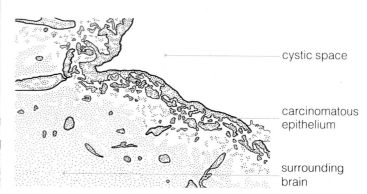

Fig. 7.30 Proptosis of the left eye due to an orbital metastasis.

This 75 year old woman presented with retro-orbital pain and a sixth nerve palsy. Later, proptosis developed, with downward and outward deviation of the globe. The CT scan showed a high density lesion in the retro-orbital space and aspiration biopsy of a lung shadow revealed adenocarcinoma.

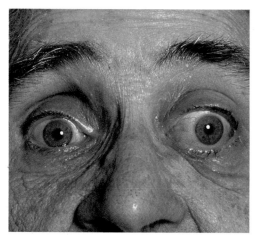
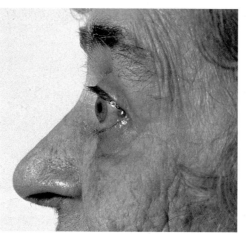

7.12

Chordoma

These rare tumours arise from primitive notochordal tissue and can occur in any age group, though most commonly between 20 and 50. They originate at any level of the spinal column, or from the skull base. The most common site in the cranial cavity is the clivus, and in the spinal column, from the sacrococcygeal region. Clivus lesions erode the sella turcica and clivus, causing compression of the optic chiasma and later the hypothalamus. Spread may take place into the nasopharyngeal space, and posteriorly into the posterior fossa (Fig. 7.33).

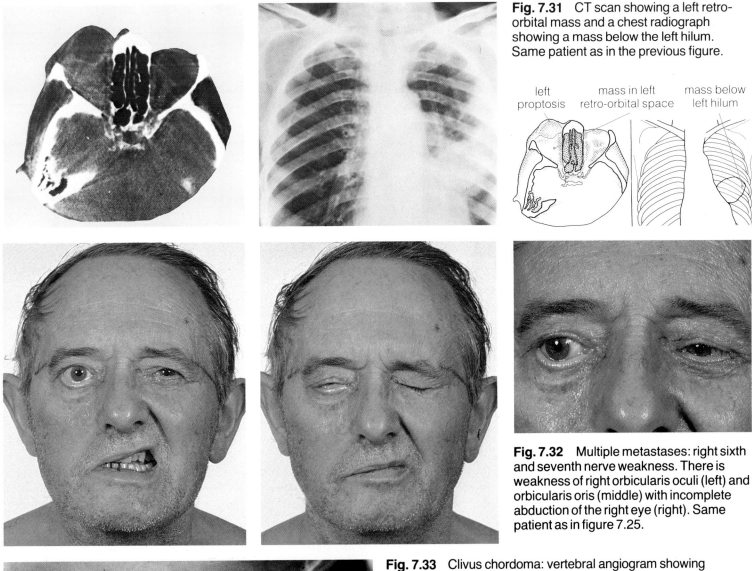

Fig. 7.31 CT scan showing a left retro-orbital mass and a chest radiograph showing a mass below the left hilum. Same patient as in the previous figure.

Fig. 7.32 Multiple metastases: right sixth and seventh nerve weakness. There is weakness of right orbicularis oculi (left) and orbicularis oris (middle) with incomplete abduction of the right eye (right). Same patient as in figure 7.25.

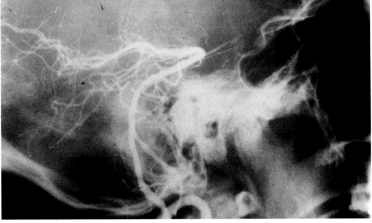

Fig. 7.33 Clivus chordoma: vertebral angiogram showing posterior displacement of the basilar artery.

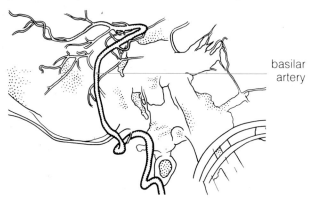

Craniopharyngioma

These are epithelial tumours arising in the region of the pituitary (Fig. 7.34). More than 50% present in childhood or adolescence. Most of them are cystic and many contain calcium. They tend to invade local structures and are liable to recur following excision. Hypothalamic disturbances, with or without evidence of raised intracranial pressure, are the most common presenting feature in childhood cases, insidious visual failure being encountered less frequently. Fundus examination reveals

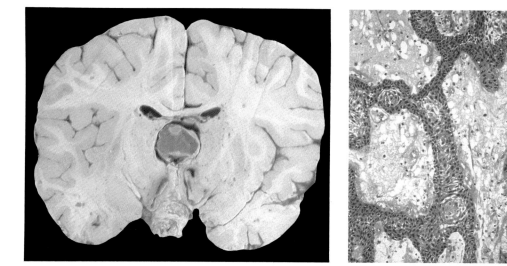

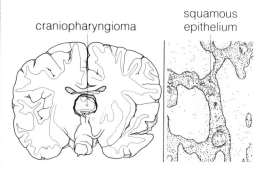

Fig. 7.34 Craniopharyngioma: brain slice showing cystic extension into the third ventricle (left); microscopic appearance (right). H&E stain, ×150.

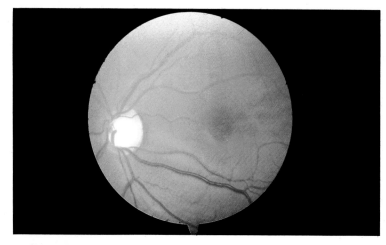

Fig. 7.35 Craniopharyngioma: fundus photograph showing optic atrophy.

This 10 year old boy presented with an 18 month history of headache. He had not complained of vision loss. Examination revealed left optic atrophy, temporal pallor of the right disc, and a left afferent pupillary defect. There were bilateral temporal field defects.

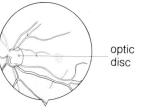

Fig. 7.36 Craniopharyngioma: skull radiograph showing areas of calcification.

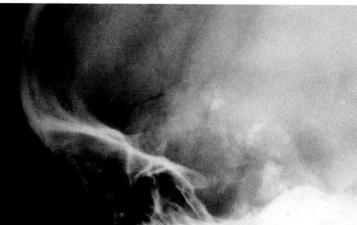

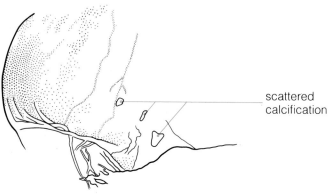

optic atrophy more frequently than papilloedema (Fig. 7.35). In adults, visual failure is the commonest presenting symptom.

Skull radiographs show destruction of the dorsum sellae, with or without suprasellar calcification (Fig. 7.36).

Angiography confirms a suprasellar mass as does the CT scan in which areas of calcification may be apparent (Figs. 7.37 & 7.38). Approximately one-third of tumours show enhancement and if they are sufficiently large, obstruction of the ventricular system may result.

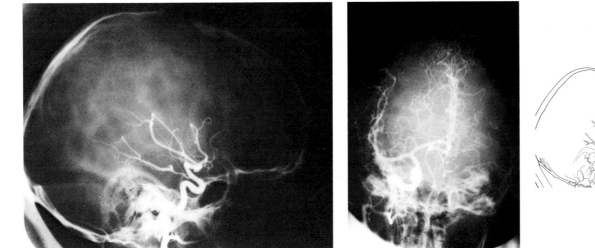

Fig. 7.37 Craniopharyngioma: carotid angiogram showing elevation of the carotid siphon (left) and the proximal segment of the anterior cerebral artery (right). Same patient as in figure 7.35.

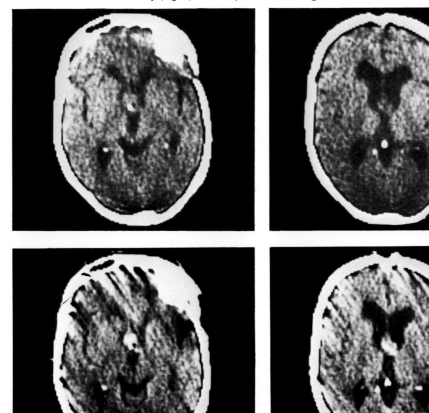

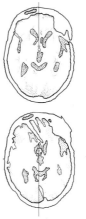
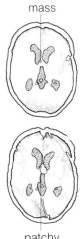

Fig. 7.38 Craniopharyngioma: CT scan at two levels showing a mass in the anterior part of the third ventricle, pre-contrast (upper) and post-contrast (lower).

This 65 year old woman had had a poor memory and difficulty in walking for three years. Examination showed a bitemporal hemianopia, dementia and bilateral pyramidal signs. A large, partly cystic, craniopharyngioma was partially removed at operation.

7.15

Pituitary Tumour

These tumours most commonly present between the ages of 20 and 40, and have an equal sex distribution. Though arising within the sella, a proportion extend through the diaphragma sella and are then liable to cause visual impairment. Chromophobe tumours are inert in an endocrinological sense, whilst acidophilic tumours may produce acromegaly and basophilic tumours, Cushing's disease. Compression of pituitary tissue, by a chromophobe tumour, can lead to hypopituitarism (Fig. 7.39).

Radiographic abnormalities of the sella are reported in between 70% and 90% of patients with pituitary tumour, consisting of enlargement with or without erosion of surrounding bone (Fig. 7.40). Upward extension of the tumour deforms the suprasellar cistern and rarely may reach the third ventricle causing obstruction of the foramen of Monro (Fig. 7.41). Enhancement is seen in some cases, either of the whole tumour, or of its capsule. Some tumours calcify, others show areas of cystic degeneration or haemorrhage. Lateral expansion may result in ophthalmoplegia, whereas upward expansion typically causes a visual defect, particularly a bitemporal hemianopia. Rarely, haemorrhage into the tumour causes it to expand

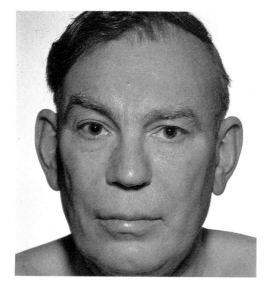

Fig. 7.39 Hypopituitarism secondary to pituitary tumour.

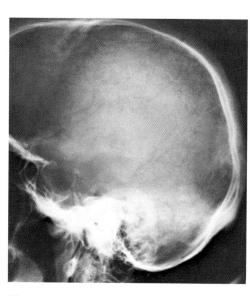

Fig. 7.40 Pituitary tumour: skull radiograph showing expanded sella.

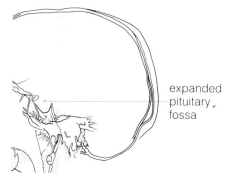

This 41 year old man had been aware of a temporal defect in the left eye for 10 years, worsening for three months. Examination showed a left afferent pupillary defect and a left temporal hemianopia. A chromophobe adenoma was subsequently removed.

expanded pituitary fossa

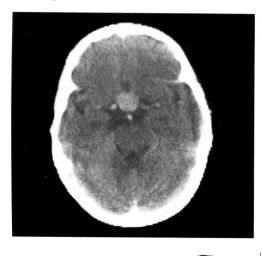 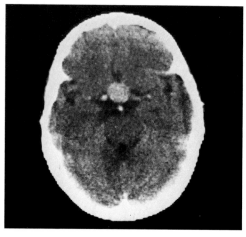 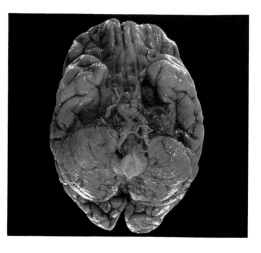

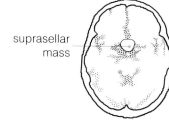

suprasellar mass

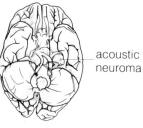

enhancing suprasellar mass

acoustic neuroma

Fig. 7.41 Pituitary tumour: CT scan showing a suprasellar mass (pre-contrast, left; post-contrast, right).

This 69 year old man had had difficulty with the vision of his left eye for several years.

Examination suggested hypopituitarism (later confirmed) together with a central defect in the left eye extending temporally and reduced visual acuity. A chromophobe adenoma was later removed.

Fig. 7.42 Acoustic neuroma (Schwannoma): inferior surface of the brain showing a left-sided acoustic neuroma occupying the cerebellopontine angle.

abruptly, pituitary apoplexy, mimicking in some cases the effects of a subarachnoid haemorrhage.

Acoustic Neuroma

These tumours, generally classified as Schwannomas, represent between 5% and 10% of all intracranial tumours. The majority present between the ages of 20 and 60, often with a long history. They usually originate from acoustic or vestibular fibres of the auditory nerve within the internal auditory meatus, later expanding into the cerebellopontine cistern (Fig. 7.42). Early symptoms include unilateral deafness and vertigo. Later, facial

numbness or pain occurs and, with large tumours, ipsilateral cerebellar signs.

Widening of the internal auditory canal is found in 70% to 90% of cases (Fig. 7.43). Computerised tomography detects these tumours with a high degree of accuracy when they have projected to a critical extent into the cerebellopontine angle (Fig. 7.44). With contrast, the tumours, often isodense on pre-contrast views, show a uniform homogeneous enhancement. Infrequently, the enhancement may be peripheral, with a central cystic component (Fig. 7.45).

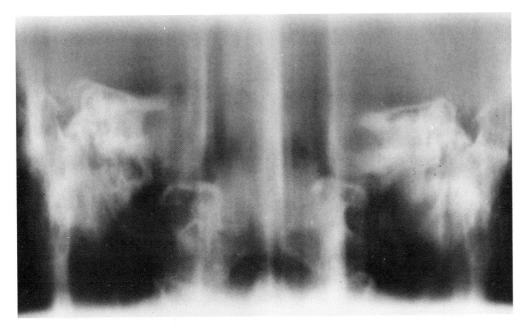

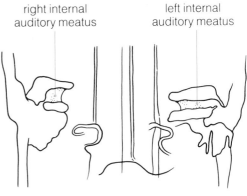

Fig. 7.43 Acoustic neuroma: skull radiograph showing expansion of the internal auditory canal.

right internal auditory meatus

left internal auditory meatus

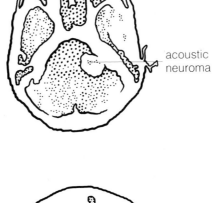

acoustic neuroma

Fig. 7.44 Acoustic neuroma: CT scan showing a uniformly enhancing mass in the cerebellopontine angle.

This 68 year old woman presented with a five month history, initially of facial pain and numbness, followed by deafness and tinnitus. Her balance had deteriorated. Examination showed nystagmus, and right fifth, seventh and eighth nerve palsies.

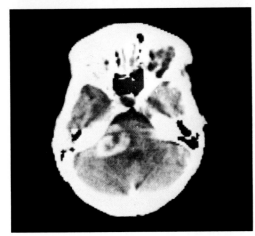

ring enhancement in acoustic neuroma

Fig. 7.45 Acoustic neuroma: CT scan showing ring enhancement of mass in the left cerebellopontine angle.

This 69 year old woman had been aware of left-sided deafness for several months. Her balance had altered and she had developed pressure sensations in the temples. Examination showed nystagmus, left deafness and slight gait ataxia.

Colloid Cyst

These are rare tumours, usually presenting between the ages of 20 and 50 and almost exclusively situated within the third ventricle. They have a smooth wall encapsulating colloid or gelatinous contents (Fig. 7.46). They may present with dementia, with focal neurological disturbances, including loss of posture, or with headache and features of raised intracranial pressure (Fig. 7.47).

Meningioma

These tumours represent some 17% of all intracranial tumours, with a peak incidence in the middle decades of life. They are slightly more common in women, and are sometimes an incidental finding at post mortem examination.

Typically, they are solid, irregular but circumscribed growths, readily separable from adjacent brain tissue (Fig.

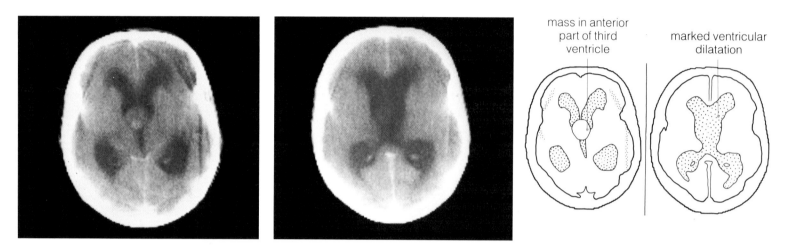

Fig. 7.46 Colloid cyst: CT scan at two levels showing a colloid cyst of the third ventricle and associated hydrocephalus.

This 25 year old male with a past history of a behavioural disorder was admitted unconscious. Within 24 hours he had lost all brain stem reflexes. Post mortem examination showed severe tonsillar and uncal herniation with brain swelling. The third ventricle was occupied by a colloid cyst.

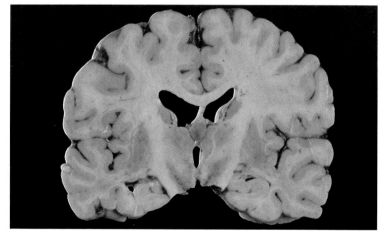

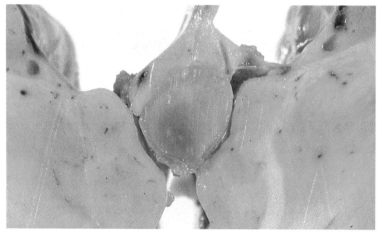

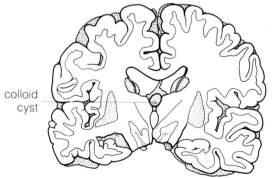

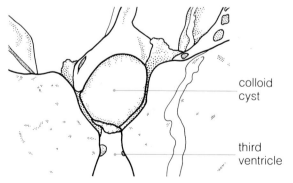

Fig. 7.47 A coronal brain slice showing a colloid cyst in the anterior part of the third ventricle occluding the foramina of Monro.

7.48, left). They arise from the meninges, usually the arachnoid endothelium. Their histology varies, with fibrous, vascular, or cellular components predominating. Cells resembling those seen in arachnoid endothelium may be found, containing small foci of calcification – psammoma bodies (Fig. 7.48, right). The tumours tend to be highly vascular, sometimes involving adjacent bone or dural sinuses. They tend to occur at particular sites, and their symptomatology is determined by their anatomical position.

Plain skull radiographs may reveal bone erosion, hyperostosis or, in 30% to 60% of cases, areas of calcification. Abnormal vascular channels are sometimes seen in the region of the tumour (Fig. 7.49). Technetium scanning detects up to 90% of supratentorial meningiomas (Fig. 7.50).

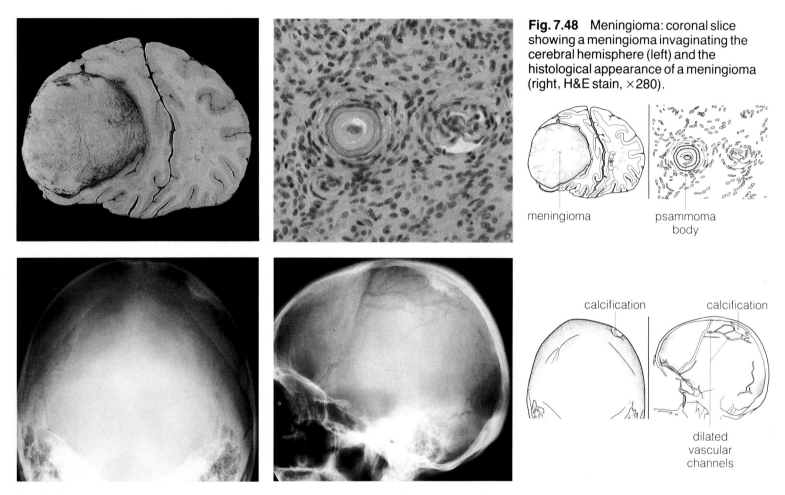

Fig. 7.48 Meningioma: coronal slice showing a meningioma invaginating the cerebral hemisphere (left) and the histological appearance of a meningioma (right, H&E stain, ×280).

meningioma

psammoma body

calcification

calcification

dilated vascular channels

Fig. 7.49 Meningioma: skull radiograph showing an area of calcification and dilated vascular channels.

This 31 year old woman gave an eighteen month history of difficulty using the right arm, and occasional dragging of the right leg. She had had periodic headaches. Examination revealed papilloedema and mild right-sided pyramidal signs.

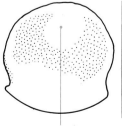
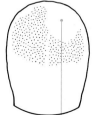

Fig. 7.50 Meningioma: technetium scan showing a large convexity meningioma.

Same patient as in figure 7.49.

convexity meningioma

convexity meningioma

Angiography characteristically demonstrates an abnormal vascular pattern with dense staining, beginning in the early arterial phase and persisting into the venous phase (Fig. 7.51). Computerised tomography detects these tumours with a high degree of accuracy, though in some instances, differentiation from a malignant glioma may not be possible on radiographic criteria alone. Most commonly the tumours appear as high density, homogeneous, circumscribed lesions, but a minority are of low density. Adjacent oedema is relatively slight. Following contrast

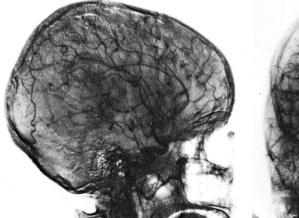
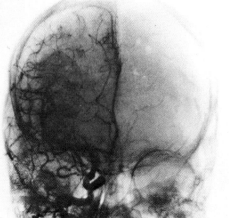
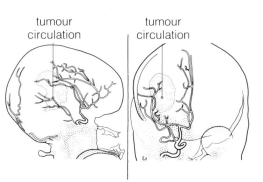

Fig. 7.51 Meningioma: angiograms showing abnormal circulation in an intraventricular meningioma.

This 50 year old woman had had vague headaches for four months and altered facial sensation on the right. Examination showed right facial numbness and a mild left hemiparesis. At operation, a large intraventricular meningioma was removed.

Fig. 7.52 Meningioma: CT scan at four levels showing a left convexity meningioma with marked enhancement. Same patient as in figure 7.49.

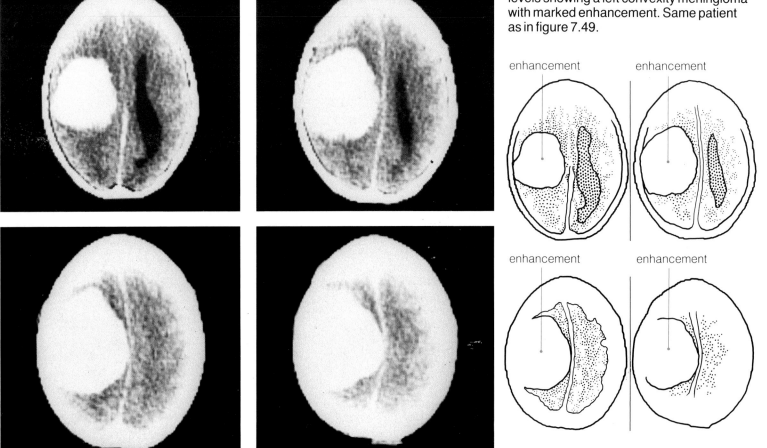

injection, rapid, dense but short-lived enhancement is seen (Fig. 7.52).

Sphenoidal-wing meningiomas, and those arising within the orbit, tend to produce an ophthalmoplegia, often with mild proptosis and involvement of fifth nerve function (Fig. 7.53). When sufficiently large, the tumours expand into the middle cranial fossa and may then present with epilepsy (Fig. 7.54).

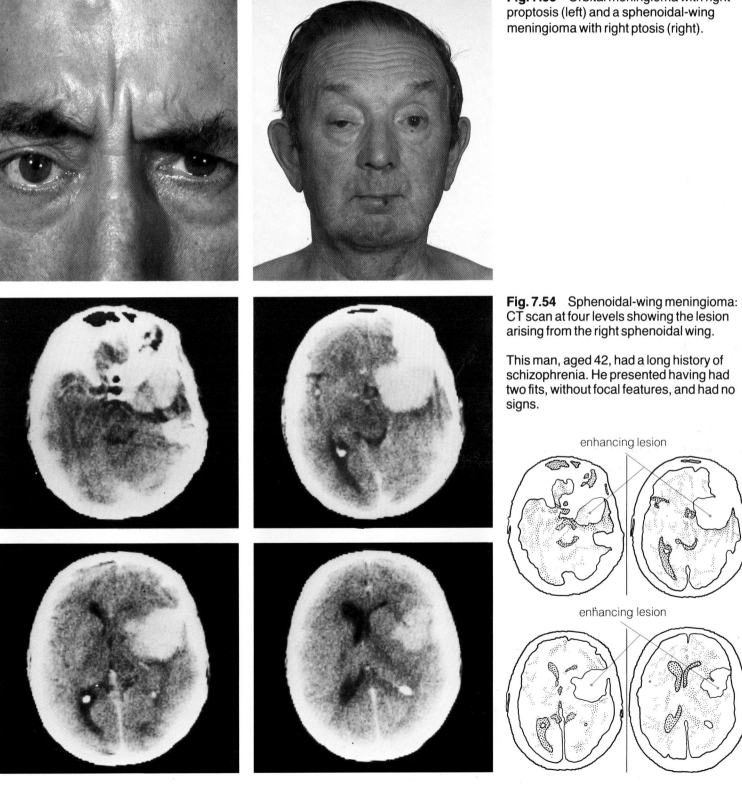

Fig. 7.53 Orbital meningioma with right proptosis (left) and a sphenoidal-wing meningioma with right ptosis (right).

Fig. 7.54 Sphenoidal-wing meningioma: CT scan at four levels showing the lesion arising from the right sphenoidal wing.

This man, aged 42, had a long history of schizophrenia. He presented having had two fits, without focal features, and had no signs.

enhancing lesion

enhancing lesion

Tumours arising from the olfactory groove may compress the olfactory nerve, producing anosmia, or compress one or both optic nerves. Visual failure may be conspicuous in such cases (Figs. 7.55 & 7.56).

Parasagittal meningiomas tend to present with focal neurological deficit, particularly of the leg, or with epilepsy, sometimes of Jacksonian type (Fig. 7.57). Intraventricular meningiomas are rare (Fig. 7.58). Menin-

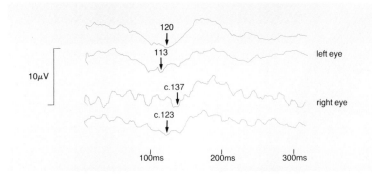

Fig. 7.55 Olfactory groove meningioma: visual evoked responses measured before (left) and after (right) removal of the tumour, showing lessening in latency and restoration of amplitude

of the P2 deflection. This 33 year old woman presented with rapidly progressive bilateral visual failure, with predominantly infero-nasal field defects.

Fig. 7.56 Olfactory groove meningioma. CT scan showing tumour with marked contrast enhancement: pre-contrast (left) and post-contrast (right). Same patient as in figure 7.55.

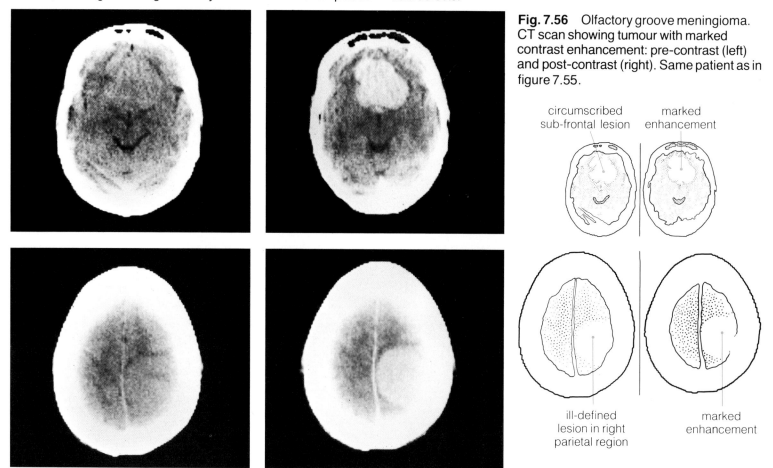

Fig. 7.57 Parasagittal meningioma. CT scans showing a right parasagittal lesion with enhancement: pre-contrast (left) and post-contrast (right).

This 39 year old man had developed distal weakness of the left leg six months previously. One month before admission he developed Jacksonian seizures beginning in the leg, and radiating to the trunk, arm and face. There were left-sided pyramidal signs maximal in the foot.

gioma also occur in the posterior fossa, arising from the tentorium, the clivus, around the internal auditory meatus, or in the region of the foramen magnum (Fig. 7.59).

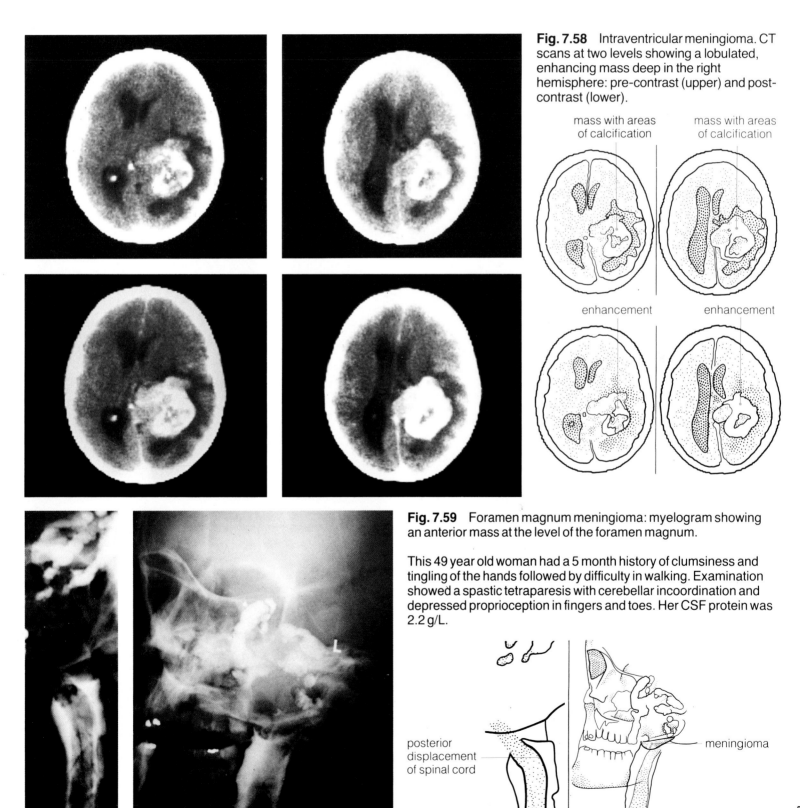

Fig. 7.58 Intraventricular meningioma. CT scans at two levels showing a lobulated, enhancing mass deep in the right hemisphere: pre-contrast (upper) and post-contrast (lower).

mass with areas of calcification   mass with areas of calcification

enhancement   enhancement

Fig. 7.59 Foramen magnum meningioma: myelogram showing an anterior mass at the level of the foramen magnum.

This 49 year old woman had a 5 month history of clumsiness and tingling of the hands followed by difficulty in walking. Examination showed a spastic tetraparesis with cerebellar incoordination and depressed proprioception in fingers and toes. Her CSF protein was 2.2 g/L.

posterior displacement of spinal cord

meningioma

Although computerised tomography has proved of remarkable value in the diagnosis of intracranial tumour, it cannot invariably distinguish benign tumours, such as meningiomas, from malignant lesions. If it is used for this purpose, as many as 5% of intracranial masses may be misidentified (Fig. 7.60).

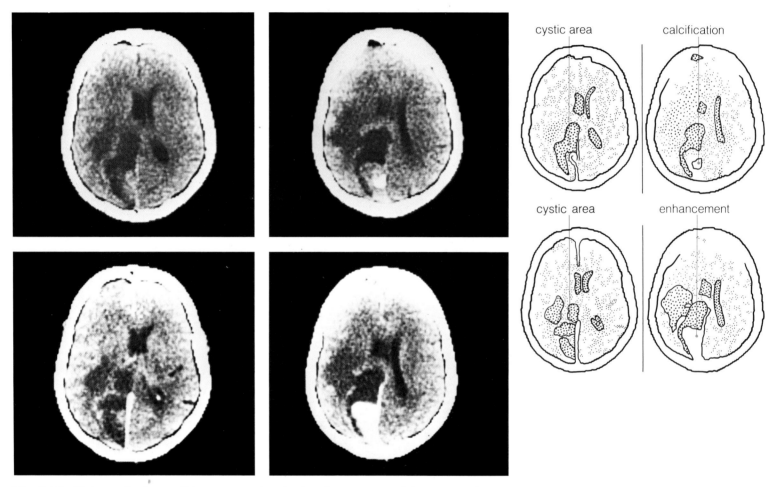

Fig. 7.60 Falx meningioma. CT scan at two levels showing a lesion alongside the falx, with an area of calcification within it, a cystic space anteriorly, and prominent enhancement: pre-contrast (upper) and post-contrast (lower).

This 64 year old woman presented with the relatively sudden onset of dysphasia, dysgraphia and disturbed vision. She had had occipital headaches. Her signs suggested a left parietal lesion. Her CT scan was interpreted as showing a glioma. Her disability changed little over the next three years, and serial scanning raised the suspicion that the lesion was a meningioma, a suspicion verified at craniotomy.

8. Miscellaneous Disorders I: Developmental Disorders, Hydrocephalus, Benign Intracranial Hypertension and Disorders of Higher Cortical Function

Developmental Disorders

Microcephaly and megalencephaly refer to abnormally small and large brains respectively. Both may be associated with mental retardation, particularly the former. In prosencephaly, abnormal fusion exists between the two lateral hemispheres, sometimes involving also the basal ganglia. Generally there is partial or complete agenesis of the corpus callosum and the lateral ventricles are fused to a varying degree (Figs. 8.1 & 8.2).

Agenesis of the corpus callosum, sometimes incomplete, may be associated with abnormalities of the ventricular system and of the cerebral hemispheres. The

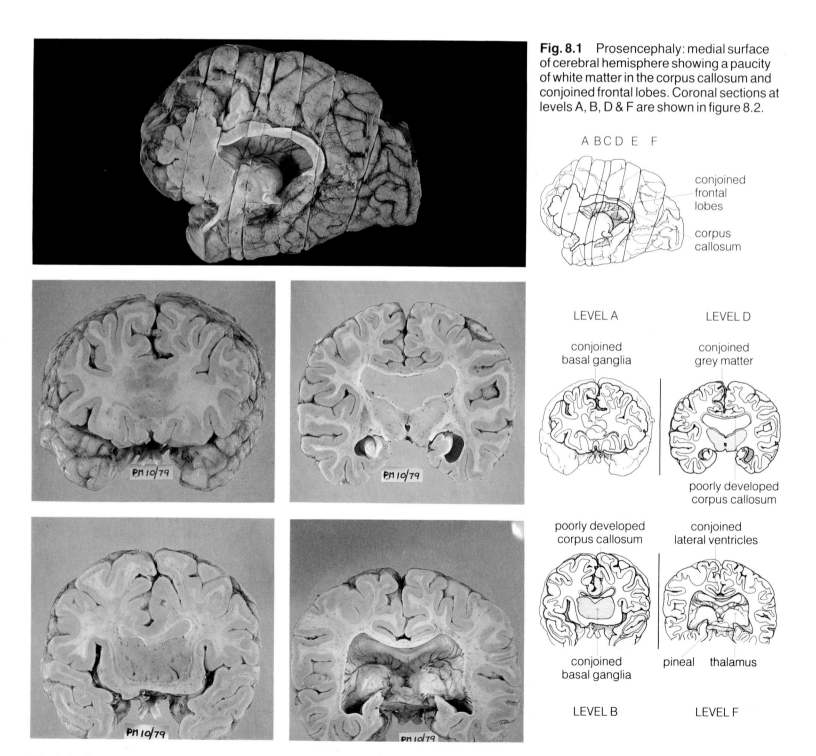

Fig. 8.1 Prosencephaly: medial surface of cerebral hemisphere showing a paucity of white matter in the corpus callosum and conjoined frontal lobes. Coronal sections at levels A, B, D & F are shown in figure 8.2.

A B C D E F

conjoined frontal lobes

corpus callosum

LEVEL A

conjoined basal ganglia

LEVEL D

conjoined grey matter

poorly developed corpus callosum

poorly developed corpus callosum

conjoined lateral ventricles

conjoined basal ganglia

pineal   thalamus

LEVEL B

LEVEL F

Fig. 8.2 Prosencephaly: coronal sections at A, B, D and F showing fused basal ganglia, a single lateral ventricle and a poorly developed corpus callosum.

8.2

disorder can generally be diagnosed in life by CT scanning or air encephalography (Fig. 8.3).

Agyria consists of a reduction in the number of secondary gyri associated with an increased depth of grey matter. The affected brain is usually small though the lateral ventricles are relatively large (Figs. 8.4 & 8.5). The abnormality may be confined to one hemisphere, resulting in a contralateral hemiplegia, or it may be incomplete (pachygyria).

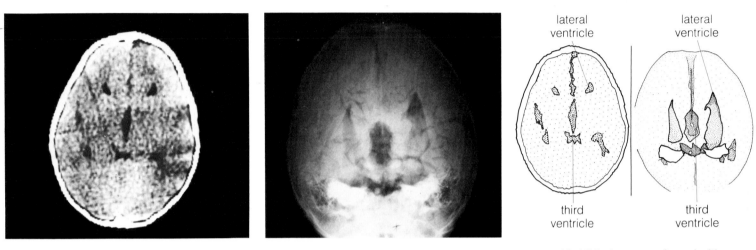

Fig. 8.3 Agenesis of the corpus callosum: CT scan (left) and an air encephalogram (right) showing abnormal separation of the lateral ventricles.

The CT scan is of a three year old child who was referred with a history of recurrent vomiting. His mother had Gorlin's syndrome, an autosomal dominant disorder comprising basal cell carcinoma, facial and gonadal abnormalities and various radiological changes, including agenesis of the corpus callosum.

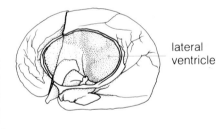

Fig. 8.4 Agyria: lateral (left) and medial (right) aspects of the brain showing lack of cortical gyri. There was an associated aqueduct stenosis causing ventricular dilatation.

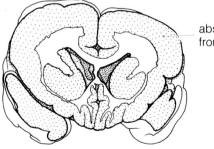

Fig. 8.5 Agyria: coronal slice of cerebral hemisphere showing lack of gyri except in the hippocampal region.

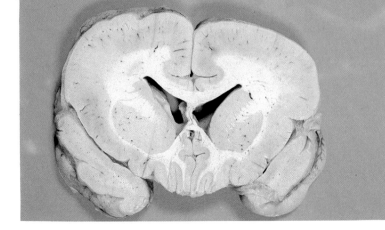

Micropolygyria refers to any type of abnormally small convolutional pattern, most characteristically pre-natal in origin. The abnormality may be focal or extend to much of the lateral cortical surface. Various patterns of altered cortical architecture are described (Fig. 8.6) with four layers comprising a superficial level, a cellular level, a third layer largely composed of myelinated fibres and the fourth a mixture of nerve cells and fibres. The changes may be unilateral, in which case the pyramidal tract derived from the normal hemisphere may hypertrophy, displacing the inferior olive (Fig. 8.7).

Porencephaly

This term has been loosely applied to any cystic cavity communicating with the subjacent lateral ventricle, though, more strictly, it has been used to describe a cavity communicating with one of the ventricles and lined by ependyma (Figs. 8.8 & 8.9). The cavity may be found in any part of the brain and the underlying ventricle is often dilated. Similar cystic spaces may be acquired as a result of cerebral softening secondary to ischaemic damage (Fig. 8.10).

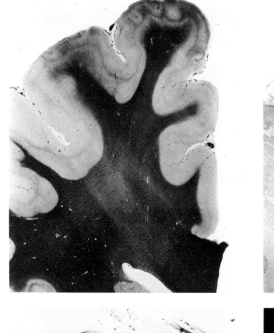
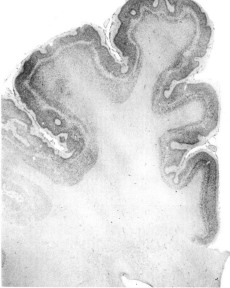
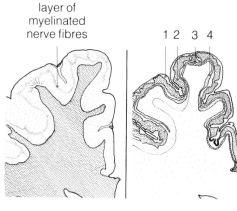

Fig. 8.6 Micropolygyria: coronal section, right hemisphere, showing altered cortical pattern (left, Loyez myelin stain, ×2.5) and a section showing the four cortical nerve cell layers (right, Thionin, ×2.5).

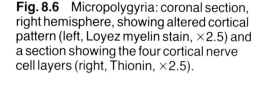

layer of myelinated nerve fibres

1 2 3 4

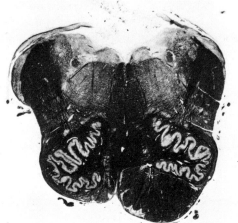
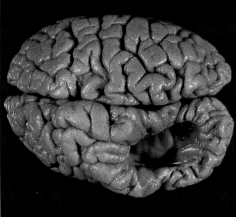
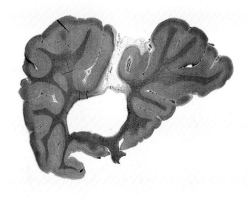

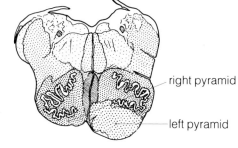

Fig. 8.7 Micropolygyria: medulla showing a small right, and a hypertrophied left, pyramid. Weigert PAL, ×2.5.

right pyramid

left pyramid

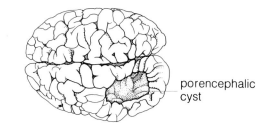

Fig. 8.8 Porencephaly: a large funnel-shaped defect in the left parieto-occipital region communicating with the posterior horn of the left lateral ventricle.

porencephalic cyst

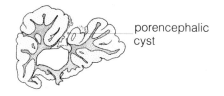

Fig. 8.9 Porencephaly: sagittal section through the parieto-occipital region of the left hemisphere showing a porencephalic cyst. Haematoxylin Van Gieson stain.

The patient was a 7 year old boy with severe mental handicap and epilepsy.

porencephalic cyst

Arachnoid Cyst

Most of these cysts are the result of a congenital malformation of the leptomeninges, though some authors have preferred to consider them as due to a maldevelopment of the cerebral hemisphere producing a form of arachnoid diverticulum. The cysts most commonly arise in the region of the Sylvian fissure. In infants, they may act as a space-occupying lesion, but in adults they are often asymptomatic (Fig. 8.11).

Epidermoid Cyst

These probably originate during foetal life, are usually pial and generally midline. They may contain areas of bone or cartilage. Their symptomatology depends on their site, though ventricular dilatation is a common manifestation of their particular position (Fig. 8.12).

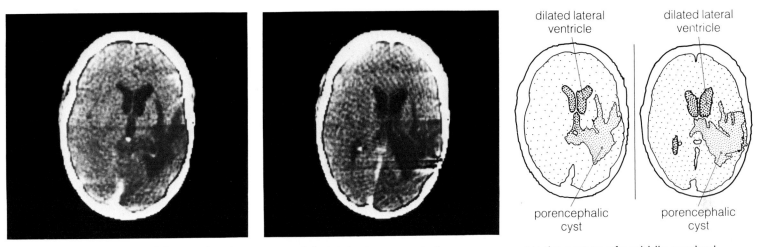

Fig. 8.10 Porencephaly: CT scan showing an area of diminished density in the posterior temporal region, communicating with an expanded lateral ventricle.

This 37 year old man had developed a right temporal haematoma 5

years before, consequent to the rupture of a middle cerebral aneurysm. The aneurysm was clipped and the haematoma evacuated. The patient subsequently developed temporal lobe seizures. Examination showed a left homonymous hemianopia and a memory defect.

Fig. 8.11 Arachnoid cyst: CT scan at two levels showing a cyst occupying the right middle cranial fossa.

This 58 year old man was admitted with dyspnoea and severe headache. His blood pressure rose from 140/90 to 200/150. He had bilateral retinal infarctions and haemorrhages.

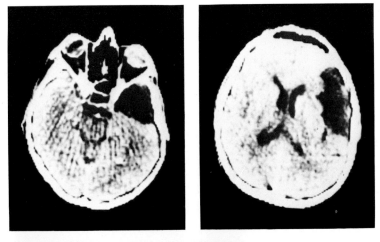

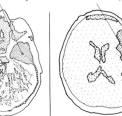

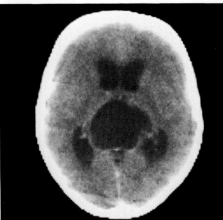

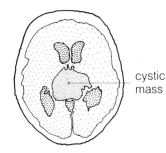

Fig. 8.12 Epidermoid cyst: CT scan showing a large irregular low density lesion with a higher density rim lying in the suprasellar region.

This 34 year old woman had had weakness and ataxia of the left arm for several months, followed by involvement of the other limbs and dysarthria. Her affect was inappropriate and she had mild bilateral pyramidal and cerebellar signs. At craniotomy, an epidermoid cyst was partially excised.

Intracranial Calcification

This commonly results from a disorder of calcium metabolism, or from certain infections, for example toxoplasmosis (Fig. 8.13). Extensive calcification, particularly of the basal ganglia may not have a discoverable cause and is sometimes associated with microcephaly (Fig. 8.14).

Tuberous Sclerosis

This condition is inherited as an autosomal dominant, and involves a number of organs besides the brain. The multiple nodules, or tubers, are scattered throughout the cerebrum, appearing as slightly pale, hardened areas sometimes containing calcium (Fig. 8.15). These areas

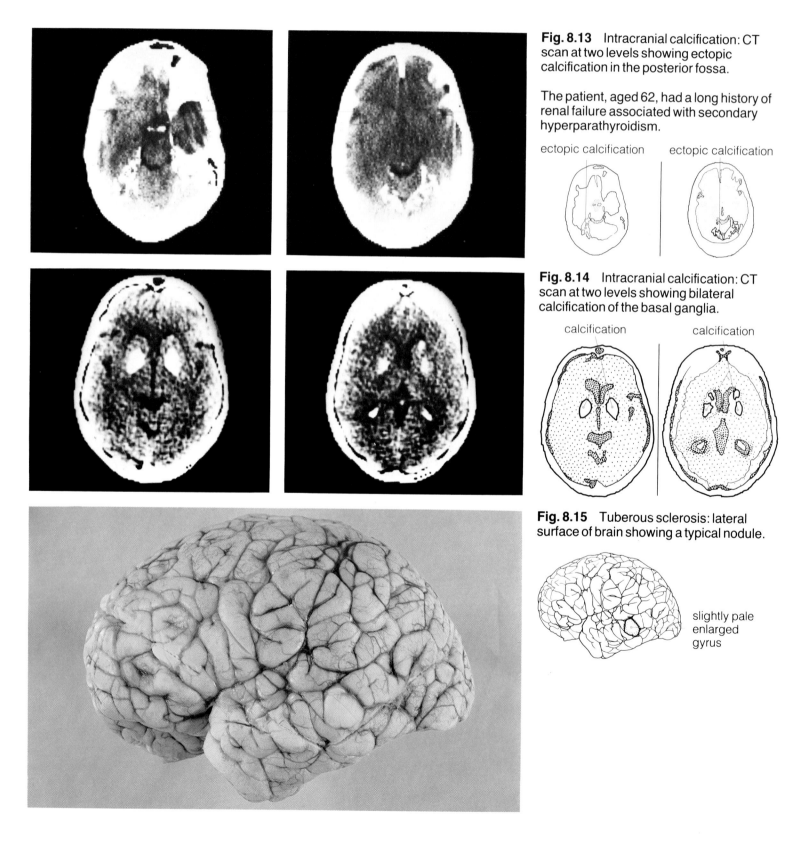

Fig. 8.13 Intracranial calcification: CT scan at two levels showing ectopic calcification in the posterior fossa.

The patient, aged 62, had a long history of renal failure associated with secondary hyperparathyroidism.

ectopic calcification   ectopic calcification

Fig. 8.14 Intracranial calcification: CT scan at two levels showing bilateral calcification of the basal ganglia.

calcification   calcification

Fig. 8.15 Tuberous sclerosis: lateral surface of brain showing a typical nodule.

slightly pale enlarged gyrus

contain an increased number of astrocytic nuclei (Fig. 8.16) and often bizarre-shaped cells.

Nodules in the periventricular region are liable to project into the ventricles, producing the so-called 'candle-guttering' appearance (Fig. 8.17, left). The skull radiograph will demonstrate calcified nodules whilst CT scanning indicates their periventricular distribution (Fig. 8.17, right). Malignant transformation of the nodules occurs, more especially in those around the ventricles (Fig. 8.18). Lesions in other organs are common. Those in

Fig. 8.16 Tuberous sclerosis: area of astrocytic overgrowth replacing grey matter.

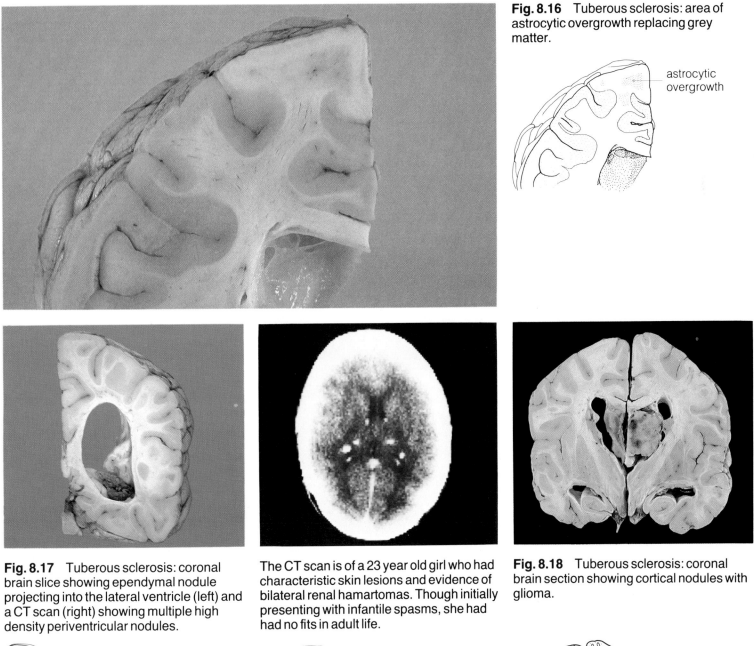

astrocytic overgrowth

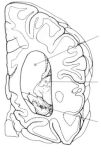

Fig. 8.17 Tuberous sclerosis: coronal brain slice showing ependymal nodule projecting into the lateral ventricle (left) and a CT scan (right) showing multiple high density periventricular nodules.

lateral ventricle

ependymal nodule

choroid plexus

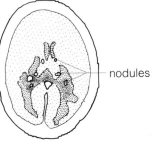

The CT scan is of a 23 year old girl who had characteristic skin lesions and evidence of bilateral renal hamartomas. Though initially presenting with infantile spasms, she had had no fits in adult life.

nodules

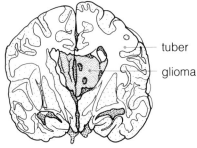

Fig. 8.18 Tuberous sclerosis: coronal brain section showing cortical nodules with glioma.

tuber

glioma

the heart consist of collections of fatty tissue, or mixtures of cells resembling those in the conduction system with fibrous tissues and fat. The facial lesions have the characteristic appearance of adenoma sebaceum (Fig. 8.19).

Encephalocoeles

These refer to anomalies in which a defect of the cranium, more commonly occipital than frontal, is associated with herniation of the underlying brain and meninges. There may be associated hydrocephalus. The mildest form of the disorder, spina bifida occulta, is asymptomatic.

Dandy-Walker Syndrome

This describes the association of hydrocephalus, a posterior fossa cyst and hypoplasia of the cerebellar vermis. When substantial, the roof of the cystic fourth ventricle extends upwards through the tentorial notch (Fig. 8.20). Malformations of the brain and other organs are frequently associated. The skull is abnormally shaped, with the lateral sinuses and their confluence situated in an unusually high position (Fig. 8.21).

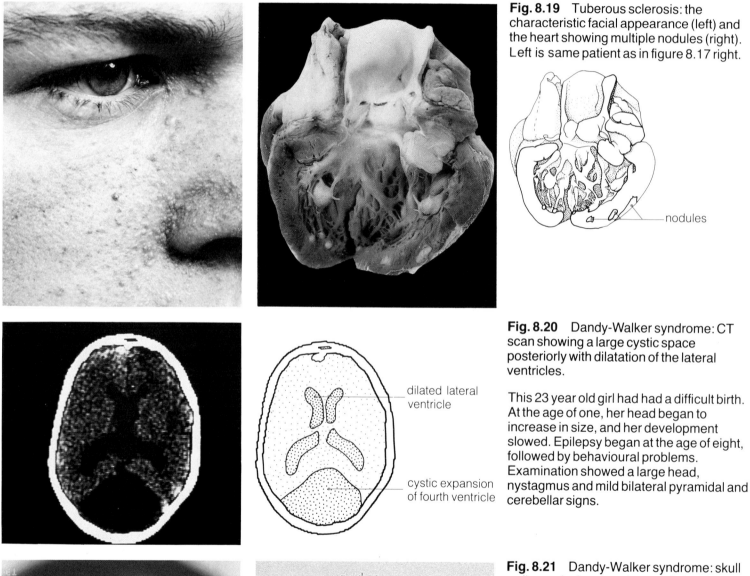

Fig. 8.19 Tuberous sclerosis: the characteristic facial appearance (left) and the heart showing multiple nodules (right). Left is same patient as in figure 8.17 right.

nodules

Fig. 8.20 Dandy-Walker syndrome: CT scan showing a large cystic space posteriorly with dilatation of the lateral ventricles.

This 23 year old girl had had a difficult birth. At the age of one, her head began to increase in size, and her development slowed. Epilepsy began at the age of eight, followed by behavioural problems. Examination showed a large head, nystagmus and mild bilateral pyramidal and cerebellar signs.

dilated lateral ventricle

cystic expansion of fourth ventricle

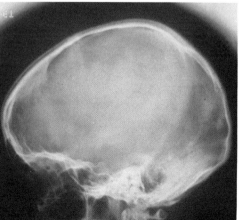
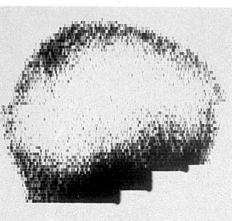
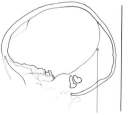
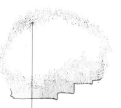

Fig. 8.21 Dandy-Walker syndrome: skull radiograph showing abnormal site of lateral sinus (left) and a technetium scan showing unusually high confluence of the sinuses (right). Same patient as in figure 8.20.

lateral sinus   confluence of sinuses

8.8

Hydrocephalus

This can theoretically result from over-production of CSF, obstruction to its flow, or failure of absorption. In practice, obstruction to flow is the commonest mechanism, most frequently at the level of the cerebral aqueduct. Aqueductal malformations have been divided into four types, comprising narrowing without gliosis, reduplication of the aqueduct, occlusion or obstruction by a neuroglial membrane and gliosis of the aqueduct (Fig. 8.22). The condition usually causes an insidious increase in intracranial pressure in early life, but occasionally presents in adults. Progressive destruction of white matter occurs, particularly in the periventricular region, result-ing in a pyramidal disturbance which predominates in the lower limbs often with incontinence due to interruption of bladder fibres.

In adults, hydrocephalus most commonly results from meningeal inflammation secondary to infection or sub-arachnoid haemorrhage. Normal pressure hydrocephalus (more accurately, intermittently raised pressure hydrocephalus) is usually associated with pathological abnormalities of the leptomeninges sometimes involving the arachnoid granulations. Classically such patients present with a triad of dementia, incontinence and a curious gait disorder. The CT scan in such patients may reveal ventricular dilatation alone (Fig. 8.23) or in association with

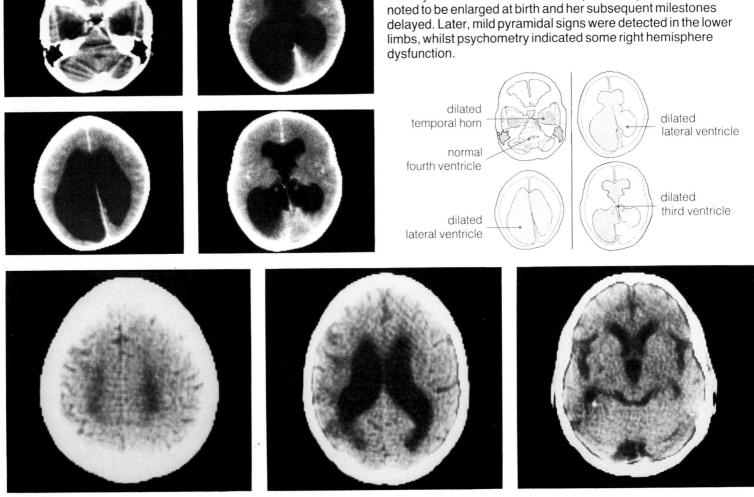

Fig. 8.22 Aqueduct stenosis: CT scan at four levels showing dilated lateral and third ventricles.

This 5 year old child had had a forceps delivery. Her head was noted to be enlarged at birth and her subsequent milestones delayed. Later, mild pyramidal signs were detected in the lower limbs, whilst psychometry indicated some right hemisphere dysfunction.

Fig. 8.23 Normal pressure hydrocephalus: CT scan at three levels showing dilated lateral ventricles and Sylvian fissures with normal cortical sulci.

This 57 year old man presented with an episode of altered awareness. Examination showed an abnormal gait, with an ataxic element, and bilateral extensor plantar responses. His affect was inappropriate and his insight limited.

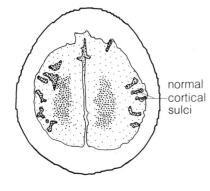

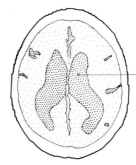

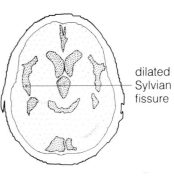

8.9

widened cortical sulci. Radioactive isotope injected into the cisterna magna typically refluxes into the ventricular system with little uptake over the cerebral convexities, though the results of this test do not predict which patients will respond to ventriculo-atrial shunting (Fig. 8.24). Intracranial pressure recording reveals intermittent high pressure, or B waves, and it is when these occupy at least 5 per cent of every 24 hour period that response to shunting occurs. Rarely, protein secreted by an intracranial tumour may be a factor behind alterations in the arachnoid granulations and subsequent hydrocephalus

(Fig. 8.25). Patients may benefit dramatically from ventriculo-atrial shunting, though a substantial number develop subdural haematoma as a complication of this procedure (Fig. 8.26).

Anoxic Brain Damage

Hypoxia in the foetus, or during the neonatal period may result in mental retardation or cerebral palsy. The associated pathological changes include either cortical damage or deep lesions principally affecting the basal ganglia and periventricular white matter. The cortical lesions may

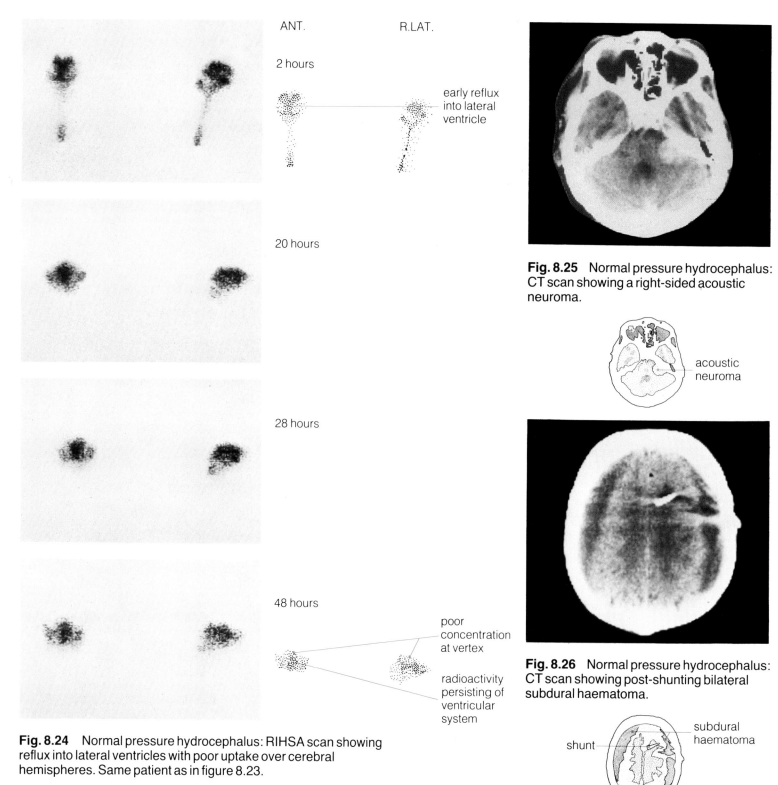

ANT.   R.LAT.

2 hours

early reflux into lateral ventricle

20 hours

28 hours

48 hours

poor concentration at vertex

radioactivity persisting of ventricular system

Fig. 8.24 Normal pressure hydrocephalus: RIHSA scan showing reflux into lateral ventricles with poor uptake over cerebral hemispheres. Same patient as in figure 8.23.

Fig. 8.25 Normal pressure hydrocephalus: CT scan showing a right-sided acoustic neuroma.

acoustic neuroma

Fig. 8.26 Normal pressure hydrocephalus: CT scan showing post-shunting bilateral subdural haematoma.

shunt   subdural haematoma

show a watershed distribution (Fig. 8.27). Where the cortical damage is unilateral, and involves the motor strip, hemiatrophy of the contralateral limbs is the consequence (Fig. 8.28).

Benign Intracranial Hypertension

Although this condition has been described in association with post-infectious polyneuritis, with certain drugs, for example corticosteroids and nalidixic acid, and following ear infections, the majority of cases are of unknown aetiology. The pathogenesis of the condition is thought to be related to impaired resorption of CSF through the arachnoid villi, sometimes with sinus thrombosis. The condition predominates in women, and usually arises in the second to fourth decades of life. Characteristically it produces raised intracranial pressure without focal deficit. Headache is the commonest presenting symptom. Visual complaints include transient obscurations and diplopia secondary to a sixth nerve palsy. Papilloedema (Fig. 8.29) is invariably accompanied by enlarged blind spots.

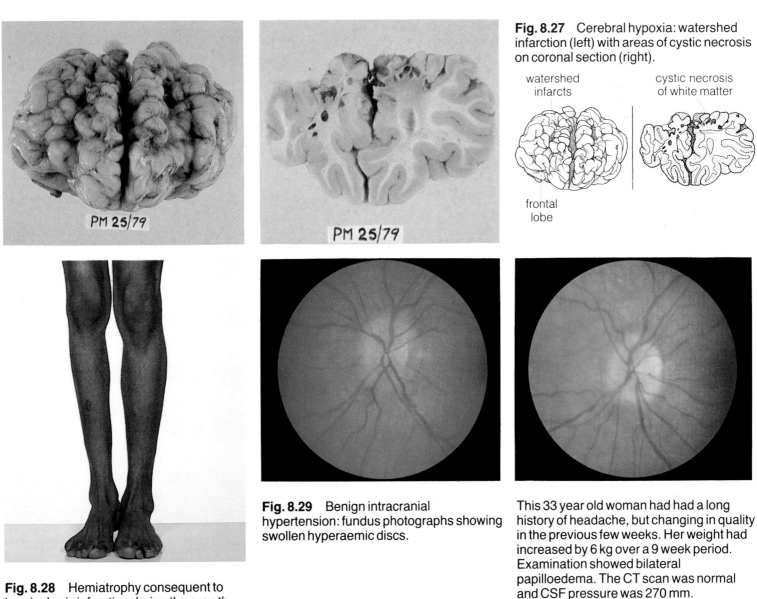

Fig. 8.27 Cerebral hypoxia: watershed infarction (left) with areas of cystic necrosis on coronal section (right).

watershed infarcts

cystic necrosis of white matter

frontal lobe

PM 25/79

PM 25/79

Fig. 8.28 Hemiatrophy consequent to hemispheric infarction during the growth period.

Fig. 8.29 Benign intracranial hypertension: fundus photographs showing swollen hyperaemic discs.

This 33 year old woman had had a long history of headache, but changing in quality in the previous few weeks. Her weight had increased by 6 kg over a 9 week period. Examination showed bilateral papilloedema. The CT scan was normal and CSF pressure was 270 mm.

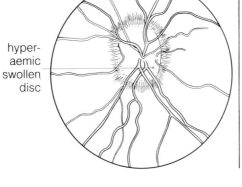

hyper-aemic swollen disc

hyper-aemic swollen disc

Sixth nerve palsies reflect false localising signs secondary to raised intracranial pressure.

Fluorescein angiography shows increased vascularity of the optic disc with later leakage of dye from the disc surface (Fig. 8.30). Radiological studies fail to reveal evidence of a focal lesion, though CT scanning may indicate narrowing of the ventricular system (Fig. 8.31).

The management of this condition is vexatious. Many cases remit spontaneously. Repeated lumbar puncture has been used, as have acetazolamide and corticosteroids.

In more chronic cases, particularly where transient obscurations of vision occur, decompression of the optic nerve within the orbit has been used to preserve vision (Fig. 8.32).

Disorders of Higher Cortical Function

Dysphasia is the most commonly encountered disorder of higher cortical function. Non-fluent dysphasia describes restricted speech output, produced slowly, articulated badly and lacking normal grammatical content. Fluent,

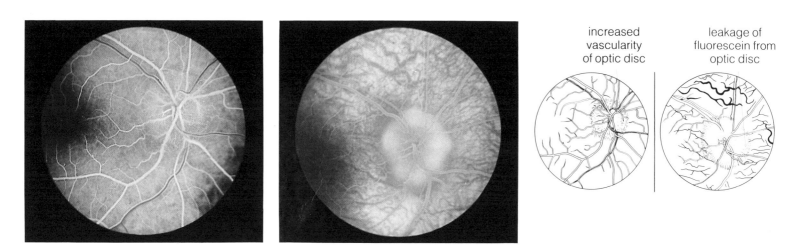

Fig. 8.30 Benign intracranial hypertension: fluorescein angiography showing increased vascularity of the disc (left) with leakage of dye from the optic disc (right).

This 13 year old girl had had non-specific bifrontal headaches for several months. Examination showed bilateral papilloedema. CT scan was normal. CSF pressure was 230 mm.

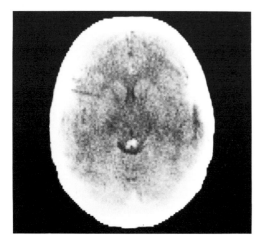
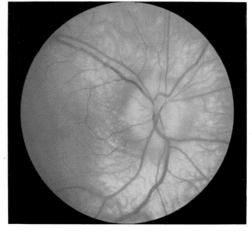
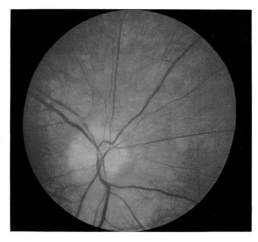

Fig. 8.31 Benign intracranial hypertension: CT scan showing small lateral ventricles.
Same patient as in figure 8.29.

Fig. 8.32 Benign intracranial hypertension: fundus photographs showing the appearance of the right optic disc

before (left) and after (right) optic nerve decompression.
Same patient as in figure 8.29.

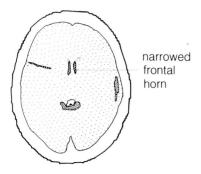
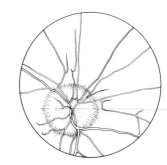

dysphasic speech is produced without difficulty and often shows a normal rhythm with retained grammatical structure. The content is defective, however, with frequent word substitutions (paraphasias). Verbal paraphasias describe substitutions by a word often related in meaning (eg. glass for cup) and literal paraphasias describe replacement of sounds in otherwise correct words (eg. spate for spade).

Fluent dysphasia is associated with lesions of the temporo-parietal region whereas non-fluent dysphasia is associated with disturbances of Broca's area (Fig. 8.33). Patients who are dysphasic display similar problems in writing (Fig. 8.34). Naming difficulties occur in all types of dysphasia. Speech problems in right-handed individuals are almost always due to left hemisphere lesions, whereas in left-handed individuals, some 40 per cent are associated with right hemisphere lesions.

Focal abnormalities of the non-dominant parietal cortex are liable to produce an impairment of the body image, with a tendency to neglect the defective limbs or even deny their abnormality. Associated disturbances include dressing apraxia, geographical disorientation and constructional apraxia (Fig. 8.35).

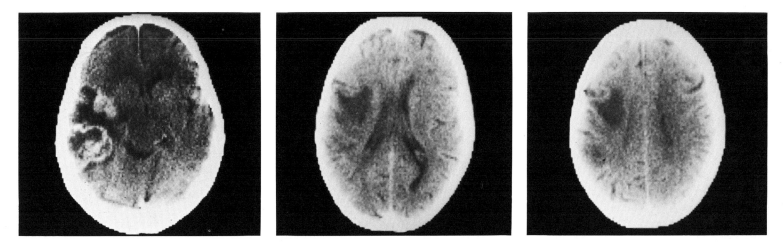

Fig. 8.33 Dysphasia: CT scans in a patient with fluent dysphasia (left) and with non-fluent dysphasia (middle & right).

(Left) This 58 year old man gave an ill-defined history of difficulty in speaking. Examination showed a relatively fluent dysphasia with poor comprehension and repetition. Biopsy of the left hemisphere mass showed a grade 4 astrocytoma.

(Middle & right) This 73 year old woman was admitted following the onset of dysphasia with right-sided weakness. There was a history of hypertension and atrial fibrillation. She had good auditory and reading comprehension but a severe non-fluent dysphasia with poor lip and tongue movement to command. CT scan showed a left hemisphere infarct.

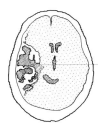 left temporo-parietal mass

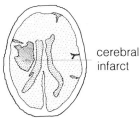 cerebral infarct

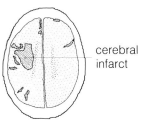 cerebral infarct

Fig. 8.34 Dysphasia: specimen of writing in a patient with left hemisphere glioma. He was asked to write, 'The Quick Brown Fox Jumps Over the Lazy Dog.' This shows dysphasic errors and right-sided neglect.

This 62 year old man could give little history, though he was aware that his speech had dramatically altered. Examination showed a fluent dysphasia with naming difficulty and poor comprehension. CT scan (Fig. 8.33, left) showed a left temporo-parietal mass. Biopsy indicated a grade 4 astrocytoma.

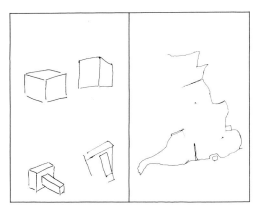

Fig. 8.35 Examples of a patient's attempts to copy diagrams, and to draw a map of the United Kingdom. The latter shows left-sided neglect.

This 64 year old woman had a right parieto-occipital grade 3 astrocytoma.

8.13

A number of disconnection syndromes are described, resulting from lesions of the association pathways of the cerebrum. Dyslexia without dysgraphia, for example, results from a lesion of the left occipital cortex together with the splenium of the corpus callosum (Fig. 8.36). Agnosia and apraxia are complex disturbances. The former defines an impaired capacity to recognise objects, for example by means of vision, in the absence of a primary disturbance of that function. The latter group of conditions refers to a deficiency of skilled motor activity in the absence of a primary disturbance of motor function. One type of apraxia results from an extensive lesion of the corpus callosum, more usually due to infarction than tumour (Fig. 8.37).

Psychological defects may result from brain surgery, for example callosal section. Pre-frontal leucotomy is now performed rarely. It is likely to result in frontal lobe lesions together with degeneration of the dorsomedial nucleus of the thalamus due to interruption of frontothalamic projecting fibres (Fig. 8.38).

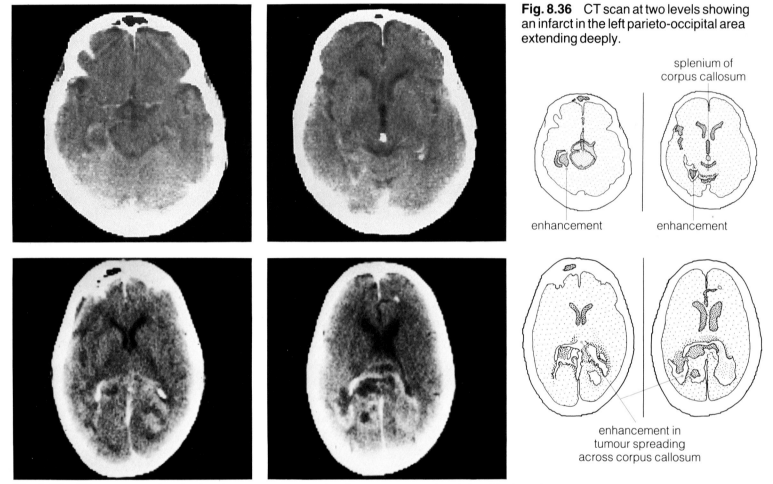

Fig. 8.36 CT scan at two levels showing an infarct in the left parieto-occipital area extending deeply.

splenium of corpus callosum

enhancement   enhancement

enhancement in tumour spreading across corpus callosum

Fig. 8.37 CT scan at two levels showing a tumour crossing the corpus callosum.

This 78 year old man was admitted with a 3 month history of increasing right-sided weakness, clumsiness and speech difficulty. Examination showed a drowsy patient with evidence of a substantial left hemisphere lesion. His mental state precluded assessment of a possible apraxia.

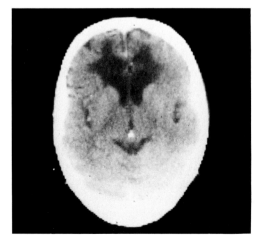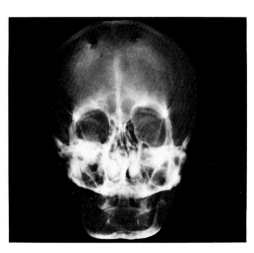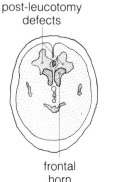

Fig. 8.38 CT scan and skull radiograph of a patient with previous leucotomy.

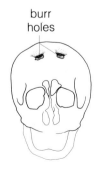

post-leucotomy defects   burr holes

frontal horn

9. Miscellaneous Disorders II: Epilepsy, Meningitis and other Inflammatory Disorders

EPILEPSY

Epilepsy is a common disorder, affecting some 0.5% of the population at some time in their lives. It is best considered a symptom, reflecting in some instances a metabolic disorder (for example, hypoglycaemia), in others a structural condition (for example, cerebral abscess), and in some being idiopathic in origin. The condition can be divided into generalised epilepsy, either grand or petit mal, and the focal epilepsies, the most common of which is temporal lobe epilepsy (complex partial seizures).

Petit mal is the best example of an idiopathic, non-structural, epilepsy. It appears between the ages of about 7 and 15, is never associated with a structural brain abnormality, and does not lead to changes on the CT scan. It is succeeded by grand mal epilepsy in adults in some 50% of cases. Typically the EEG shows generalised paroxysms of spike and wave discharge at around 3½ Hz (Fig. 9.1). Similar changes occur in some 40% of patients' siblings, when examined during the critical age range. Grand mal epilepsy has a number of causes, with structural abnormalities of the brain becoming a more important factor with increasing age. The focal epilepsies, whether temporal lobe, motor or sensory, are much more closely correlated with focal brain lesions.

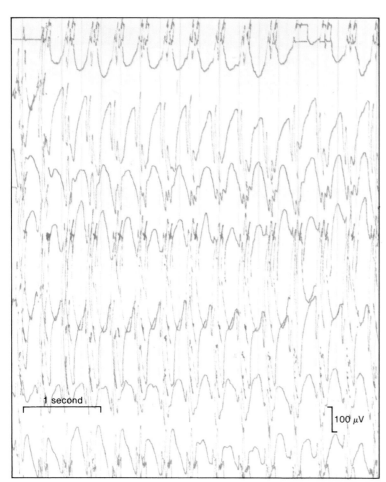

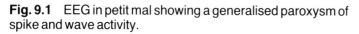

Fig. 9.1 EEG in petit mal showing a generalised paroxysm of spike and wave activity.

This 8 year old boy was having frequent absence attacks. Several occurred during the recording in which he was unresponsive with eyelid flickering for periods of up to 20 seconds.

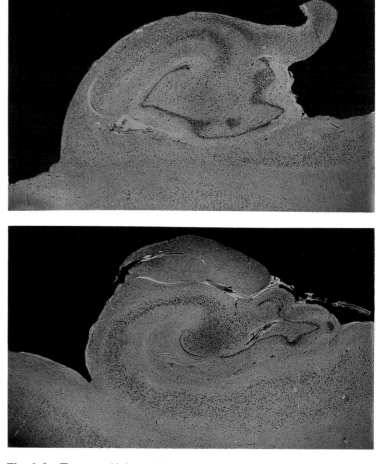

Fig. 9.2 Temporal lobe epilepsy: the pathological changes of Ammon's horn sclerosis (upper) and a control section (lower). Thionine Blue stain, ×10.

In this case, the pathological changes occurred in an elderly patient with atherosclerosis. Similar changes are found in epilepsy.

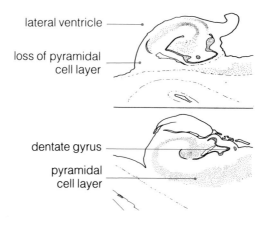

Temporal lobe epilepsy may follow uncontrolled febrile convulsions in early life. Pathological changes consequent to febrile convulsion, and thought to predispose to later temporal lobe epilepsy, are those of Ammon's horn sclerosis (Fig.9.2). The EEG in temporal lobe epilepsy may show a focal spike discharge over the relevant temporal lobe (Fig.9.3). CT scanning shows abnormalities in many patients, the proportion depending on the definition of seizure type and the presence or absence of neurological deficit (Fig.9.4). In some cases of temporal lobe epilepsy, the responsible lesion is outside the temporal lobe.

The drugs commonly used for grand mal or temporal lobe epilepsy include phenobarbitone, phenytoin, carbamazepine, primidone, sodium valproate and clonazepam. Phenytoin is metabolised by liver microsomal enzymes which became saturated at a critical dosage. Further increments in dosage result in rapid increases in serum levels with consequent intoxication, manifesting as drowsiness, ataxia and sometimes involuntary movements. Gum hypertrophy commonly occurs (Fig.9.5). Petit mal epilepsy is treated with either ethosuximide or sodium valproate.

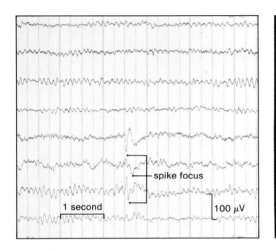

Fig. 9.3 Temporal lobe epilepsy: EEG showing a spike focus in the left anterior to mid-temporal region (arrows).

This 53 year old woman had abruptly developed attacks of a momentary abnormal feeling in some of which brief twitching of the right arm and leg had been observed. They were followed sometimes by dysphasia. Her CT scan was normal.

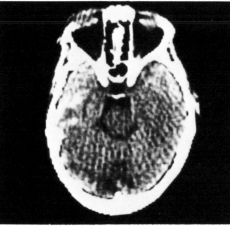

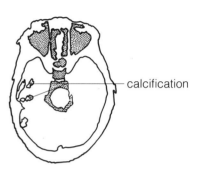

Fig. 9.4 Temporal lobe epilepsy: CT scan showing a calcified area in the left temporal lobe, possibly an arterio-venous malformation.

This 55 year old man had an 18 year history of episodes of a brief feeling of fear, sometimes with dysphasia, followed by loss of awareness. The neurological examination was normal.

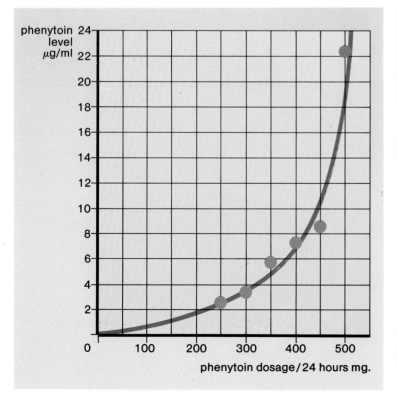

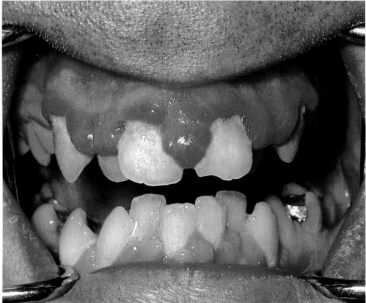

Fig. 9.5 Graph of phenytoin levels according to dosage in one patient (left) and the gum hypertrophy that commonly occurs with phenytoin therapy (right).

CNS INFECTION AND INFLAMMATORY DISORDERS

Meningitis

Inflammation of the meninges may be the result of an infective agent (bacterial, viral or fungal), the consequence of neoplastic infiltration, or may follow chemical irritation, for example with myodil used in myelography.

VIRAL MENINGITIS

This is an acutely evolving illness, with fever, malaise and signs of meningeal irritation but with little or no alteration of the conscious level. Some patients with enterovirus infection develop an erythematous rash, and additional symptoms may include sore throat, gastrointestinal disturbance or muscle pain. The CSF shows a moderately elevated protein concentration with a lymphocytic pleocytosis and a normal glucose concentration. Rarely polymorphonuclear cells predominate, and occasionally, particularly with mumps, the glucose concentration is moderately depressed. A specific agent, most commonly an enterovirus, is found in up to 70% of cases.

BACTERIAL MENINGITIS

At post-mortem, pus is found in the basal cisterns and over the cerebral convolutions. The pia over the brain base are cloudy with opalescent streaks surrounding the cortical veins over the hemisphere convexity (Fig.9.6).

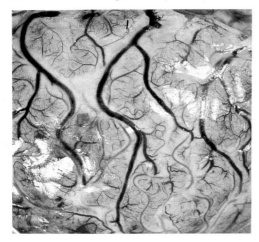

Fig. 9.6 Bacterial meningitis: lateral surface of the cerebral hemisphere showing purulent exudate.

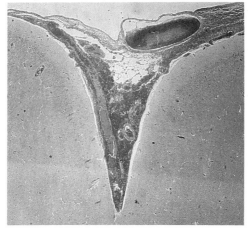

Fig. 9.7 Bacterial meningitis: section showing exudate in the subarachnoid space of a cerebral sulcus H & E stain, ×8.

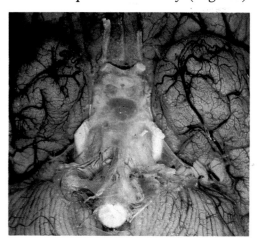

Fig. 9.8 Tuberculous meningitis: inferior brain surface showing exudate in basal cisterns.

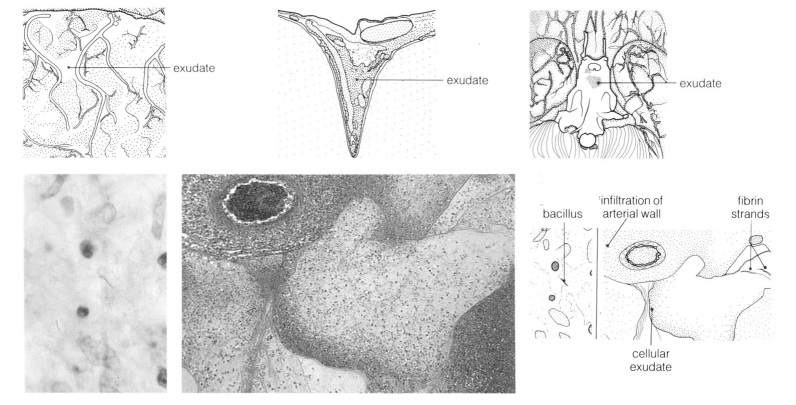

Fig. 9.9 Tuberculous meningitis: exudate containing an acid-fast bacillus (left, Ziehl-Neelsen stain, x 950) and exudate in the subarachnoid space, showing an abundance of fibrin, the copious cellular exudate, and infiltration of the arterial wall predominantly by mononuclear cells (right, H & E stain, ×60).

The patient, aged 81, had had backache, epigastric pain and vomiting for 1 week, followed by confusion and pyrexia. There was neck stiffness. CSF showed 165 lymphocytes, a protein of 3.06 g/L and a glucose of 0.5 mml/L. The patient died 4 days after commencing anti-tuberculous therapy.

Microscopy reveals polymorphonuclear and mononuclear cells with macrophages between the pia and arachnoid. A fibrinous exudate is present, extending into the depths of the cortical sulci (Fig.9.7). The commonest agents are pneumococcus, meningococcus and *Haemophilus influenzae*. The predominant organism varies according to the age of the patient.

The disease causes fever, lethargy, headache and signs of meningeal irritation, but the illness is far more profound than viral meningitis, with fulminating forms causing death within 24 hours. Signs of meningeal irritation may be lacking in the neonate, in the elderly and in deeply unconscious patients. A petechial rash is particularly associated with meningococcal meningitis, but occurs in only 50% of cases, and can also complicate other bacterial infections, including, rarely, *E. coli*. Associated conditions include sore throat, otitis media and pneumonia. Acute brain swelling may develop, particularly with *Haemophilus* infection.

The cerebrospinal fluid pressure is usually elevated. The protein concentration is raised in most patients, though seldom above 10g/L. The cell count, predominantly polymorphonuclear, may reach 100,000/mm^3. Rarely the count is barely raised, or even normal. Glucose concentration is depressed, often to immeasurable levels. Early treatment is vital, though paradoxically, patients with a short history tend to have a worse prognosis.

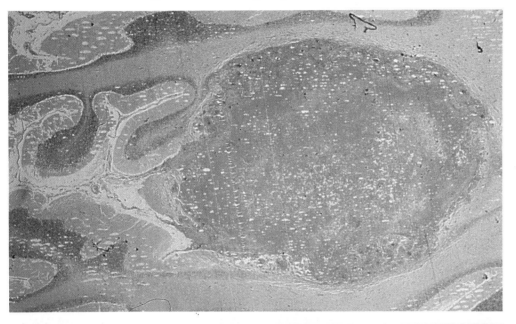

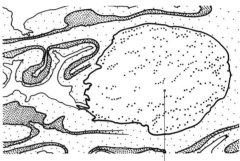

Fig. 9.10 Tuberculoma: section of cerebellum showing a well-demarcated tuberculoma composed largely of caseous material. H & E stain, ×7.

tuberculoma

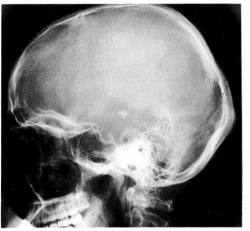

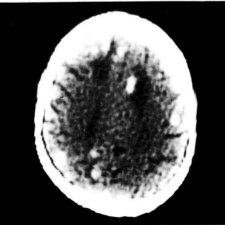

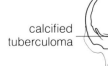

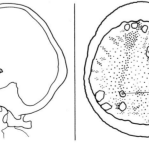

calcified tuberculoma

multiple tuberculomata

Fig. 9.11 Tuberculoma: skull radiograph showing a calcified tuberculoma (left) and a CT scan showing multiple high density tuberculomata with surrounding oedema (right).

This 20 year old man (right) had been treated three years previously for pulmonary and possibly meningeal tuberculosis. His epilepsy began then and continued, with a brief feeling of nervousness followed by generalised convulsions. There were no localising signs. The CT scan had been performed one year after his initial presentation.

TUBERCULOUS MENINGITIS

Typically this is of subacute onset. It is usually considered to be the consequence of rupture of a tuberculous focus (Rich's focus) from the brain into the subarachnoid space, though other sources have been suggested, including a primary focus in the choroid plexus. It is always associated with primary disease elsewhere in the body, often not clinically apparent.

Macroscopic examination shows a greenish-grey opacity of the meninges spreading over the cerebral convexities and occupying the basal cisterns (Fig.9.8). If the disease has lasted several weeks, microscopy reveals an exudate of fibrin-containing lymphocytes, plasma cells and epithelioid cells, with varying numbers of bacteria (Fig.9.9).

Annual notification in England and Wales amounts to some 100 cases, with a mortality around 30%. Following malaise, fever, headache and muscle pain, signs of meningeal irritation appear, with drowsiness and subsequently focal neurological abnormalities including cranial nerve palsies and hemiplegia. The majority have a normal chest radiograph, many a normal skin test; a history of tuberculous disease, or contact with the disease, is often lacking.

The protein concentration of the CSF is almost always elevated, though not usually over 5g/L, and the cell count tends to lie between 25 and 500 cells/mm^3. In acute onset cases, the cell count may be higher and may have a significant proportion of polymorphonuclear cells. Rarely, the

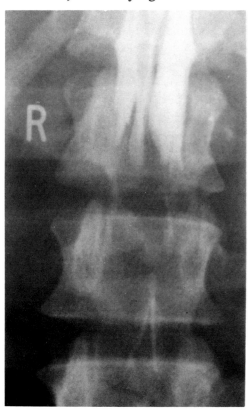

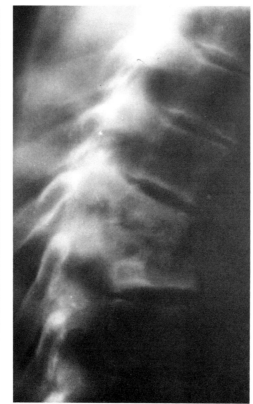

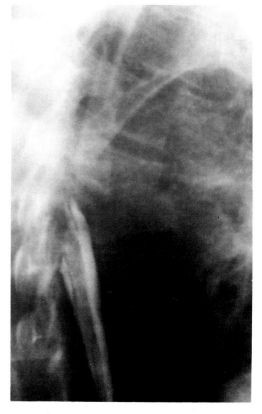

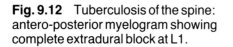

Fig. 9.12 Tuberculosis of the spine: antero-posterior myelogram showing complete extradural block at L1.

This 29 year old man had a two week history of back pain followed by lower limb weakness. Examination showed a spastic paraparesis. Laminectomy revealed a paraspinal abscess, histology of which showed typical tuberculous features.

Fig. 9.13 Tuberculosis of the spine: plain radiograph showing collapse of D7 and D8 (left) and myelogram showing complete block at the same level due to an extradural mass (right).

This 59 year old man had had back pain for several months followed by weakness and altered sensation in the lower limbs. He had a past history of pulmonary tuberculosis. CSF protein was 1.98 g/L. At thoracotomy an extra-dural abscess was excised with histology consistent with tuberculosis.

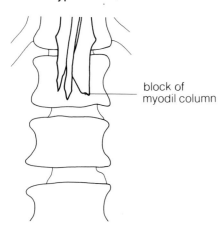

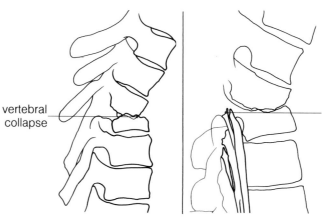

cellular reaction is lacking initially, probably due to depressed tuberculin sensitivity. The glucose concentration is depressed, though less so than with pyogenic meningitis. In cases where the diagnosis is uncertain, a radioactive bromide partition test can be used to demonstrate an abnormal blood/CSF barrier. Complications include cranial nerve palsies, hemiplegia, optic atrophy, hydrocephalus and epilepsy. Treatment is usually with streptomycin, isoniazid and rifampicin, with single or double therapy continuing for 18 to 24 months.

Tuberculomata once accounted for one-third of intracerebral tumours in Great Britain and are still common in third world countries. Many cases in this country are in the Asian population, primarily in children and young adults. In children they tend to arise below the tentorium, and in adults, above, principally in the frontoparietal lobes. They are multiple in up to one-third of cases.

Histologically there is a central caseating core surrounded by a collagen capsule containing epithelioid cells, lymphocytes and giant cells (Fig.9.10). Organisms are found on microscopy in about 70%. Some 30 to 50% of patients have extracranial tuberculosis and a similar proportion have a history of previous infection. The most common presentation is with signs of raised intracranial pressure, including papilloedema. Seizures occur in at least 50% of cases but fever is uncommon and only one-third have hemiparesis. The most common CSF abnormality is a raised protein concentration. Skin testing may

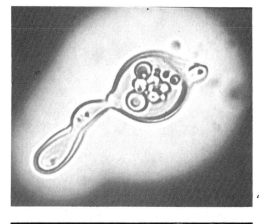

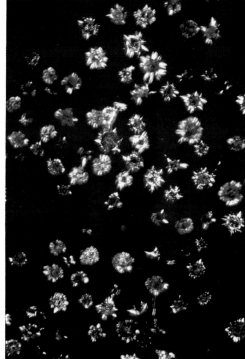

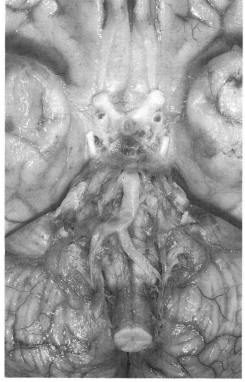

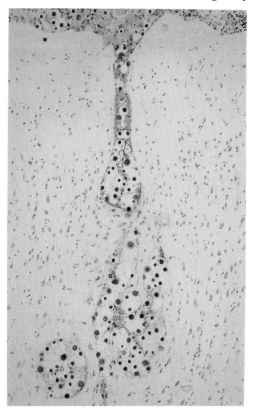

Fig.9.15 Cryptococcal meningitis: opacity of the basal leptomeninges (left) and section showing cryptococci distending the perivascular space of a cortical blood vessel (right). Nissl stain, x 40.

Case (right) is the same patient as in figure 9.14.

Fig.9.14 Cryptococcal meningitis: *Cryptococcus neoformans*. Nigrosin preparation, ×120 (upper) and buffered cresyl violet under polarized light, x 110. (lower).

The patient, aged 70, had a 6 weeks' history of fever, and a 4 week history of headache with anorexia, memory loss and subsequent diplopia. Examination showed left 6th and 7th cranial nerve palsies with signs of meningeal irritation. Cryptococci were isolated from the CSF.

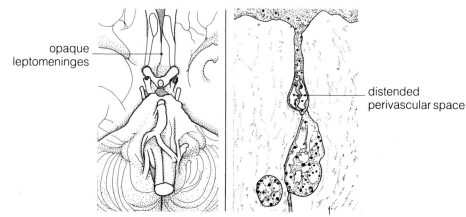

opaque leptomeninges

distended perivascular space

9.7

be negative and the ESR is usually normal. An abnormal chest radiograph occurs in up to 50% of patients; calcification on the skull radiograph is found in 5% (Fig.9.11, left). CT scanning is the most sensitive radiological technique, with low or high density areas sometimes with ring or diffuse enhancement and adjacent oedema (Fig.9.11, right). Treatment is usually medical rather than surgical.

Tuberculous disease of the spine most frequently affects the thoracic region (Pott's paraplegia). Spinal cord involvement is secondary to abscess formation (Figs.9.12 & 9.13), granulation tissue in the epidural space, angulation of the cord secondary to vertebral collapse or infarction due to occlusion of nutrient vessels.

CRYPTOCOCCAL MENINGITIS

Cryptococcus neoformans is an ovaloid body measuring 2 to 15μm surrounded by a polysaccharide capsule (Fig. 9.14). Access to the meninges is usually via the respiratory tract. Macroscopically, numerous cystic spaces up to 3 mm in diameter occupy mainly the superficial cortical layers, sometimes also following perforating vessels, and are surrounded by a granulomatous reaction (Fig. 9.15).

The disease is slightly more common in men and usually presents in adults with signs of meningeal irritation, or, less commonly, with signs of raised intracranial pressure, epilepsy or focal neurological deficit. Many of the patients have disorders of the immune system. The CSF is usually

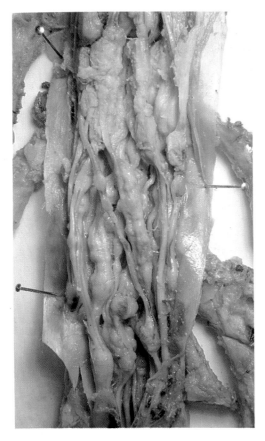

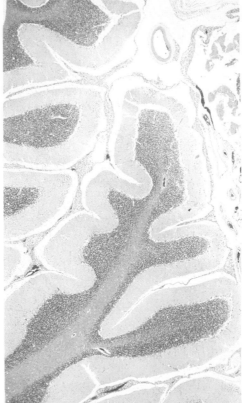

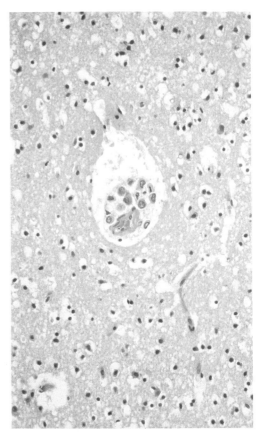

Fig. 9.16 Carcinomatous meningitis: roots of cauda equina thickened by carcinoma cells.

Fig. 9.17 Carcinomatous meningitis: cerebellum showing leptomeningeal carcinomatosis (left, ×10) and invasion, along Virchow-Robin space (right, x 250). H&E stain.

This 55 year old man developed an anaplastic carcinoma of the bladder. Two months later, he presented with headache, then numbness of the hands, diplopia, dysarthria and ataxia. Examination showed dysarthria, nystagmus, left 6th and right 7th nerve palsies, bilateral limb ataxia, areflexia and gait ataxia.

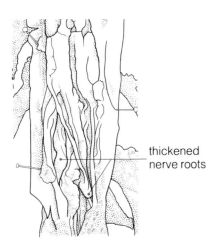

thickened nerve roots

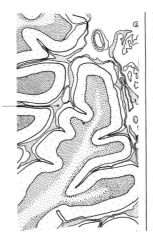

carcinoma cells in leptomeninges

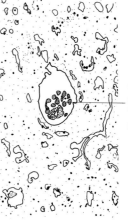

carcinoma cells in Virchow-Robin space

abnormal, with changes similar to those seen in tuberculous meningitis. The chest radiograph is abnormal in approximately 40% of cases, and the CT scan may detect low density lesions. Therapy is probably best with a combination of amphotericin B, flucytosine and miconazole, but mortality remains around 30%.

CARCINOMATOUS MENINGITIS

In this condition a diffuse infiltration of the leptomeninges by carcinomatous cells occurs (Figs.9.16 & 9.17). A similar condition develops in some leukaemic patients. The primary carcinomas most commonly responsible are those of the breast and bronchus. The initial symptoms are usually non-specific, with headache and back or limb pain. Later, a combination of cranial nerve and spinal root lesions appears, often with alteration of the conscious state.

The most commonly affected cranial nerves are the seventh, fifth and third (Figs.9.18 & 9.19). Optic nerve involvement leads to a rapidly progressing visual failure. Spinal root manifestations include focal weakness or sensory loss, particularly in the lower limbs, with areflexia. CSF changes include an increased protein concentration, an increased cell count and a depressed glucose concentration. Malignant cells in the CSF are found in the majority, though multiple examinations may be required. Radiotherapy together with intrathecal cytotoxic agents may delay progression temporarily.

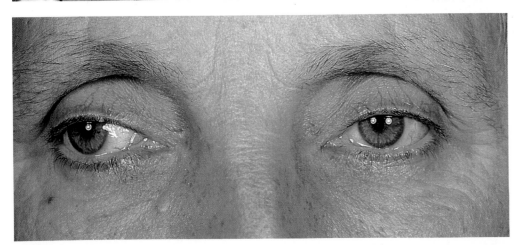

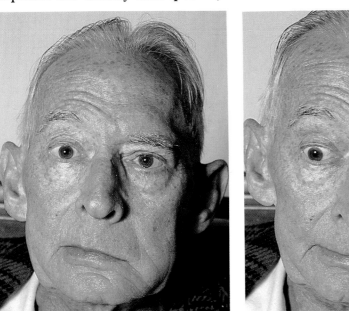

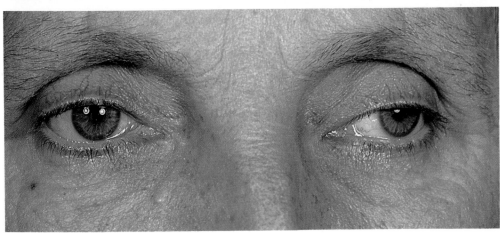

Fig. 9.18 Carcinomatous meningitis: left lower motor neurone facial weakness (left) with reduced abduction of right eye due to 6th nerve palsy (right).

This 75 year old man had a myeloproliferative disorder. He presented with pain in the left ear, left deafness, diplopia, facial weakness and loss of use of the hands. Examination showed left 7th and 8th, and right 6th nerve involvement with global limb weakness and depressed reflexes. CSF examination revealed a marked pleocytosis.

Fig. 9.19 Carcinomatous meningitis: bilateral medial rectus weakness with slight left ptosis.

This 58 year old woman had developed carcinoma of the breast 2 years previously. Within a year, there was evidence of bone and hepatic metastases. Three weeks previously she had developed intermittent diplopia, ptosis and vertigo. Examination showed a variable left ptosis, incomplete adduction of both eyes, depression of limb reflexes and some gait ataxia. Her CT scan showed parenchymal metastases.

Cerebral Abscess

Intracranial abscess most commonly results from a pulmonary source, with septic emboli initiating the pathological process. Contiguous sites to the brain responsible for abscess formation include infection of the ear or paranasal sinuses. Entry may occur via a skull fracture. In up to 20% of cases the source is not apparent.

Initially an area of septic encephalitis develops with focal necrosis, haemorrhage, polymorphonuclear infiltration and surrounding oedema. Later encapsulation occurs, with a layer of granulation tissue surrounded by collagen (Figs.9.20 & 9.21). Infection in the middle ear cavity spreads upwards to pierce overlying bone and dura before penetrating the temporal lobe (Figs.9.22 & 9.23).

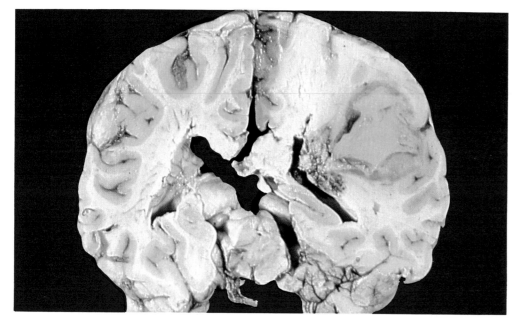

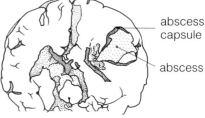

Fig. 9.20 Cerebral abscess: abscess in the right cerebral hemisphere.

This 24 year old man had Fallot's tetralogy He gave a history of right-sided headache over three weeks. There were no abnormal neurological findings. The patient died 24 hours after admission.

abscess capsule

abscess

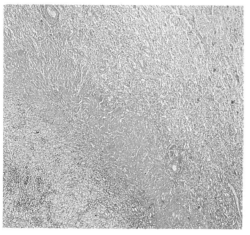

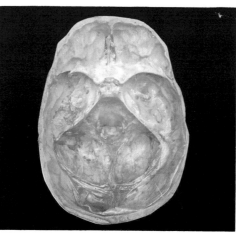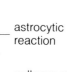

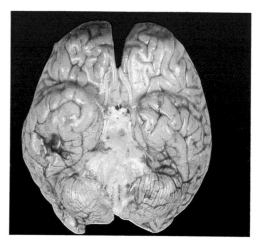

Fig. 9.21 Cerebral abscess: an abscess surrounded by collagen and inflammatory cells. Masson's trichrome stain, ×30.

Fig. 9.22 Cerebral abscess: perforation of dura in the floor of the right middle cranial fossa (left) with penetration of the overlying

temporal lobe (right): basal meningitis can be seen.

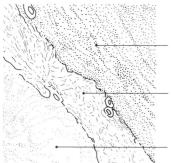

astrocytic reaction

collagenous wall

purulent material

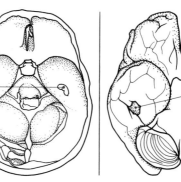

perforation in dura

site of entry into right temporal lobe

purulent exudate

9.10

In one series of 107 abscesses, four were associated with Fallot's tetralogy (Fig.9.24).

Presentation may be with fever, drowsiness and generalised seizures without focal deficit, or alternatively with signs of a mass lesion without clear evidence of intracranial sepsis.

Angiography reveals an avascular mass, whilst technetium scanning is abnormal in virtually all cases of developed abscess; the EEG generally shows a focal slow-wave disturbance. By the time the abscess has matured, CT scanning reveals a low density core surrounded by an enhancing capsule (Fig.9.25, left). Rupture into the ventricular system leads to ependymitis, revealed on the scan by enhancement in the walls of the ventricular system (Fig.9.25, right). The abscess is surrounded by oedema, though less prominently than at the stage of cerebritis.

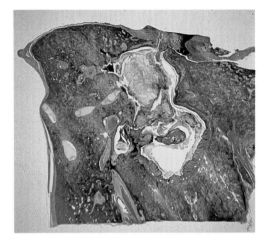

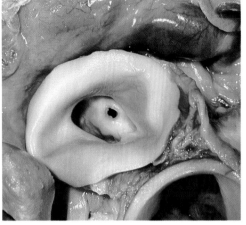

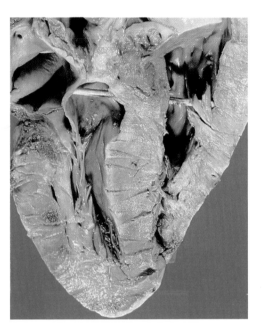

Fig. 9.23 Cerebral abscess: section showing site of perforation from the middle ear to the middle cranial fossa and adherent temporal lobe. Haematoxylin & Van Gieson stain, ×3.

Fig. 9.24 Cerebral abscess: Fallot's tetralogy with pulmonary stenosis (left) and right ventricular hypertrophy and ventricular septal defect (right).

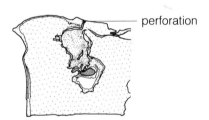
perforation

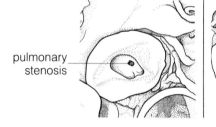
pulmonary stenosis

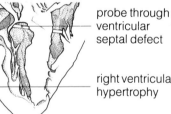
probe through ventricular septal defect

right ventricular hypertrophy

Fig. 9.25 Cerebral abscess: CT scan showing a left thalamic abscess (left) with ependymal enhancement due to an associated ventriculitis (right).

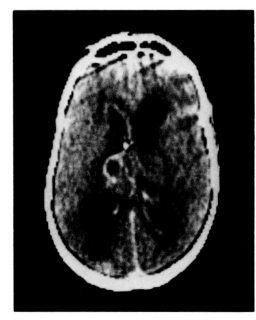

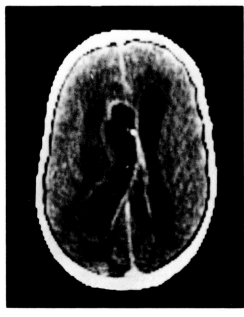

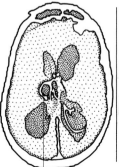

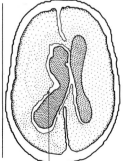

abscess

enhancement in wall of lateral ventricle

Corticosteroids may influence the enhancement pattern. Blood-borne abscesses tend to be multiple (Fig.9.26).

Antibiotic therapy, with or without corticosteroids, is preferred at the stage of cerebritis, with surgery the treatment of choice when the abscess has become encapsulated.

Subdural Empyema

Subdural or extradural abscesses follow meningitis, neurosurgical procedures or frontal sinus infection (Fig.9.27). They may coincide with intracerebral abscess.

The CT scan shows a low density, or occasionally isodense, extracerebral lesion with compression of the underlying brain (Fig.9.28).

Hydatid Disease

This condition is due to infestation by the cystic stage of *Taenia echinococcus (Echinococcus granulosus)*. The cyst is unilocular with a double wall, from the inner layer of which capsules are budded off. Heads of worms are produced from the inner walls of the capsules (Fig.9.29). The cysts most commonly occur in the liver and lungs.

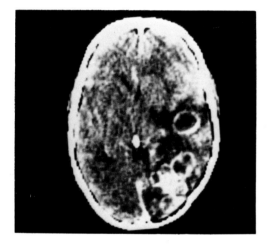
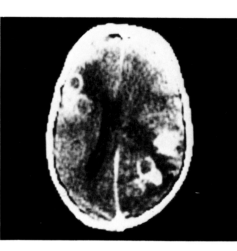
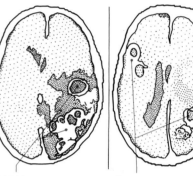

Fig. 9.26 Cerebral abscess: CT scan at two levels showing multiple abscesses in the left frontal and right parietal lobes.

This 42 year old man developed multiple abscesses due to infection with *Nocardia spp.* following renal transplantation.

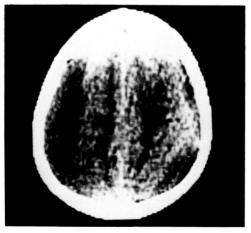
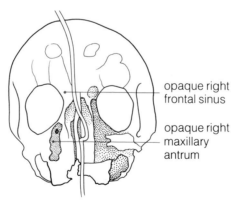

Fig. 9.27 Subdural empyema: skull radiograph showing pus in the right frontal and maxillary sinuses.

This 13 year old boy had a six day history of fever, right frontal headache, irritability and declining consciousness. Examination showed bilateral papilloedema.

opaque right frontal sinus

opaque right maxillary antrum

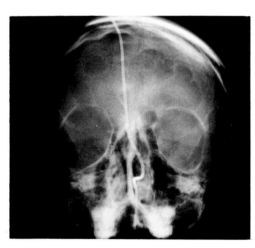
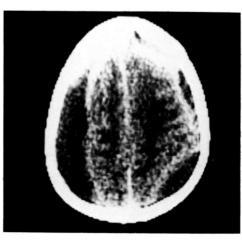

Fig. 9.28 Subdural empyema: CT scan showing bilateral subdural empyema, pre-contrast (left) and post-contrast (right).

Same patient as in figure 9.27.

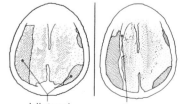

bilateral subdural empyema

membrane enhancement

abscesses

abscesses

Involvement of the brain may be asymptomatic or may produce epilepsy (Fig.9.30).

Cysticercosis

The CNS is infested in 60 to 90% of patients with cysticercosis, the encysted stage of the pork tapeworm, *Taenia solium*. The cysts, usually multiple, may be asymptomatic, but are a common cause of epilepsy in endemic areas, for example, India. The seizures are often focal, and are associated with a CT scan abnormality in approximately 90% of cases (Fig.9.31). Areas of calcification are seen on the skull radiograph in 11 to 35% of cases. The diagnosis may be facilitated by scanning following labelling of the lesion by indium-113 attached to anti-cysticercus antibody. The same antibodies labelled with [131]In have been used for treatment.

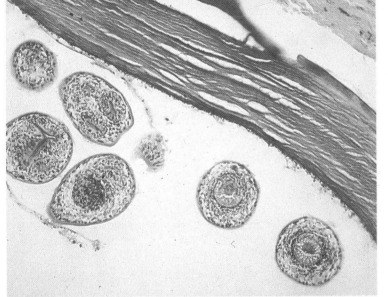

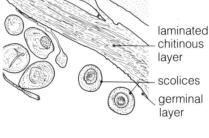

Fig. 9.29 Hydatid disease: wall of cyst with laminated chitinous layer and inner germinal layer, surrounding scolices with invaginated heads.

laminated chitinous layer
scolices
germinal layer

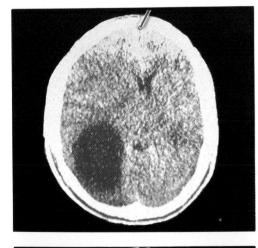

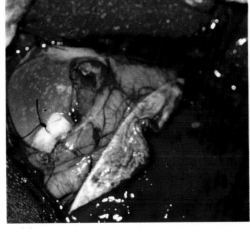

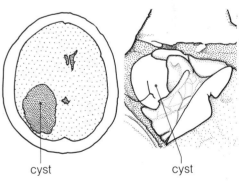

Fig. 9.30 Hydatid disease: cyst revealed on CT scan (left) and at craniotomy (right).

cyst   cyst

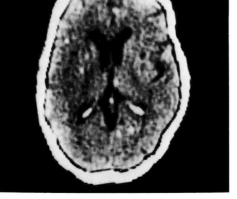

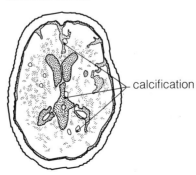

Fig. 9.31 Cysticercosis: CT scan showing calcified areas.

calcification

Syphilis

This condition is caused by the organism *Treponema pallidum*. Following primary infection, invasion of the central nervous system may occur, probably from three to eighteen months later. This initial pathological event is a meningitis, occurring in some 25% of cases having a previous primary infection, and usually asymptomatic. Subsequent symptomatic manifestations of the disease include meningovascular syphilis, optic atrophy, tabes dorsalis and general paralysis of the insane, perhaps occurring in around 5% of those with a previous syphilitic history. Congenital neurosyphilis displays similar manifestations, together with a number of stigmata affecting other systems, including defective teeth and interstitial keratitis (Fig. 9.32). Meningeal reaction is common to all forms of neurosyphilis, together with disease of the parenchyma of varying degree and uncertain aetiology. Overlap of the clinical groups is considerable.

CSF changes include a pleocytosis, with an average, for example of 25 to 50 cells in tabes and general paralysis, an elevated protein concentration, sometimes reaching 1.5 g/L, and an elevated IgG concentration. The FTA – ABS

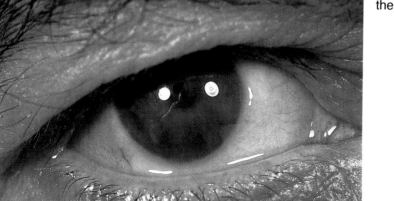

Fig. 9.32 Congenital syphilis: interstitial keratitis, with clouding of the right cornea.

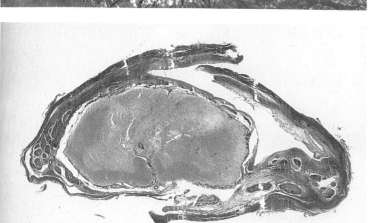

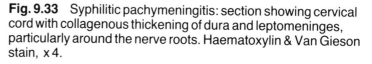

Fig. 9.33 Syphilitic pachymeningitis: section showing cervical cord with collagenous thickening of dura and leptomeninges, particularly around the nerve roots. Haematoxylin & Van Gieson stain, x 4.

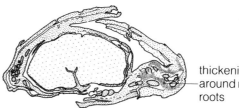

thickening around nerve roots

Fig. 9.34 Meningovascular syphilis: cerebral artery showing intimal hyperplasia. H & E stain, x 60.

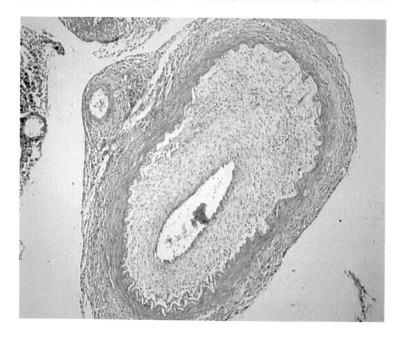

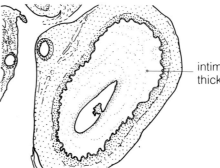

intimal thickening

and TPI serological tests are positive in almost all cases of neurosyphilis.

Spinal syphilis embraces a number of clinical syndromes, with pathological changes of arachnoiditis and endarteritis of spinal vessels coinciding (Fig.9.33). In meningovascular syphilis, an endarteritis of cerebral vessels with infiltration of media and adventitia by inflammatory cells and intimal hyperplasia results in vascular occlusion (Heubner's endarteritis) (Fig.9.34). Presentation may be with stroke-like syndromes in relatively young individuals (Fig. 9.35).

General paralysis was once common. It accounted for 1,539 deaths in England and Wales in 1925, for example. It is more frequent in men and usually presents between the ages of 30 and 50, most commonly between 5 and 20 years after the initial infection.

The brain is covered by thickened meninges, with ependymitis, ventricular dilatation and cortical atrophy (Fig.9.36), most marked in the frontal and parietal lobes.

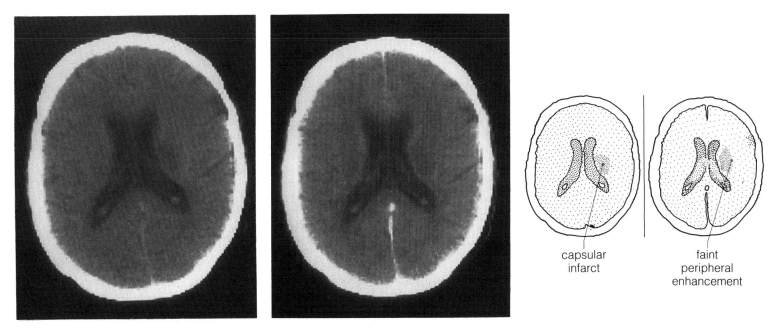

capsular infarct

faint peripheral enhancement

Fig. 9.35 Menovascular syphilis: CT scan showing infarct in right internal capsule (pre-contrast, left) with faint peripheral enhancement (post-contrast, right).

This 38 year old man presented with three attacks of left-sided weakness, the last persisting. Examination confirmed a left hemiparesis. The CSF contained 32 lymphocytes with positive TPHA and FTA. He made a good, though incomplete, recovery.

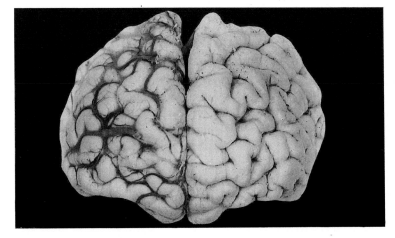

Fig. 9.36 General paralysis: normal frontal lobes (left) with leptomeninges removed on the right . Frontal lobes in GPI (right)

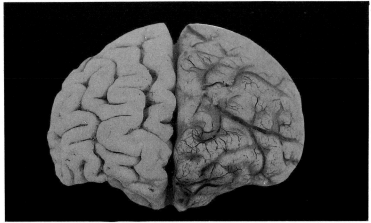

with widened sulci (the leptomeninges have been removed on the left) and cloudy leptomeninges.

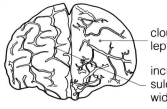

cloudy leptomeninges

increased sulcal width

9.15

Microscopy shows loss of cortical lamination with a reduction in the nerve cell population. Spirochaetes can be found in the cortex (Fig.9.37).

The condition produces alteration of judgement, sometimes involving consideration of grandiose schemes. Intellectual function deteriorates, then a number of specific neurological signs and symptoms appear, including dysarthria, tremor and epileptic fits. Some 50% of cases have Argyll Robertson pupils (Fig.9.38) with meiosis and fixation to light, but an intact near response.

Tabes dorsalis characteristically comprises lightning pains, ataxia, Argyll Robertson pupils and loss of tendon reflexes. Macroscopic changes in the dorsal columns comprise a greyish discoloration with atrophy. Microscopically there is leptomeningitis, atrophy of the dorsal roots and degeneration of part, or the whole, of the dorsal col-

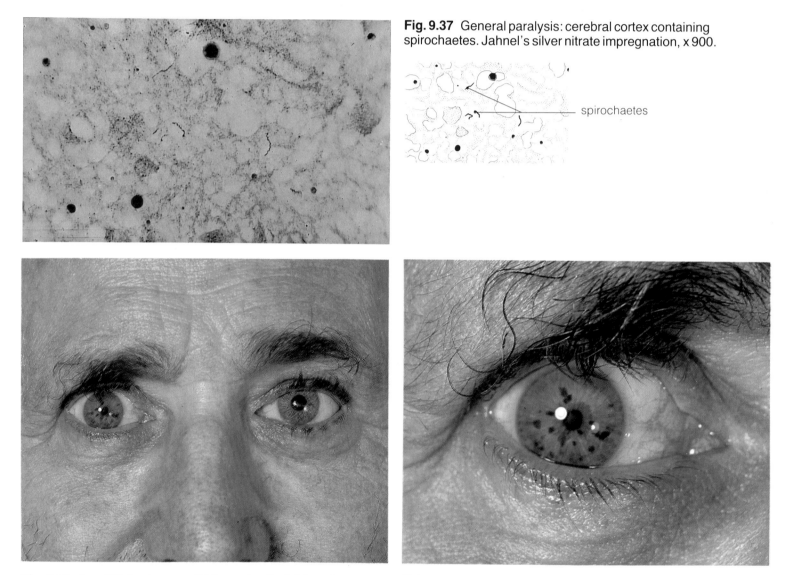

Fig. 9.37 General paralysis: cerebral cortex containing spirochaetes. Jahnel's silver nitrate impregnation, x 900.

spirochaetes

Fig. 9.38 Argyll Robertson pupil. The patient's right pupil was small, slightly irregular and fixed to light though reacting to a near stimulus. The left eye is artificial.

This 69 year old man had presented at the age of 43 with numbness of the right leg. Examination showed a glass eye on the left (the eye had been enucleated at the age of six following an injury), a right Argyll Robertson pupil, lower limb areflexia and depressed pin prick sensation in the right leg. The CSF contained 39 lymphocytes with positive serology. Subsequently he had numerous gastric crises.

umns (Fig. 9.39). The condition again is more common in men and most commonly appears between the ages of 30 and 50. Probably some 70% declare themselves between 5 and 20 years after the initial infection. Lightning pains occur in at least 90% of cases and predominate in the lower limbs. Sensory loss to all modalities develops, rather patchily over the legs, inner arm and chest with depressed reflexes and an ataxic gait. Abnormal pupils occur in the majority. Visceral crises may develop, with paroxysmal abdominal pain associated with intractable vomiting being the most common. With loss of pain sensation, trophic ulcers may occur, together with gross destruction of joint architecture (Charcot joint) (Figs. 9.40 & 9.41).

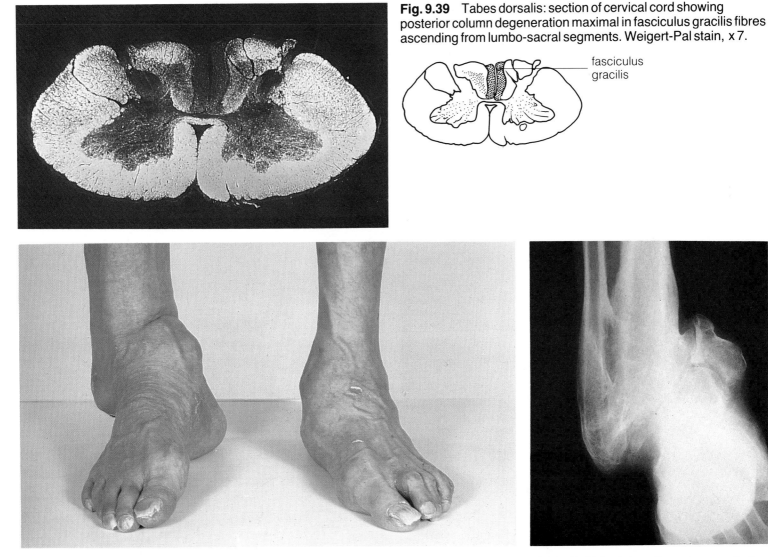

Fig. 9.39 Tabes dorsalis: section of cervical cord showing posterior column degeneration maximal in fasciculus gracilis fibres ascending from lumbo-sacral segments. Weigert-Pal stain, x 7.

fasciculus gracilis

Fig. 9.40 Tabes dorsalis: deformity of the right ankle due to a Charcot joint.

This 60 year old man developed difficulty in walking with incoordination. The deformity of his right ankle had followed a painless fracture. He had Argyll Robertson pupils, lower limb areflexia, distal sensory loss in the lower limbs, and an ataxic gait. CSF and blood TPHA were positive.

Fig. 9.41 Tabes dorsalis: antero-posterior radiograph of the right ankle showing gross deformity.

Same patient as in figure 9.40.

Optic atrophy commonly occurs in tabes secondary to a chronic inflammatory reaction in the pia mater of the intracranial optic nerve and chiasm. Visual failure is usually gradual and tends to affect the peripheral field.

Poliomyelitis

The causative virus gains access to the central nervous system via the nasopharynx or alimentary tract. The major sites of pathological change are the ganglion cells of the spinal cord, particularly of the anterior horns (Fig.9.42), though the brain stem, and even the cerebrum, do not escape.

The disease predominates in children, particularly under the age of ten, and principally occurs in countries of temperate climate. It shows a seasonal prevalence, most cases appearing in the later summer and autumn. Following vaccination programmes, the disease has become almost extinct in developed countries.

A preparalytic stage, with fever, malaise and headaches, is followed by a rapidly evolving lower motor neurone weakness, often asymmetrical, and predominantly in the lower limbs. Slow recovery occurs over several months, leaving various deformities such as abnormal foot posture, kyphoscoliosis and flail joints. The CSF shows an inflammatory reaction with polymorphonuclear leucocytes predominating initially.

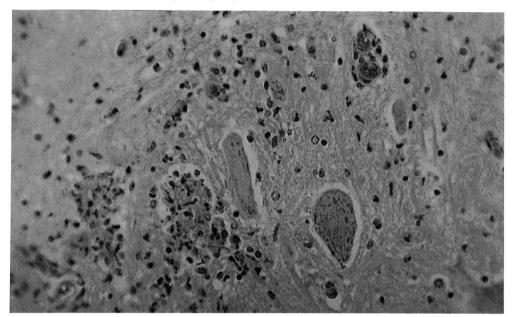

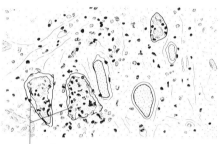

Fig. 9.42 Poliomyelitis: part of anterior horn from a four-day-old case. Some necrotic nerve cells are surrounded by polymorphonuclear leucocytes, lymphocytes and microglia. H & E stain, x 300.

nerve cells surrounded by cellular reaction

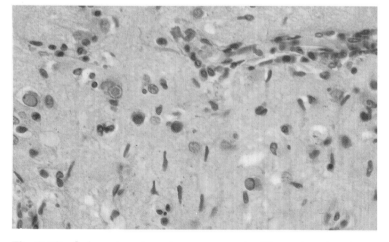

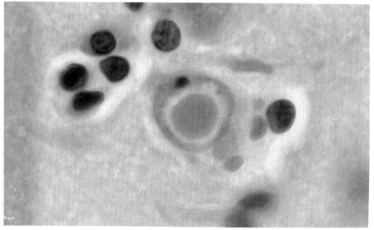

Fig. 9.43 Subacute sclerosing panencephalitis: cortex showing an intranuclear inclusion body and perivascular lymphocytic cuffing (left, Haematoxylin & Van Gieson stain, x 500) and a high power view of an inclusion body (right, Lendrum's Phloxine Tartrazine stain, x 1500).

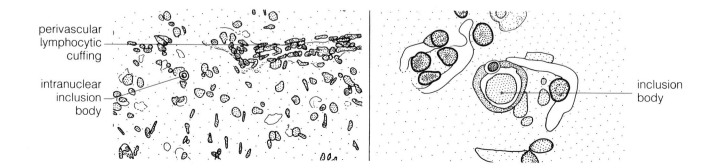

perivascular lymphocytic cuffing

intranuclear inclusion body

inclusion body

Subacute Sclerosing Panencephalitis

This disease follows measles infection after a mean interval of 5 years. The grey matter shows loss of nerve cells with astrocytic proliferation, microglial reaction and perivascular lymphocytic cuffing (Fig.9.43, left). The white matter reveals loss of myelinated fibres with astrocytic proliferation. Nerve cells contain homogeneous rounded inclusion bodies in the nucleus or in the nucleus and the cytoplasm (Fig.9.43, right).

The condition is confined to children and adults under 25 years. Behaviour disorder is followed by dementia, myoclonus and incoordination. Eventually mutism is associated with decorticate postures. It affects between 1 to 3 children per million, particularly those who have had measles before the age of two. Most patients die within 3 years, though a small proportion survive longer and, rarely, remissions and relapses appear. High measles antibody levels occur in serum and CSF with oligoclonal banding in the latter absorbable by measles antigen.

Acute Haemorrhagic Leucoencephalitis

This condition usually shortly follows an upper respiratory tract infection. There is a rapid decline in the conscious level with or without paralysis, and an inflammatory reaction in the CSF. Most patients die within a few days. The brain is swollen with numerous haemorrhages in the cerebral white matter, sometimes also involving

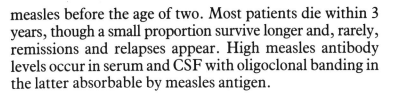

Fig. 9.44 Acute haemorrhagic leucoencephalitis: coronal brain slice showing swelling of white matter on the right with petechial haemorrhages.

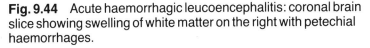

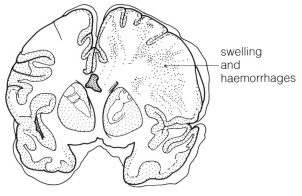

swelling and haemorrhages

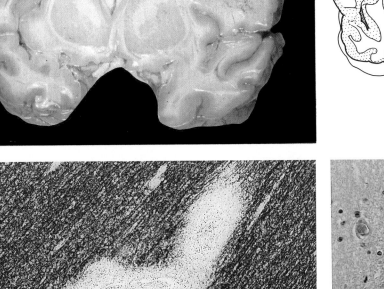

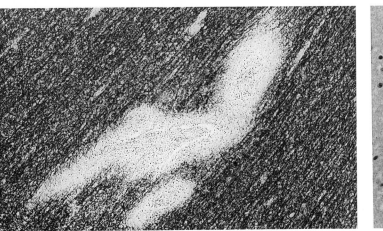

Fig. 9.45 Post-vaccinal encephalomyelitis: cerebral white matter showing perivenular demyelination (left, Myelin stain, x 20) and cellular reaction in the Virchow-Robin space and in the parenchyma around the venule (right, H&E stain, x 200).

perivenular demyelination

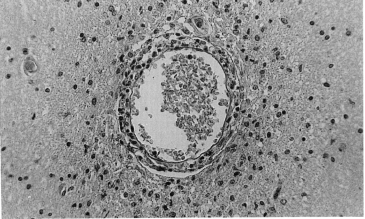

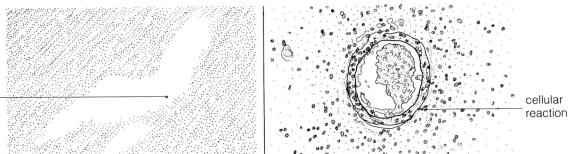

The patient, aged 15, was admitted in coma, 16 days after smallpox vaccination, having had 6 days progressive malaise and stupor. Examination showed a flaccid paresis of the lower limbs with urinary retention and neck stiffness. He died 24 hours later.

cellular reaction

brain stem and cerebellum (Fig.9.44). There is vessel necrosis with perivascular oedema and polymorphonuclear reaction.

Post-vaccinal Encephalomyelitis

This condition follows vaccination against rabies or smallpox, or an acute exanthematous illness, particularly measles, chicken pox or rubella, or a relatively trivial upper respiratory tract infection. The pathological changes include perivenous demyelination, with lesser axonal disruption; the areas are surrounded by microglial cells with astrocytic enlargement (Fig.9.45).

Symptoms usually begin abruptly, with coma and convulsions predominating in some cases and cerebellar symptomatology in others. The CSF tends to show an inflammatory reaction but may be normal in 20% of cases. Relapses occasionally occur.

Creutzfeldt-Jakob Disease

This condition, also called subacute spongiform encephalopathy, is rare. It tends to arise in late middle life, has an equal sex distribution, and usually leads to the patient's death within 3 years. The annual mortality rate for England and Wales is 0.09 per million. The disease is transmissible to animals and, rarely, human to human transmission has been recorded. Pathological features include nerve cell loss, astrocytic proliferation and a spongiform appearance due to dilatation of nerve cell processes.

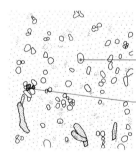

Fig. 9.46 Creutzfeldt-Jakob disease: section showing neuronal loss with astrocytic proliferation and spongiform vacuolation of the parenchyma. Haematoxylin & Van Gieson stain, x 350

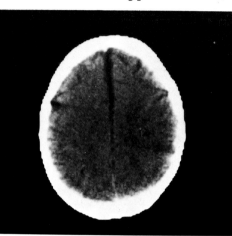

Fig. 9.47 Creutzfeldt-Jakob disease: CT scan showing mild frontal atrophy.

The patient, aged 67, had a month's history of an altered mental state with dysphasia. Examination showed severe dysphasia and disorientation. Myoclonic jerks developed and the patient deteriorated rapidly. Autopsy confirmed the clinical diagnosis.

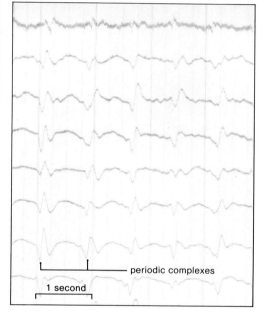

— periodic complexes

1 second

Fig. 9.48 Creutzfeldt-Jakob disease: EEG (position 8) showing periodic complexes at approximately 1.25 Hz.

Same patient as in figure 9.47.

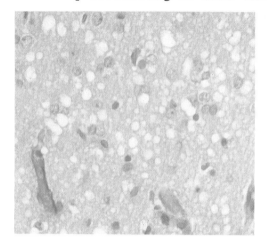

spongiform vacuolation

astrocytic proliferation

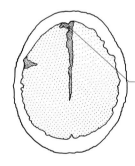

enlarged inter-hemispheric fissure

Fig. 9.49 Herpes simplex encephalitis: coronal brain section showing haemorrhagic necrosis of cortex and white matter of the right temporal and left parietal lobes.

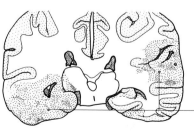

haemorrhagic necrosis

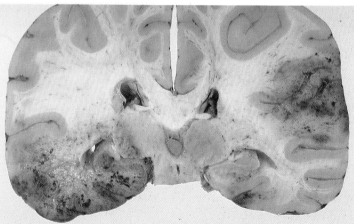

(Fig.9.46). The illness tends to be non-specific in its initial manifestations but is soon followed by signs of progressive dementia, with pyramidal and extra-pyramidal signs. Involvement of the cerebellum or spinal cord may be conspicuous. Later, the patient becomes mute with decorticate posturing, fits or myoclonic jerks. Radiological investigation may be unrewarding, though some degree of cortical atrophy with or without ventricular dilatation is common (Fig.9.47). The EEG may show generalised, synchronous high voltage polyphasic complexes at a frequency of 1 to 2 per second, or spike wave complexes around 70 to 75 per minute. These occur in cases with myoclonus or in the terminal stages of the disease (Fig. 9.48).

Herpes Simplex Encephalitis

This is probably the commonest cause of encephalitis, particularly of the necrotising variety. The condition particularly affects the temporal lobe, though other parts of the cerebrum, and also the brain stem, may be affected. The involvement may be predominantly unilateral with haemorrhage, oedema and necrosis of the affected part (Figs.9.49 & 9.50).

Generally the onset is acute with a rapidly evolving focal neurological deficit, together with evidence, in the majority, of raised intracranial pressure. The CSF frequently contains an excess of red cells, in addition to non-specific

Fig. 9.50 Herpes simplex encephalitis: intranuclear inclusion in nerve cell. H & E stain, x 250.

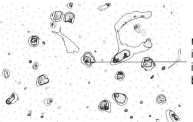

rounded
intranuclear
inclusion
body

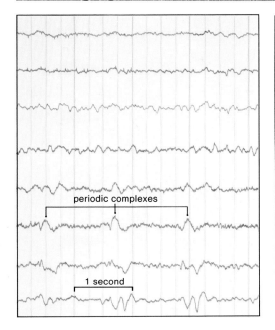

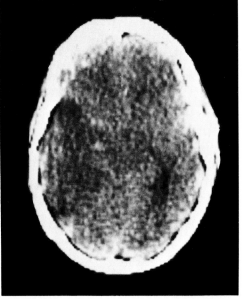

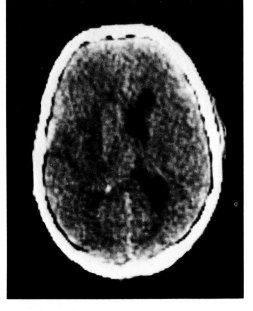

Fig. 9.51 Herpes simplex encephalitis: EEG showing periodic polyphasic complexes every 1½ seconds maximal in the left occipital region.

periodic complexes

1 second

Fig. 9.52 Herpes simplex encephalitis: CT scan at two levels showing a low density area in the left temporoparietal region.

This was a 21 year old man with an initial suspected diagnosis of meningitis who later developed a fixed dilated left pupil and a right hemiparesis. CSF contained 340 cells, 90% lymphocytes, and the diagnosis was confirmed by temporal lobe biopsy.

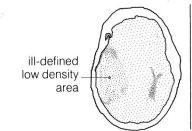
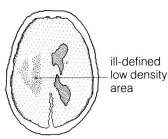

ill-defined
low density
area

ill-defined
low density
area

changes indicative of an acute inflammatory process. The EEG may show characteristic periodic complexes, usually maximal over the frontotemporal lobes (Fig. 9.51), and the technetium scan is frequently positive. The CT scan usually demonstrates a low density area in the fronto-temporal regions with mass effect, haemorrhagic elements, but little or no enhancement (Fig. 9.52). Though these radiological features are suggestive, diagnosis can only be firmly established in the acute stage by brain biopsy. There is some evidence that treatment with anti-viral agents, such as acyclovir, lessens mortality, and reduces the otherwise considerable residual morbidity.

Herpes Zoster Infection

Classically this causes a skin eruption on one side of the trunk in the distribution of a spinal sensory root. In reality, the condition may affect a limb, or some of the cranial nerves.

Ophthalmic zoster is far more common than eruptions in the second or third division of the trigeminal nerve. Corneal involvement may lead to keratitis or ulceration. Occasionally there are associated lesions of the optic or oculomotor nerves (Fig.9.53).

Geniculate zoster is associated with the name of Ramsay Hunt; the ear becomes red and swollen in association with a facial palsy (Fig.9.54). At times, mixed lesions appear,

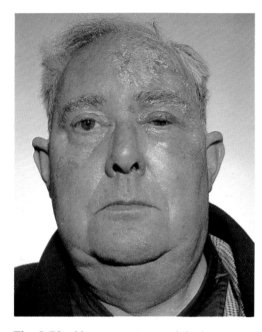

Fig. 9.53 Herpes zoster: rash in the distribution of the ophthalmic division of the left trigeminal nerve.

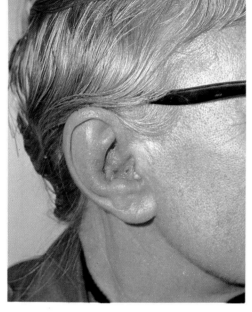

Fig. 9.54 Herpes zoster. Ramsay Hunt syndrome showing vesicles around the

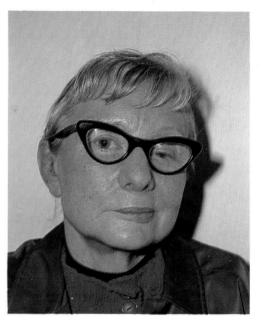

right external auditory meatus (left) in association with a right facial paresis (right).

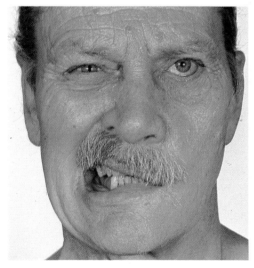

Fig. 9.55 Herpes zoster. Ramsay Hunt syndrome: left facial paresis.

This 58 year old man developed left facial weakness without taste loss or hyperacusis. Examination showed a severe left facial weakness and vesicles over the left hard palate.

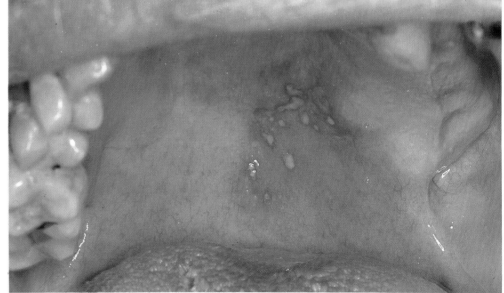

Fig. 9.56 Herpes zoster. Ramsay Hunt syndrome: vesicles on the hard palate.

Same patient as in figure 9.55.

for example, a facial palsy in association with a rash over the palate (Figs.9.55 & 9.56).

Spinal zoster begins with malaise then abnormal sensations such as burning or shooting pains in a dermatomal distribution. After three to four days vesicles appear followed by scabbing, sometimes with subsequent scar formation. Almost all cases are unilateral. Thoracic segments are involved most commonly (perhaps in 70% of cases). In the cervical region, the third and fourth segments are affected far more commonly than other segments whilst lower sacral involvement is uncommon (Fig.9.57).

In association with the spinal syndrome, motor root or spinal cord involvement may occur. With recovery there may be post-herpetic neuralgia. Sometimes parts of the involved dermatome become anaesthetic, occasionally predisposing to trophic ulceration (Fig.9.58).

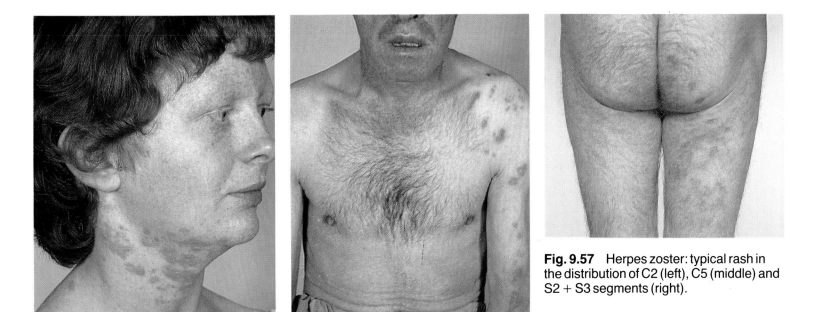

Fig. 9.57 Herpes zoster: typical rash in the distribution of C2 (left), C5 (middle) and S2 + S3 segments (right).

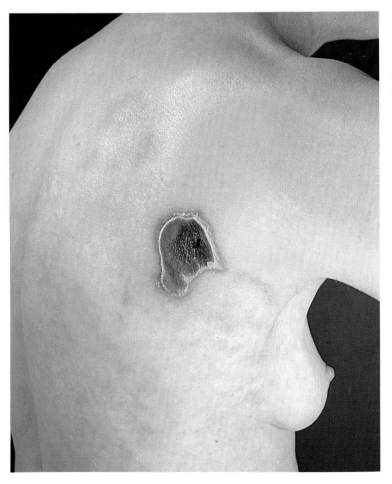

Fig. 9.58 Herpes zoster: trophic ulcer in the distribution of dermatome affected by previous rash.

The patient had had shingles previously. During an episode of lobar pneumonia she applied a hot poultice to an anaesthetic area thereby producing a trophic ulcer.

9.23

Sarcoidosis

This condition can affect the nervous system in a number of ways. Most common is involvement of cranial nerves or the peripheral nervous system. Of the former, seventh nerve paralysis is particularly frequent. With the latter, there may be peripheral motor or sensory involvement, sometimes with segmental sensory change over the trunk. Central nervous system disease is less common and tends to pursue a more progressive course. Signs of meningeal infiltration may appear with CSF abnormalities including a raised protein concentration and a lymphocytic pleocytosis. Ocular lesions are common in sarcoidosis, including uveitis, chorioretinitis and optic nerve abnormalities. Iridoplegia may develop, sometimes progressing to a tonic pupil syndrome (Fig.9.59).

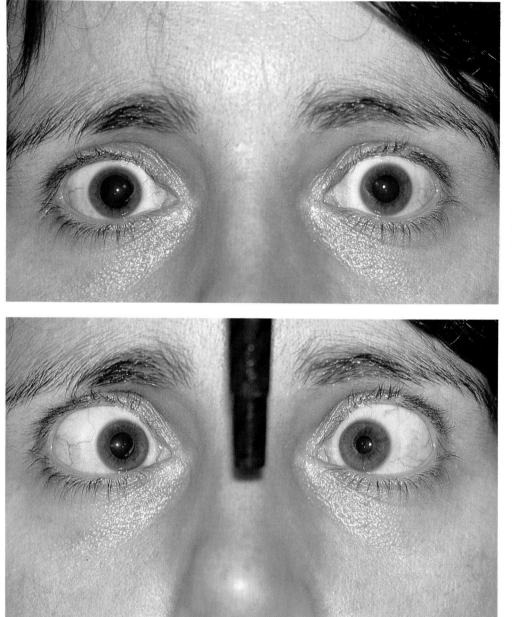

Fig. 9.59 Sarcoidosis: partial right iridoplegia with dilated pupil (upper) and incomplete near response (lower).

This 30 year old woman gave a history of a generalised rash, followed by malaise, muscle pain and blurred vision. She had noticed paraesthesiae in the face and abdomen. Examination showed a right iridoplegia, bilateral facial weakness and sensory loss, depressed limb reflexes and distal sensory loss. CSF contained 14 lymphocytes and a protein of 1.8g/L. Liver and Kveim biopsy were positive. Her condition dramatically responded to steroids though a right tonic pupil developed.

10. Multiple Sclerosis, other Demyelinating Disorders and Cerebellar Disorders

MULTIPLE SCLEROSIS

This is a relatively common condition in the mainland United Kingdom, with a prevalence varying between 40 and 60 per 100,000. Its incidence increases in the Northern Hemisphere with distance from the Equator, being most commonly encountered in Iceland and the Shetlands. A similar gradation probably exists with increasing distance in the Southern Hemisphere from the Equator. It is generally considered to result from an acquired insult to the nervous system, perhaps a slow-virus infection, encountered in the first few years of life, in individuals genetically susceptible to the disease. Studies of histocompatibility antigens have indicated that some determinants, particularly A3, B7 and DW2 are more common in multiple sclerosis (MS) than in a control population.

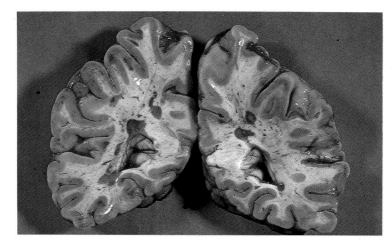
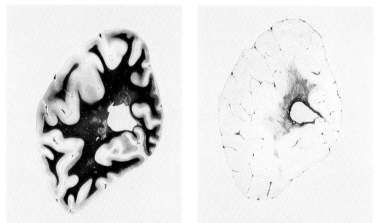

Fig. 10.1 Multiple sclerosis: coronal brain section showing numerous plaques of demyelination particularly in the periventricular area (left) and plaques in relation to the occipital horn of the lateral ventricle, with corresponding gliosis (middle, Heidenhain's myelin stain and right, Holzer preparation).

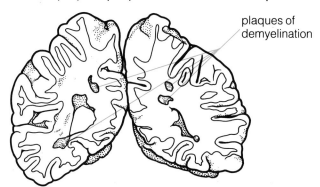

plaques of demyelination

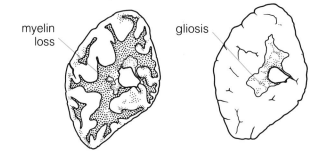

myelin loss

gliosis

Fig. 10.2 Multiple sclerosis: plaques of demyelination involving optic nerves and chiasm. Heidenhain's myelin stain.

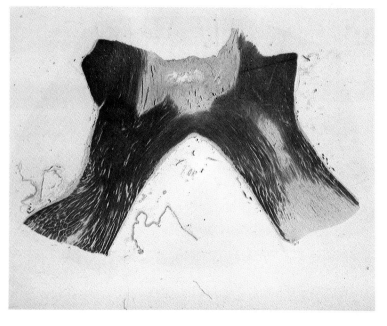

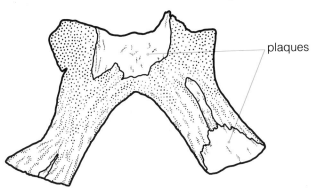

plaques

Pathologically, there is demyelination of white matter of the central nervous system, characteristically in a perivascular distribution. Certain areas, including the optic nerves, periventricular white matter, brain stem and spinal cord are particularly affected (Figs. 10.1-10.4). Later, axonal degeneration may be conspicuous.

The vast majority of cases begin between the ages of 20 and 50, with the maximum incidence in the fourth decade of life. Approximately 60% of patients are women. Signs of optic nerve involvement may be the first manifestation of the disease. An acute optic neuritis leads to vision loss, usually unilateral, in association with pain in many instances, particularly on movement of the affected eye.

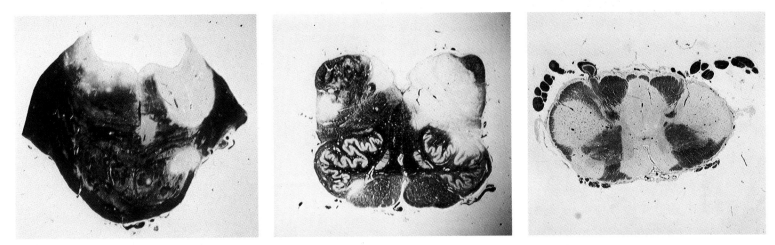

Fig. 10.3. Multiple sclerosis: plaques in the pons and middle cerebellar peduncle (left), multiple confluent plaques in the medulla at the level of the inferior olives (middle) and plaques in the cervical spinal cord (right). Heidenhain's myelin stain.

The patient, aged 60, had a ten year history of difficulty in walking and stiffness of the limbs. Examination showed a bilateral internuclear ophthalmoplegia with limb pyramidal and cerebellar signs. The CSF contained abnormal IgG ratios and oligoclonal bands.

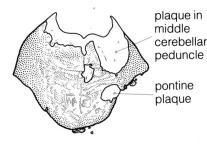

plaque in middle cerebellar peduncle

pontine plaque

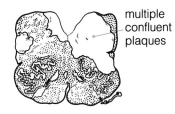

multiple confluent plaques

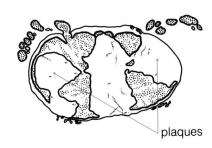

plaques

Fig. 10.4 Multiple sclerosis: myelin stain showing sharp demarcation between plaque and adjacent normal white matter.

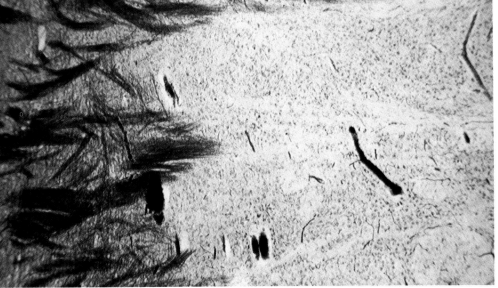

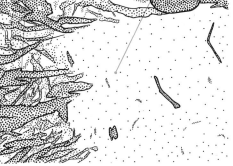

normal white matter

plaque

10.3

The optic nerve disc appearance initially may be normal, or may show an acute swelling indistinguishable from papilloedema (Fig.10.5). In the later stages of the disease, optic atrophy is common, manifesting as either temporal pallor, or a more diffuse atrophy of the optic disc (Fig.10.6). Brain stem involvement is also common, with, perhaps, oculomotor disturbances the most frequent. Lesions of the medial longitudinal bundle produce an internuclear ophthalmoplegia with impaired adduction on lateral gaze and nystagmus in the abducting eye.

Bilateral lesions are usually associated with vertical nystagmus, and, in a young individual, are highly suggestive of multiple sclerosis (Fig.10.7).

Spinal cord involvement is inevitable at some stage of the disease, producing motor, sensory or sphincteric disturbance, or a combination. Cervical cord lesions, particularly of the posterior column, may be associated with a Lhermitte phenomenon, in which neck flexion induces a strange, shock-like feeling to radiate down the spine, sometimes into the limbs.

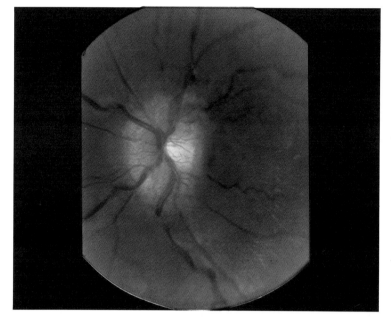

Fig. 10.5 Multiple sclerosis: acute optic neuritis with swelling of the optic nerve.

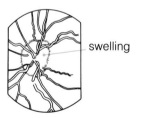

swelling

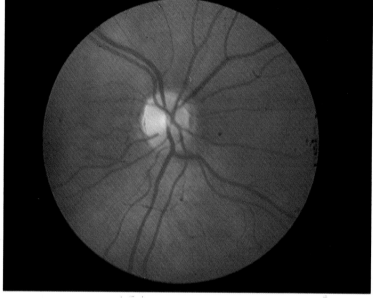

Fig. 10.6 Multiple sclerosis: optic atrophy with pallor of the optic disc, maximal on the temporal aspect.

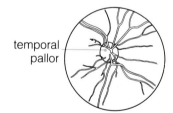

temporal pallor

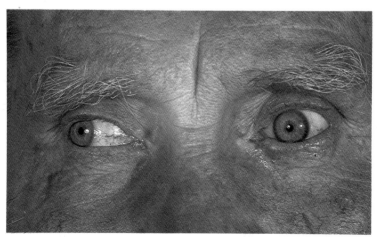

Fig. 10.7 Multiple sclerosis: failure of adduction on gaze to the right (left) and to the left (right).

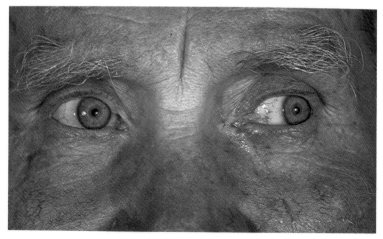

The patient, aged 60, had a ten year history of difficulty in walking and stiffness of the limbs. Examination showed a bilateral internuclear ophthalmoplegia with limb pyramidal and cerebellar signs. The CSF contained abnormal IgG ratios and oligoclonal bands.

10.4

A rarer manifestation of the disease, possibly secondary to cervical cord pathology, is the phenomenon of tonic seizures. Here, frequent, short-lived, unilateral muscle spasms occur, producing flexion at the elbow, wrist and fingers, with extension of the leg and inversion of the foot (Fig. 10.8).

Many patients with established multiple sclerosis, and some in the early stages, describe paroxysmal exacerbation or precipitation of symptoms by certain exogenous factors, including a hot bath, emotional stimuli, exercise and eating (Fig. 10.9). The phenomenon is probably the consequence of temporary conduction block in partially demyelinated nerve fibres.

Wasting is uncommon in multiple sclerosis. It most commonly reflects the effect of plaques impinging on anterior horn cells or roots but, when extensive, is almost certainly due to a central lesion with trans-synaptic degeneration (Fig. 10.10). Involvement of the retrochiasmal

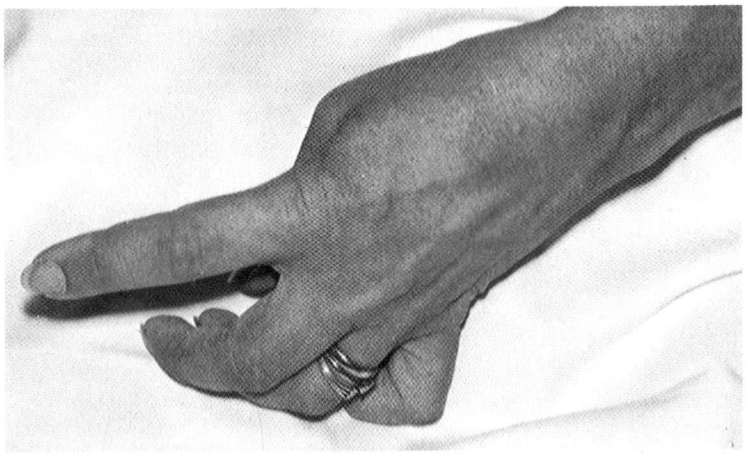

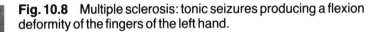

Fig. 10.8 Multiple sclerosis: tonic seizures producing a flexion deformity of the fingers of the left hand.

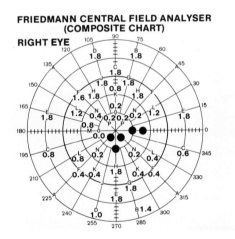

Fig. 10.9 Multiple sclerosis: Friedmann visual fields before (left) and after (right) a hot bath, during which visual acuity fell from 6/18 to less than 6/60. Filled circles indicate sites of absent response. The higher the figure the more normal the retinal response.

This man had an attack of left optic neuritis at the age of 24, followed by left-sided sensory and motor symptoms. An attack of right optic neuritis occurred two years later. Within a few years, he noticed that his vision would blur with exertion, emotional stress, hot baths, and eating. At the same time his lower limb weakness increased.

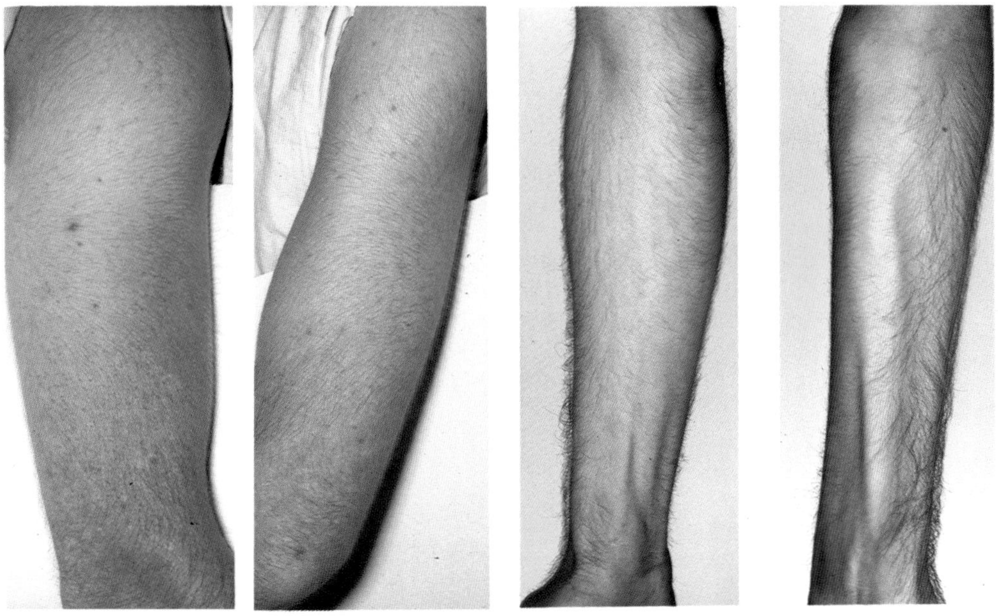

Fig. 10.10 Multiple sclerosis: conspicuous wasting of the left upper arm and forearm with the right arm as control.

In 1977, at the age of 27, this man developed diplopia with left-sided sensory symptoms. He rapidly recovered. In 1978, he developed ataxia with dysarthria, again recovering, and in 1982, severe left-sided weakness. By then, he was emotionally labile, with limited insight, and had prominent bilateral pyramidal and cerebellar signs.

visual pathway is also uncommon, with a homonymous defect being found, rather than a central scotoma due to optic nerve disease (Figs.10.11 & 10.12).

Investigation

CSF examination is of considerable value. An increased cell count, though rarely exceeding 50 cells/mm³, is frequent, particularly at the time of an acute exacerbation. A raised protein concentration has been reported in up to 75% of patients, seldom above 1 g/L. A raised IgG concentration, compared to protein or albumin, occurs in up to 80% of patients. Electrophoresis reveals oligoclonal bands in the γ_4 band in as many as 90% of definite cases (Fig.10.13).

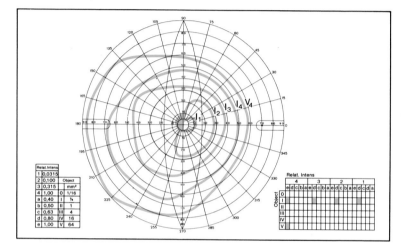

Fig. 10.11 Multiple sclerosis: visual fields showing a small paracentral homonymous hemianopia.

This woman presented at the age of 30, with attacks of vertigo. A year later, she developed altered feeling in the hands and feet,

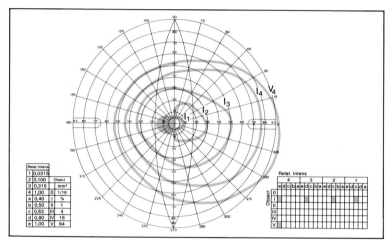

followed, after five months, by an area of vision loss to the left of fixation. For two years, she had had a positive Lhermitte phenomenon. Visual fields showed a paracentral homonymous hemianopia. The CSF:IgG ratios were abnormal.

Fig. 10.12 Multiple sclerosis: visual evoked responses showing delayed potential with left half field stimulation compared to normal potential from right half field stimulation.
Same patient as in figure 10.11.

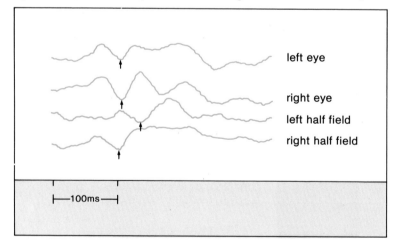

Fig. 10.13 Multiple sclerosis: CSF electrophoretic strip showing oligoclonal bands (arrows).

This 20-year-old woman had had an episode of left optic neutritis the previous year. She presented with diplopia, vertigo and lower limb paraesthesiae. Examination showed a left gaze paresis and a left internuclear ophthalmoplegia, together with bilateral limb pyramidal signs. Recovery was incomplete.

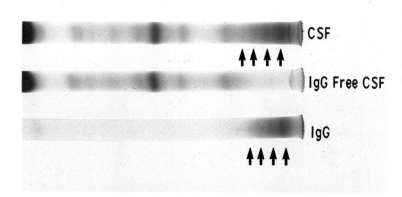

Electrophysiological investigation is helpful in identifying sites of demyelination which have not been clinically evident. Visual evoked responses (VER) are abnormal in up to 90% of definite MS cases. Most characteristic is a marked delay of the potentials with a relatively preserved wave form (Fig. 10.14). Auditory evoked responses are capable of detecting silent brain stem lesions (Fig. 10.15).

whilst somatosensory evoked responses can identify spinal cord disturbances.

Neuroradiological investigation is seldom indicated in MS, other than to exclude other diagnostic possibilities.

CT scanning may detect ventricular dilatation and sometimes reveals periventricular zones of attenuation particularly in longer standing cases (Fig. 10.16). During

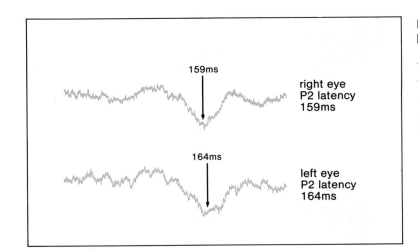

Fig. 10.14 Multiple sclerosis: visual evoked responses showing bilateral delay.

This patient presented in 1981 with blurring of vision, confined to the left eye, followed by paraesthesiae in the left face and foot. Subsequently, she had episodes of right, then left, optic neuritis, and an attack of diplopia during which an internuclear ophthalmoplegia was detected. At the time of the recording, she had mild bilateral optic atrophy.

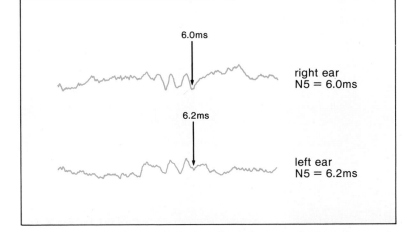

Fig. 10.15 Multiple sclerosis: auditory evoked responses showed a delayed, rather poorly defined N5 (arrow) from the left ear, with a marginally delayed N5 from the right ear.

Same patient as in figure 10.14.

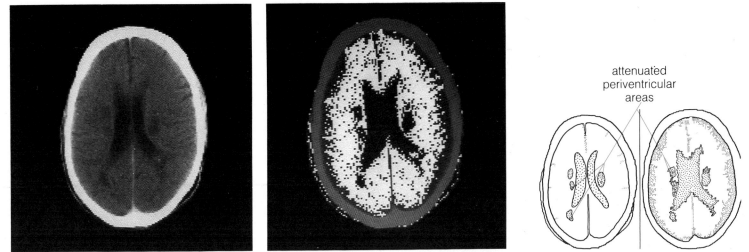

Fig. 10.16 Multiple sclerosis: CT scan showing periventricular low-density areas (left). A negative image of the scan identifies the areas more clearly (right).

Same patient as in figure 10.10.

exacerbations, enhancing lesions can be detected, often later resolving into areas of low attenuation (Fig. 10.17). Magnetic resonance imaging enables areas of demyelination to be detected more accurately than is achieved by CT scanning.

Corticosteroids may shorten the duration of acute relapses, but neither they, nor immunosuppressants appear to conspicuously influence the long term course of the disease. Manipulation of the diet, with reduction in animal fats, and supplements of unsaturated fatty acids, may marginally influence the number and severity of exacerbations.

OTHER DEMYELINATING DISORDERS

There are a number of diseases of the central nervous system in which abnormal myelin formation occurs, rather than destruction of normal myelin. The former conditions are classified as leucodystrophies and usually present in childhood. The leucodystrophies are characterised by diffuse degeneration of white matter in the centrum ovale and cerebellum, with prominent axonal

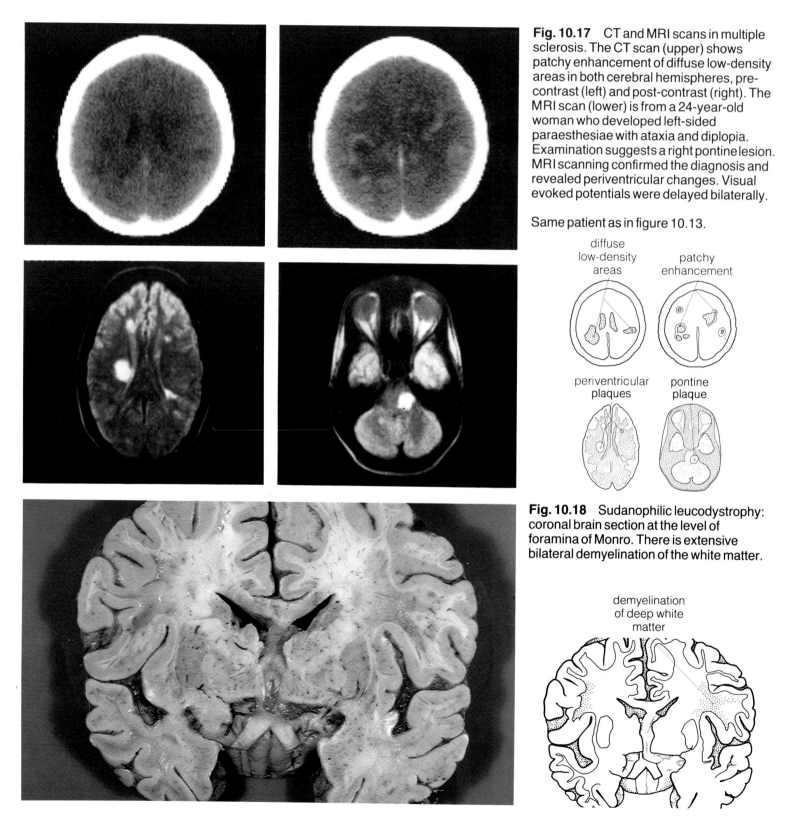

Fig. 10.17 CT and MRI scans in multiple sclerosis. The CT scan (upper) shows patchy enhancement of diffuse low-density areas in both cerebral hemispheres, pre-contrast (left) and post-contrast (right). The MRI scan (lower) is from a 24-year-old woman who developed left-sided paraesthesiae with ataxia and diplopia. Examination suggests a right pontine lesion. MRI scanning confirmed the diagnosis and revealed periventricular changes. Visual evoked potentials were delayed bilaterally.

Same patient as in figure 10.13.

diffuse low-density areas

patchy enhancement

periventricular plaques

pontine plaque

Fig. 10.18 Sudanophilic leucodystrophy: coronal brain section at the level of foramina of Monro. There is extensive bilateral demyelination of the white matter.

demyelination of deep white matter

loss and degeneration of the cerebral peduncles and pyramidal tracts (Fig.10.18). The central white matter lesions are poorly defined. Sudanophilic leucodystrophy has some similarities with diffuse cerebral sclerosis (Schilder's disease). The infantile form (Pelizaeus-Merzbacher disease) presents in infants within the first few months of life, and is inherited as a sex-linked recessive. Pathologically there are areas of diffuse demyelination with scattered foci of preserved myelin sheaths (Fig.10.19).

Alexander's disease produces mental retardation and intractable epilepsy. Hydrocephalus is common. Pathological changes include a leucodystrophy and homogeneous rod-shaped bodies arranged in a radial fashion around the walls of blood vessels and lining the pial surfaces of the brain (Figs.10.20 & 10.21).

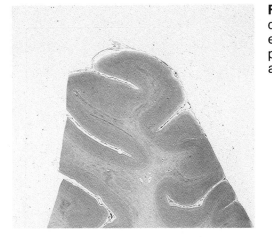

Fig.10.19 Pelizaeus-Merzbacher disease: section of occipital lobe showing extensive loss of myelin with some perivascular sparing, producing a tigroid appearance.

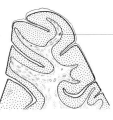

tigroid appearance of white matter

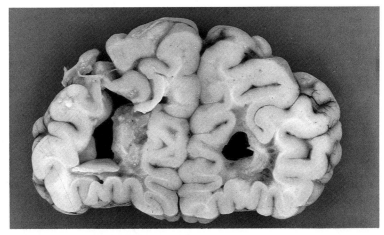

Fig.10.20 Alexander's disease: coronal section through the frontal lobes showing demyelination with cystic degeneration of deep white matter.

frontal horn

demyelination with cystic degeneration

Fig.10.21 Alexander's disease: spinal cord preparation showing hyaline bodies lining the pial surface and surrounding a penetrating blood vessel. Haematoxylin Van Gieson, ×400.

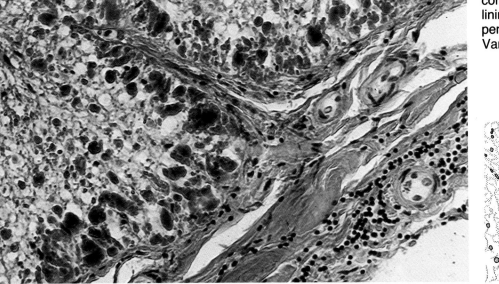

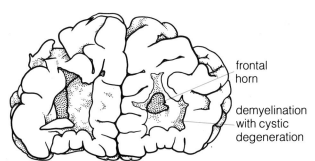

hyaline bodies

Krabbe's disease (globoid cell leucodystrophy) presents around the age of 5 months and affected infants seldom survive beyond the age of one year. Severe demyelination of white matter is seen in the cerebrum, cerebellum and spinal cord (Fig. 10.22). Vessels in the cerebral white matter are surrounded by large multinucleate cells (globoid cells) and mononuclear cells (Fig. 10.23).

In Metachromatic leucodystrophy, diffuse demyelination of the white matter of the cerebral hemispheres is associated with accumulation of metachromatic material at various sites in the central and peripheral nervous system, and in other organs (Figs. 10.24 & 10.25).

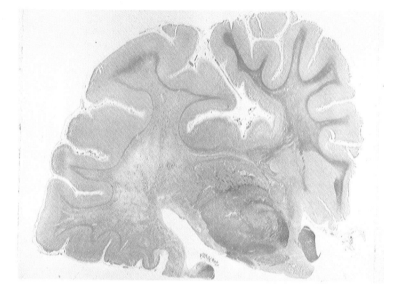

Fig. 10.22 Krabbe's disease: a section of one hemisphere through the level of the mammilary bodies stained for myelin. There is pallor of myelin staining in the white matter with preservation of the subcortical fibres. Klüver-Barrera stain.

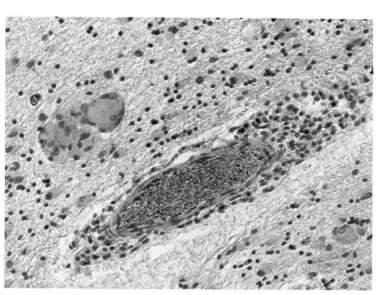

Fig. 10.23 Krabbe's disease: section showing globoid cells and perivascular cuffing with mononuclear cells. Haematoxylin van Gieson, × 330.

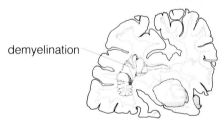

demyelination

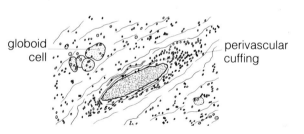

globoid cell

perivascular cuffing

Fig. 10.24 Metachromatic leucodystrophy. Coronal brain section showing yellowish discoloration of white matter (left). Cerebral cortex and white matter showing myelin loss in deep white matter with metachromatic material in the subcortical region (right, toluidine blue, × 35).

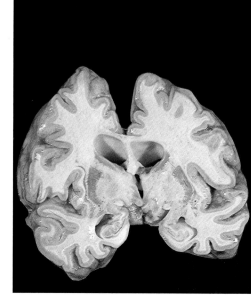

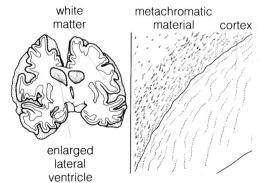

white matter

metachromatic material cortex

enlarged lateral ventricle

CONDITIONS AFFECTING CEREBELLAR FUNCTION

Cerebellar disorders result in impairment of voluntary muscle control, producing dysarthria, limb and gait ataxia and abnormalities of eye movement. The primary pathological process may be in the cerebellum itself, or the fibre pathways leading to and from it.

Olivopontocerebellar Degeneration

This condition tends to present in late middle life. Genetic factors are unusual. The condition produces a progressive cerebellar syndrome, principally affecting gait initially, followed by limb weakness, dementia, impaired sphincter control and bulbar manifestations. Histological changes include atrophy of the cerebellar cortex, olives and grey and white matter of the pons, with particular involvement of the middle cerebellar peduncle (Fig. 10.26).

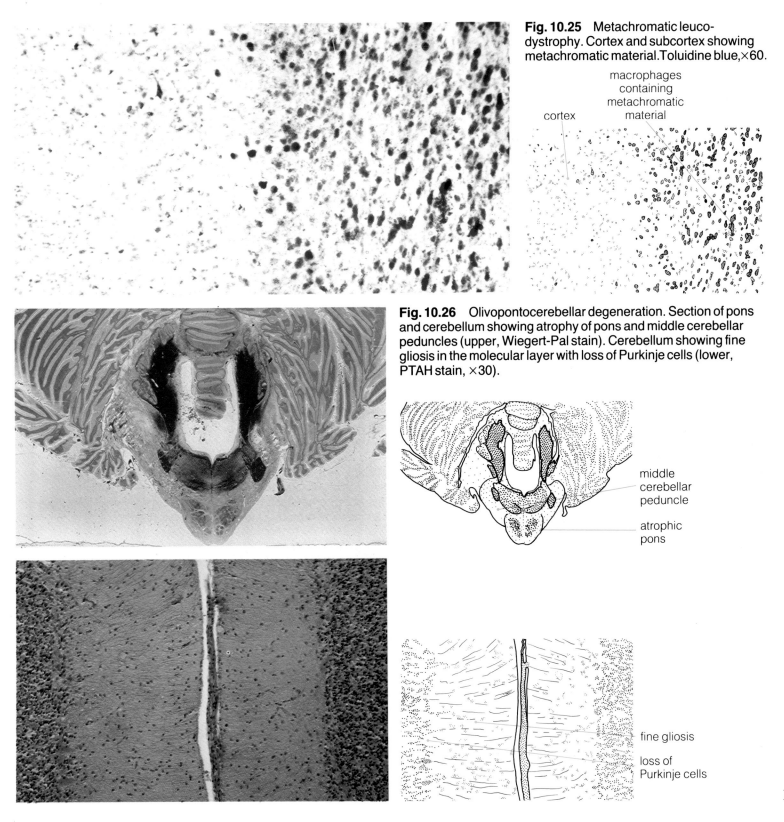

Fig. 10.25 Metachromatic leucodystrophy. Cortex and subcortex showing metachromatic material. Toluidine blue, ×60.

cortex

macrophages containing metachromatic material

Fig. 10.26 Olivopontocerebellar degeneration. Section of pons and cerebellum showing atrophy of pons and middle cerebellar peduncles (upper, Wiegert-Pal stain). Cerebellum showing fine gliosis in the molecular layer with loss of Purkinje cells (lower, PTAH stain, ×30).

middle cerebellar peduncle

atrophic pons

fine gliosis

loss of Purkinje cells

10.11

Cerebellar Degeneration

An hereditary form of cortical cerebellar degeneration occurs, with onset in some cases in children, in others in adult life. Latter cases tend to arise in the fifth decade. The course is progressive. Inheritance may be autosomal dominant, recessive or sex-linked (Figs.10.27 & 10.28).

Cortical cerebellar degeneration may occur in association with carcinoma. Gait ataxia is usually the first sign, followed by limb clumsiness and dysarthria. Some patients may display other non-metastatic neurological disorders, such as the Eaton-Lambert syndrome, peripheral neuropathy or limbic encephalitis. Pathological changes include widespread loss of Purkinje cells with lesser involvement of the neurons of the granular layer.

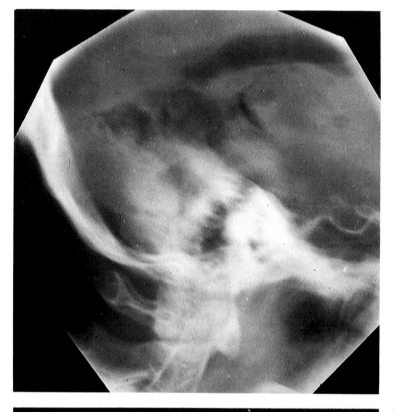

Fig. 10.27 Cortical cerebellar degeneration: air encephalogram showing expanded spaces over and between the superior cerebellar folia.

This man, aged 55, had developed gait ataxia at the age of 47. Later he was dysarthric. His father and two paternal uncles had had a similar history. Three of his siblings were affected. Examination showed dysarthria, nystagmus, bilateral cerebellar signs and severe gait ataxia.

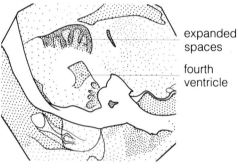

Fig. 10.28 Cerebellar degeneration: CT scan showing enlarged fourth ventricle.

This 48-year-old woman gave a three year history of progressive dysarthria and gait ataxia. Abnormalities were confined to disturbed cerebellar function with gait ataxia. Evoked response studies were normal. There was no family history.

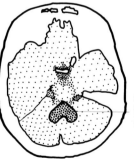

Degeneration of long tracts of the spinal cord may coexist (Fig. 10.29). Carcinoma of the bronchus and ovary are the commonest associated tumours.

Cerebellar degeneration arises in some alcoholics, frequently in association with a neuropathy. Gait disorder is followed by dysarthria and limb incoordination. Typically the lower limbs are much more severely affected. Nystagmus is often not conspicuous. Once developed, the condition rarely regresses, even with abstinence. Pathological changes include degeneration of the cerebellar cortex, particularly the superior vermis (Fig. 10.30) with lesser involvement of the hemispheres.

Ataxia may be a manifestation of myxoedema. Limb ataxia is often less prominent and nystagmus infrequent. Some cases have other neurological complications, such as carpal tunnel syndrome, deafness or myopathy (Fig. 10.31).

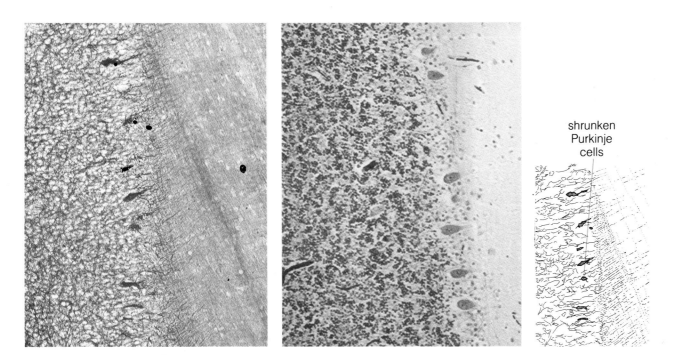

Fig. 10.29 Cortical cerebellar degeneration: no normal Purkinje cells remain (left, Bielschowsky stain). A normal control is shown (right, luxol fast blue with cresyl violet counterstain, × 70).

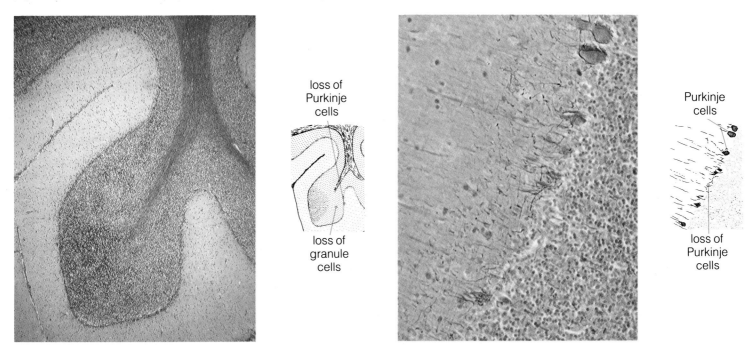

Fig. 10.30 Alcoholic cerebellar degeneration: reduction of granule and Purkinje cells with replacement gliosis. Haematoxylin-eosin and luxol fast blue, ×40.

Fig. 10.31 Myxoedema: section showing focal loss of Purkinje cells. Bielschowsky stain, ×230.

Ataxia-Telangiectasia

This condition is inherited as an autosomal recessive. The child is noted to be ataxic on commencing to walk with subsequent limb ataxia, dysarthria and involuntary movements. In addition, intellectual impairment is found, together with evidence of a peripheral neuropathy. The cutaneous telangiectasia develop from the age of 3 onwards, and are found on the conjunctivae, neck, nose and around the elbows (Fig.10.32). There is immunodeficiency, in association with depressed IgA levels, leading to recurrent respiratory tract infection and early death. There is an increased incidence of lymphoma.

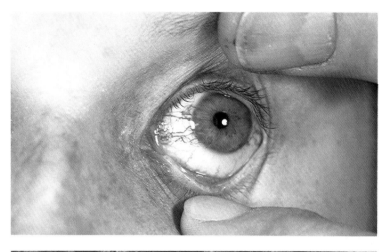

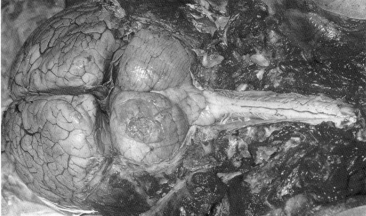

Fig. 10.32 Ataxia telangiectasia.

This 20-year-old patient had a long history of ataxia, with more recent dysphagia and dysarthria. Examination showed telangiectasia on the sclera, neck and elbows. There was nystagmus, dysarthria, titubation and severe cerebellar incoordination. Reflexes were absent with bilateral extensor plantar responses.

Fig. 10.33 Arnold-Chiari malformation: caudal displacement of the upper cervical cord has resulted in an abnormal course of the upper cervical roots.

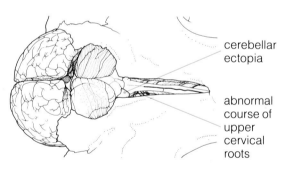

cerebellar ectopia

abnormal course of upper cervical roots

Fig. 10.34 Arnold-Chiari malformation: sagittal slice of the brain and vertebral column showing tonsillar herniation and folding of the upper cervical cord (left) and an associated myelomeningocoele (right).

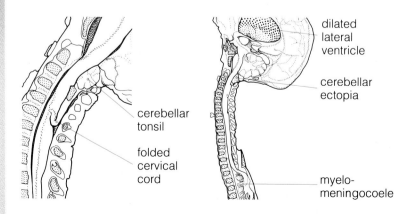

cerebellar tonsil

folded cervical cord

dilated lateral ventricle

cerebellar ectopia

myelo-meningocoele

Arnold-Chiari Malformation

This is subdivided into Type I (Fig. 10.33), in which there is herniation of the cerebellar tonsils through the foramen magnum, and Type II, where both medulla and fourth ventricle share in the displacement. There is sometimes an associated hydrocephalus. The condition is frequently associated with cystic cavitation of the spinal cord.

Type II anomalies tend to present in childhood with progressive hydrocephalus (Fig. 10.34). The Type I anomaly frequently presents in adult life, with either syringomyelia, or the features of an ataxic syndrome often with lower cranial nerve disturbances. Abnormalities of the neck may be found, either clinically or on radiological investigation (Fig. 10.35).

Myelography confirms cerebellar ectopia, and either this, or vertebral angiography, will demonstrate displacement of the posterior inferior cerebellar arteries (Figs. 10.36 & 10.37).

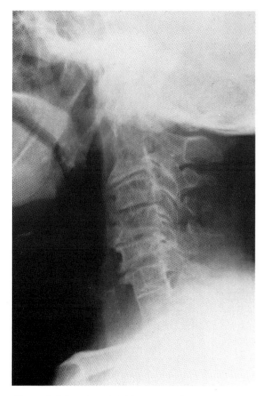

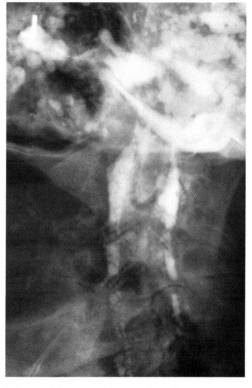

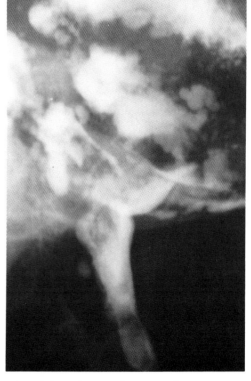

Fig. 10.35 Arnold-Chiari malformation: cervical spine radiograph showing partial fusion of the second and third cervical vertebrae.

This 72-year-old man had had a cold sensation in the left leg for two years with heaviness. Examination showed jerk nystagmus with a downbeat element on lateral gaze, possible tongue fasciculation and bilateral limb weakness and ataxia. Joint position sense was depressed in the right hand and both legs, with an ataxic gait.

Fig. 10.36 Arnold-Chiari malformation: myelogram showing a displaced loop of the posterior inferior cerebellar artery due to cerebellar ectopia. Foramen magnum decompression was performed when the the cerebellar tonsils were found extending to the upper border of C2.

Same patient as in figure 10.35.

Fig. 10.37 Arnold-Chiari malformation: myelogram showing cerebellar ectopia.

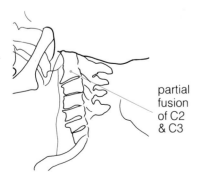

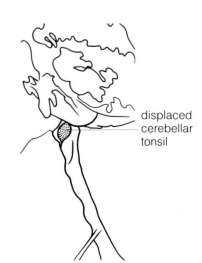

10.15

CT scanning of the foramen magnum, with metrizamide in the subarachnoid space, can also demonstrate the abnormality (Fig. 10.38).

Surgical decompression of the foramen magnum may prevent progression of the condition, though results are often disappointing.

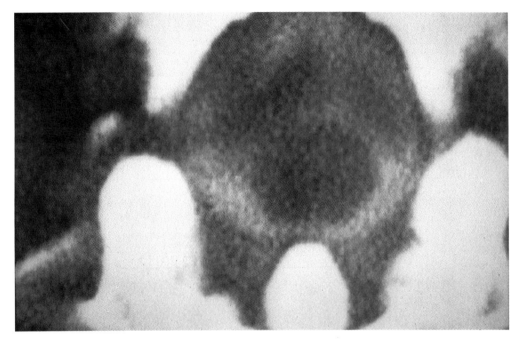

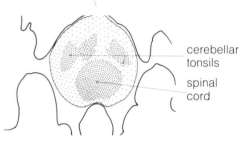

Fig. 10.38 Arnold-Chiari malformation: CT scan with metrizamide in the subarachnoid space demonstrating ectopic cerebellar tonsils.

cerebellar tonsils

spinal cord

11. Spinal Cord and Nerve Root Disorders

Cervical Spondylosis

Dorsomedial protrusion of an intervertebral disc produces spinal cord or cauda equina compression, according to the level at which it occurs, whilst dorsolateral protrusion may compress the adjacent nerve root against the lateral part of the vertebral lamina. The protrusion may consist of the annulus fibrosus itself, or herniations of the central nucleus pulposus through a defect in the annulus. In the cervical region, the C5/6 and C6/7 discs are most commonly affected where most movement in the cervical spine takes place. There are often multiple protrusions.

Oblique views of the cervical spine are particularly important for the demonstration of protrusion into the intervertebral foramen by zygapophyseal or neurocentral osteophytes (Fig.11.1). Myelography demonstrates the extent of bony or soft tissue encroachment upon the subarachnoid space, and is likely to reveal more than the changes demonstrated by plain radiographs (Fig.11.2).

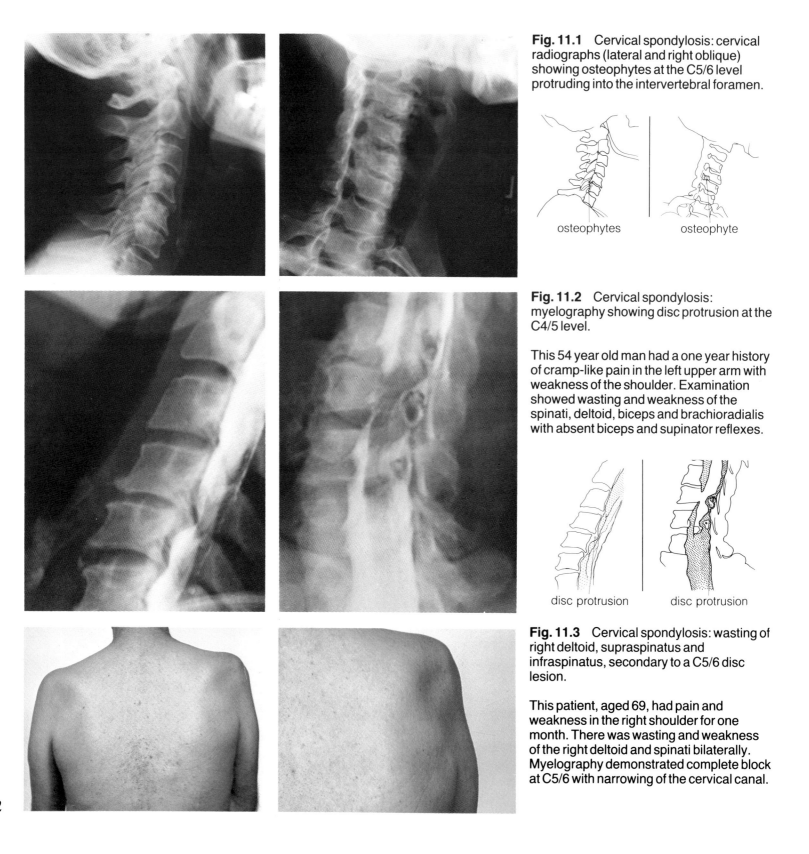

Fig. 11.1 Cervical spondylosis: cervical radiographs (lateral and right oblique) showing osteophytes at the C5/6 level protruding into the intervertebral foramen.

osteophytes   osteophyte

Fig. 11.2 Cervical spondylosis: myelography showing disc protrusion at the C4/5 level.

This 54 year old man had a one year history of cramp-like pain in the left upper arm with weakness of the shoulder. Examination showed wasting and weakness of the spinati, deltoid, biceps and brachioradialis with absent biceps and supinator reflexes.

disc protrusion   disc protrusion

Fig. 11.3 Cervical spondylosis: wasting of right deltoid, supraspinatus and infraspinatus, secondary to a C5/6 disc lesion.

This patient, aged 69, had pain and weakness in the right shoulder for one month. There was wasting and weakness of the right deltoid and spinati bilaterally. Myelography demonstrated complete block at C5/6 with narrowing of the cervical canal.

Most commonly, nerve root compression produces pain, sometimes with depression or absence of the appropriate reflexes. Severe muscle wasting and weakness is a less common clinical feature, implying nerve root involvement or effects on the anterior horn cells in the adjacent spinal cord (Fig. 11.3).

Cervical myelopathy results from compression or ischaemia of the spinal cord secondary to disc protrusion. The compressive effect is closely related to the diameter of the spinal canal, a sagittal diameter of 13 mm being considered critical. Myelography in such cases reveals partial or complete obstruction to the flow of contrast with widening of the spinal cord (Fig.11.4).

Thoracic disc protrusion is relatively rare and usually involves the lower thoracic spine. It presents with signs of cord compression, with spastic paraparesis, sensory disturbances and changes in sphincter function (Fig.11.5).

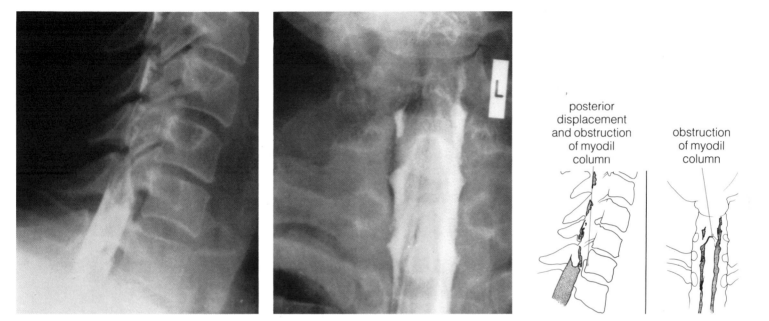

Fig. 11.4 Cervical spondylosis: myelogram, showing protrusion of the C5/6 disc with cord compression.

This 43 year old man gave a two month history of numbness of the left hand and leg, together with the right middle, ring and little fingers. His walking had deteriorated. Examination showed a spastic paraparesis, slight weakness of the hands and impaired proprioception in the left hand and foot.

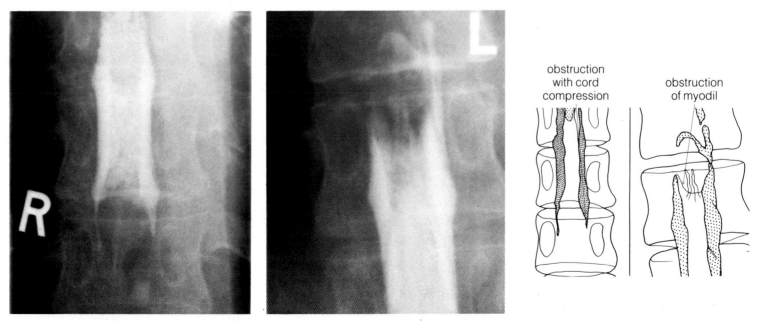

Fig. 11.5 Thoracic disc disease: myelogram showing protrusion of the D8/9 disc with cord compression.

This 42 year old man had developed numbness of the right, then left, leg fifteen months previously. His walking had deteriorated and he complained of urgency of micturition. Examination showed a spastic paraparesis and spinothalamic loss in the right leg extending to D10.

Kyphoscoliosis may occasionally result in spinal cord disorders (Figs. 11.6 & 11.7), but in most patients with spinal deformities, for example, ankylosing spondylitis, the spinal cord remains unaffected.

Lumbar Spondylosis

The most common site for protrusion of a disc in the lumbar region is at the L5/S1 level, the incidence falling as the lumbar spine is ascended. As in the cervical region, the protruded material may be annulus fibrosus or nucleus pulposus. In some instances, previous back injury predisposes to the development of the condition, but in many patients it appears to arise de novo.

Typically an acute disc prolapse produces back and limb pain with sensory, motor or mixed symptoms in the appropriate leg. The pains tend to be exacerbated by

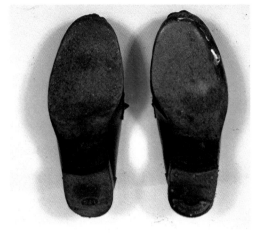

Fig. 11.6 Thoracic kyphosis: differential shoe wear.

This 60 year old man had difficulty with walking for several years with excessive wear of his left shoe. Examination showed a marked thoracic kyphosis, with a spastic paraparesis together with slight loss of muscle bulk in the left leg. Myelography showed obstruction in the upper dorsal region at the level of the kyphus.

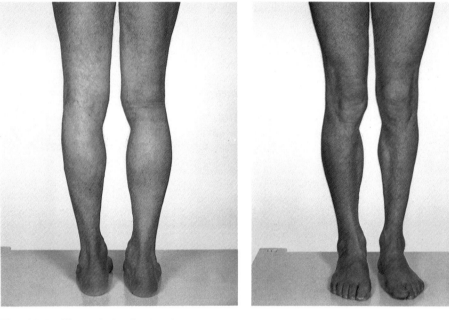

Fig. 11.7 Thoracic kyphosis: slight wasting of the left leg.

Same patient as in figure 11.6.

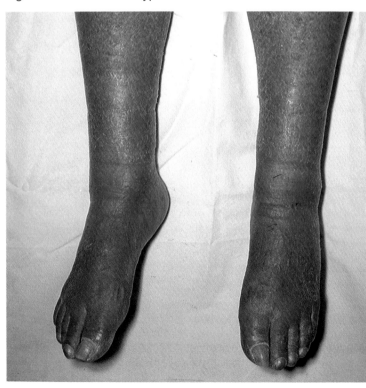

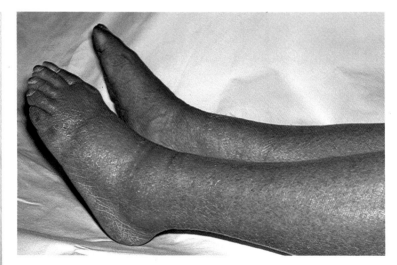

Fig. 11.8 Lumbar spondylosis: bilateral foot drop.

This 65 year old woman developed altered feeling spreading from the feet to the knees over several weeks, with difficulty in elevating the feet. There was a history of recurrent back pain. Examination showed bilateral weakness of inversion and dorsiflexion of feet and toes. The ankle jerks were absent and pin prick was depressed over the feet and shins. Myelography showed narrowing at L4/5 & L5/S1.

movement or by manoeuvres which elevate intrathecal pressure. With central disc protrusion, substantial bilateral lower limb weakness is usual, associated with disturbance of sphincter function, and urgent surgical intervention becomes necessary (Figs.11.8 & 11.9). Lateral disc protrusions compress the adjacent nerve root. Thus, with S1 root involvement, the pain is referred to the buttock, posterior thigh and calf, with altered feeling over the lateral margin of the foot and reduction or absence of the ankle jerk (Fig.11.10). Muscle weakness, though often slight, affects the glutei, hamstrings and calf muscles (Fig.11.11). Involvement of the L5 root may produce less florid signs, with motor weakness often confined to extensor hallucis longus.

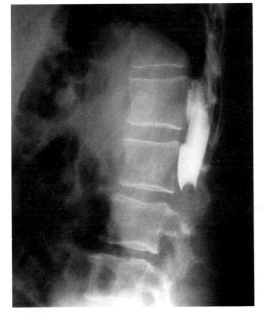

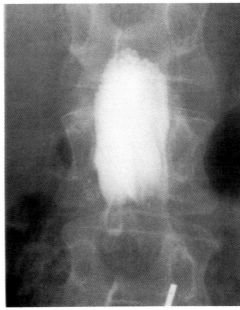

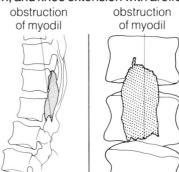

Fig. 11.9 Lumbar spondylosis: myelography showing a central disc protrusion at L2/3.

This 61 year old man presented with a week's history of back pain followed by marked lower limb weakness. Examination confirmed the weakness, maximal in hip flexion, and knee extension with areflexia.

Fig. 11.10 Lumbar spondylosis: myelography showing an L5/S1 disc protrusion on the left.

This 36 year old man had recurrent pains to the left of the lumbar spine radiating to the left leg. Examination showed slight depression of the left ankle jerk.

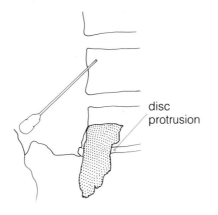

disc protrusion

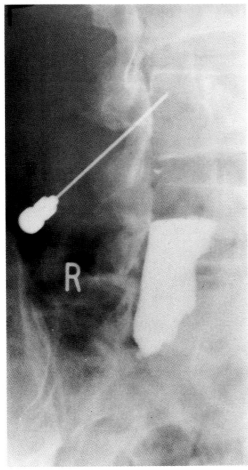

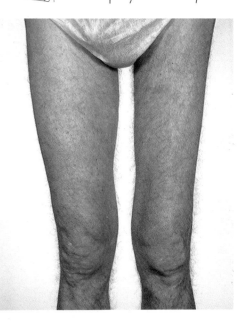

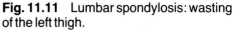

Fig. 11.11 Lumbar spondylosis: wasting of the left thigh.

This patient, aged 71, had back pain for 1 year radiating to both hips, together with weakness and numbness of the left leg. Examination showed wasting of the left thigh, weakness of left hip flexion and knee extension, an absent left knee jerk and reduced pin prick over the anterolateral thigh.

11.5

Degenerative changes in the lumbar spine in association with a congenitally small canal may lead to the clinical syndrome of intermittent claudication of the cauda equina. Symptoms are precipitated by certain postures or with exercise. Typically, numbness or paraesthesiae rather than pain radiate from foot to buttock or vice versa, with relief from rest or change in posture. Myelography demonstrates a narrow canal with osteophyte formation or superimposed disc protrusion (Fig. 11.12). Both mechanical and vascular factors have been incriminated in the causation of the symptoms and, rarely, a similar clinical picture occurs in association with severe stenosis of the terminal aorta (Fig. 11.13).

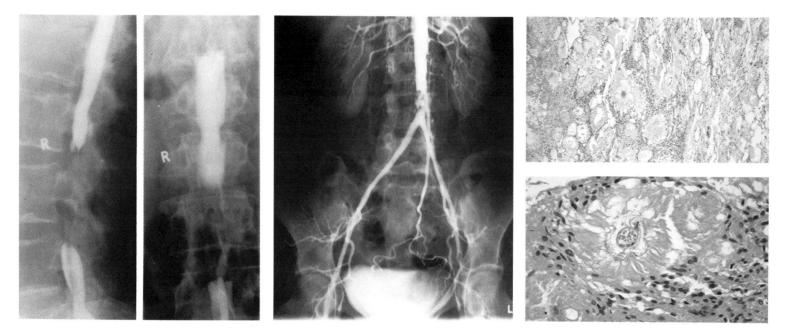

Fig. 11.12 Intermittent claudication of the cauda equina: lumbar myelography showing severe stenosis at L2/3 with lesser narrowing at L3/4 and L4/5.

This 68 year old woman had leg pain for 3 years, precipitated by walking. In addition, she experienced paraesthesiae in the buttocks when sitting after exercise. The left ankle jerk was absent.

Fig. 11.13 Intermittent claudication of the cauda equina: angiography showing narrowing of the terminal abdominal aorta.

This 30 year old woman, for 2 years, had noticed paraesthesiae spreading from the buttocks to the feet during exercise, followed by numbness and heaviness. There were no neurological signs, but a loud abdominal bruit with barely palpable femoral pulses. Bypass of her abdominal aortic stenosis relieved the symptoms.

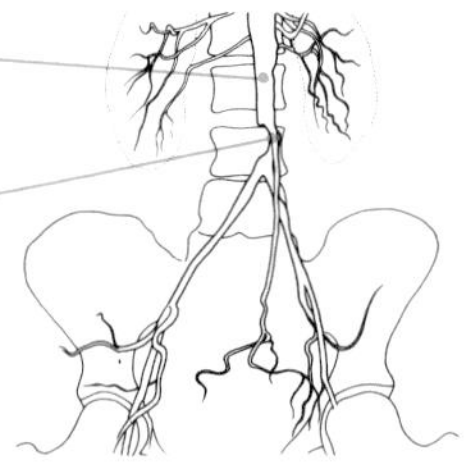

Fig. 11.14 Spinal cord myxopapillary ependymoma: ×30 (upper) and ×200 (lower).

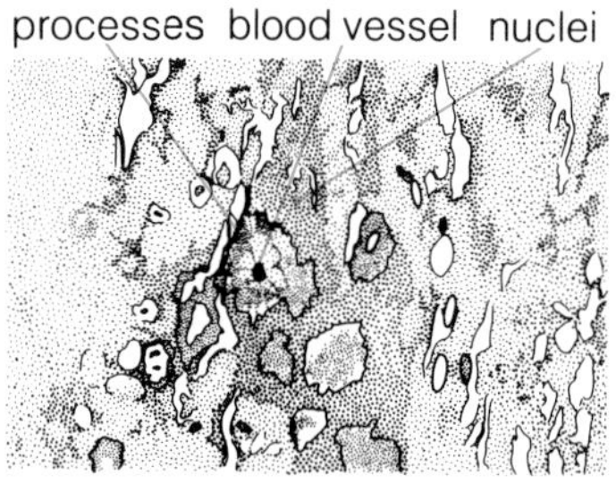

obstruction at L2/3

narrowing at L4/5

tapered lower abdominal aorta

stenosis above aortic bifurcation

tumour cell processes   central blood vessel   tumour nuclei

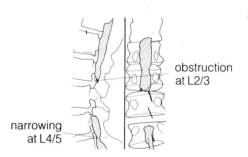

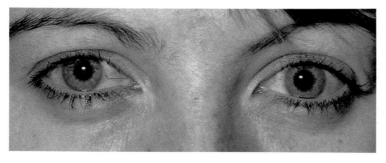

Fig. 11.15 Spinal cord tumour: right Horner's syndrome.

This 28 year old woman gave a history of altered feeling in the left thigh and clumsiness of the right leg. Examination showed a right Horner's syndrome and mild right-sided pyramidal signs in the arm and leg. Myelography showed localised expansion of the cord at C6.

Tumours of the Spinal Cord and Cauda Equina

Tumours affecting the spinal cord may arise from within its substance (intramedullary) or may compress it externally (extramedullary and either intradural or extradural).

Intramedullary tumours are less common than those in the other two sites, and are usually ependymomas or astrocytomas (Fig.11.14). Clinical presentation reflects involvement of sensory, motor and sphincter pathways (Fig.11.15) whilst extramedullary tumours may, in addition, produce signs of nerve root involvement.

For intramedullary tumours, diagnosis is established by myelography, revealing expansion of the spinal cord at the appropriate levels (Figs. 11.16 & 11.17). CT scanning, with or without contrast medium, may indicate the nature of the tumour, at least in terms of a cystic component, or the presence of an associated syringomyelia (Fig. 11.18).

MRI scanning also has the capacity to illustrate the nature of any expanding process within the spinal cord.

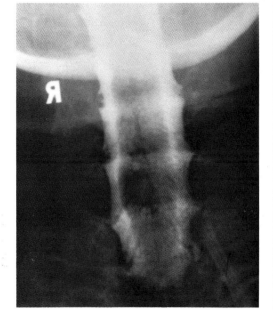
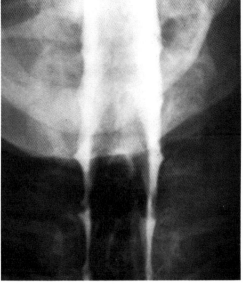
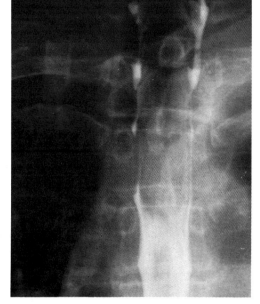

Fig. 11.16 Spinal cord tumour: myelography showing localised bulging of the cervical cord at the C6 level.

Same patient as in figure 11.15.

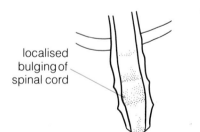

Fig. 11.17 Spinal cord tumour: myelography showing expansion of the cord between C4 and D3.

This 55 year old woman had numbness and weakness in the right leg for two years followed by burning in the left leg. She

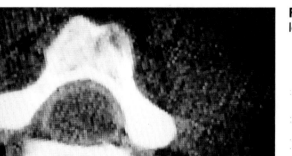

complained of frequency of micturition with occasional incontinence. Examination showed a spastic paraparesis with a pin prick level at about D4. The cord tumour displayed on myelography proved to be an ependymoma.

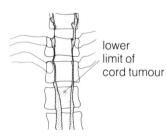

Fig. 11.18 Spinal cord tumour: CT scan showing a large central low-density area in the spinal cord.

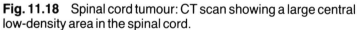
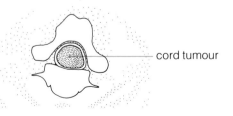

Meningioma

These account for up to one-third of primary intraspinal tumours and are much more common in women. They tend to arise in patients over the age of 40. Thoracic meningiomas are most common, followed by those in the cervical region. They usually originate in the region of the nerve roots, and have a globular shape. They sometimes invade the dura but rarely the bone (Fig.11.19). Plain radiographs may show erosion of the inner surface of the pedicles, though far less frequently than in the case of neurofibromas. Myelography reveals an intradural mass (Figs.11.20 & 11.21).

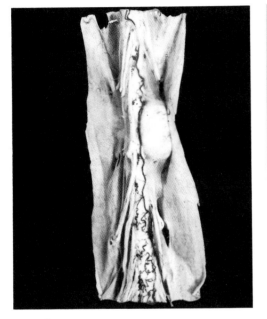

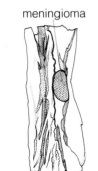

Fig. 11.19 Meningioma: dorsal aspect of the thoracic cord showing a right-sided meningioma.

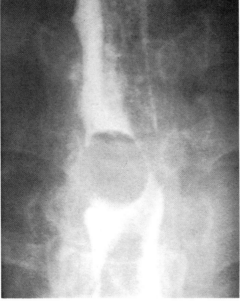

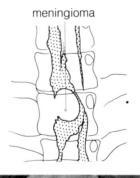

Fig. 11.20 Thoracic meningioma: myelography showing a filling defect in the mid-dorsal region.

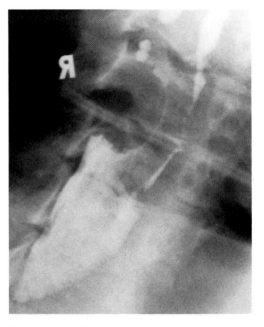

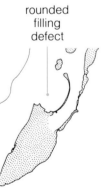

Fig. 11.21 Cervical meningioma: myelography showing a filling defect at C5 on the right.

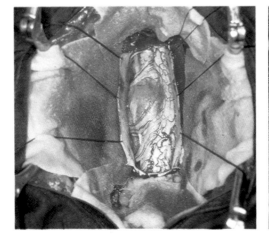

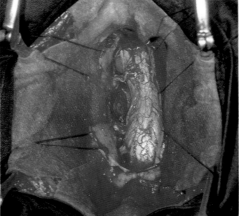

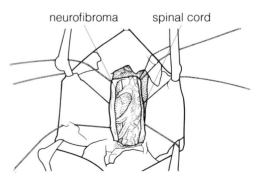

Fig. 11.22 Neurofibroma: operative views before (left) and after (right) removal.

Neurofibroma

Von Recklinghausen's disease, neurofibromatosis, is inherited as an autosomal dominant, and comprises cutaneous neurofibroma, schwannoma and café-au-lait pigmentation (Figs.11.22 & 11.23). With increasing numbers of café-au-lait patches, the diagnosis becomes more likely (Fig.11.24). Neurofibroma may be visible within the iris (Fig.11.25), and there is an increased incidence of ependymoma, astrocytoma and optic nerve glioma.

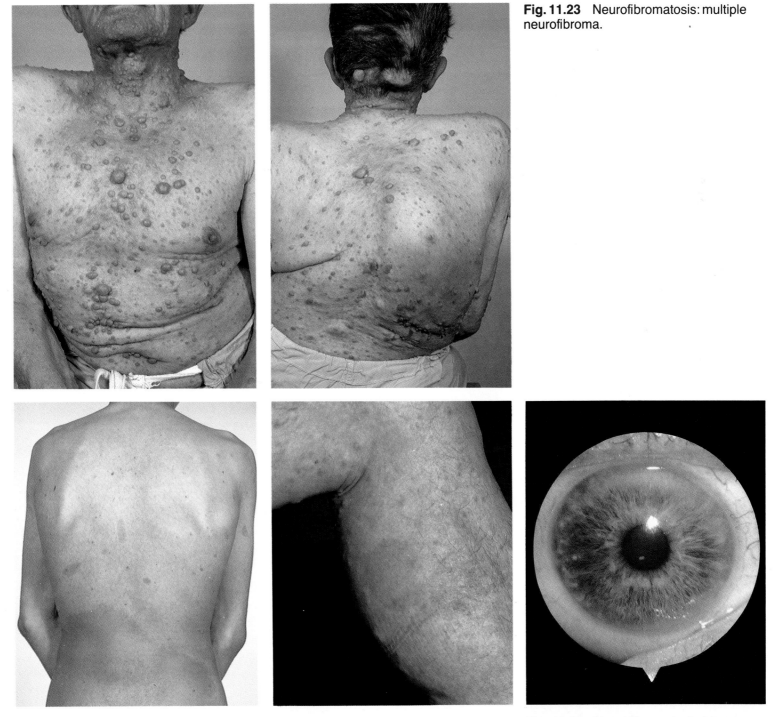

Fig. 11.23 Neurofibromatosis: multiple neurofibroma.

Fig. 11.24 Neurofibromatosis: café-au-lait pigmentation on the back and the leg.

Fig. 11.25 Neurofibromatosis: iris neurofibromata.

Spinal neurinomas, or schwannomas, are more often iso-lated than occurring as part of the generalised disease. Their incidence is roughly similar to that of spinal meningioma, reaching a peak in the fourth and fifth decades. They arise from nerve roots, most commonly sensory, at cervical, dorsal or lumbar level. Some tumours invade the foramen (Fig. 11.26), whilst others stay within the intradural space, or extend extradurally (Fig. 11.27).

They most commonly present with pain, either local or radicular (Fig.11.28), followed by manifestations of sensory and motor root and cord involvement. The CSF protein is usually elevated but may be normal in approximately 15% of cases. Lumbar neurofibroma is more difficult to diagnose as the physical signs are less conspicuous (Fig.11.29).

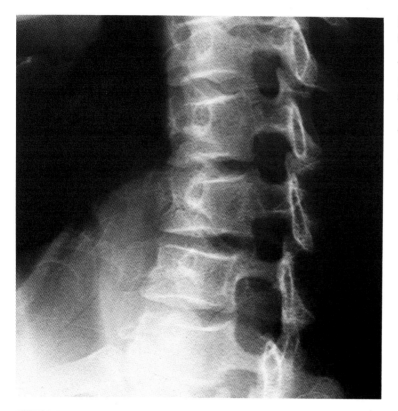

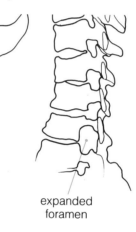

Fig. 11.26 Cervical neurofibroma: cervical radiograph showing a marked expansion of the C6/7 intervertebral foramen.

This 45 year old man had neck and right shoulder pain for six months. Examination showed depression of the left biceps and supinator reflexes.

expanded foramen

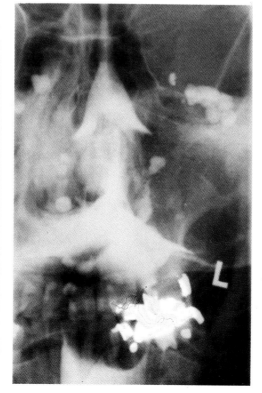

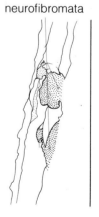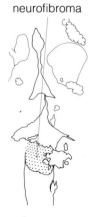

Fig. 11.27 Myelogram showing a left-sided extradural mass at C6/7 and intradural masses at C5 (left) and at the foramen magnum (right).

Same patient as in figure 11.26.

neurofibromata   neurofibroma

Extradural Tumours

Extradural metastases most commonly originate from primary tumours of the breast, lung, prostate and kidney. They have been reported to occur in 5% of patients with systemic cancer who have a post-mortem examination. Almost two-thirds occur in the thoracic region. Pain, either local or in a radicular distribution, is usually the first symptom though by the time of presentation most patients have motor and sensory symptoms and at least half have sphincter disturbances. Myelography reveals severe or complete block at the appropriate level (Fig.11.30). There is some evidence that radiotherapy is as successful as surgical decompression, particularly for patients with lymphoma. At least 30% of patients survive twelve months.

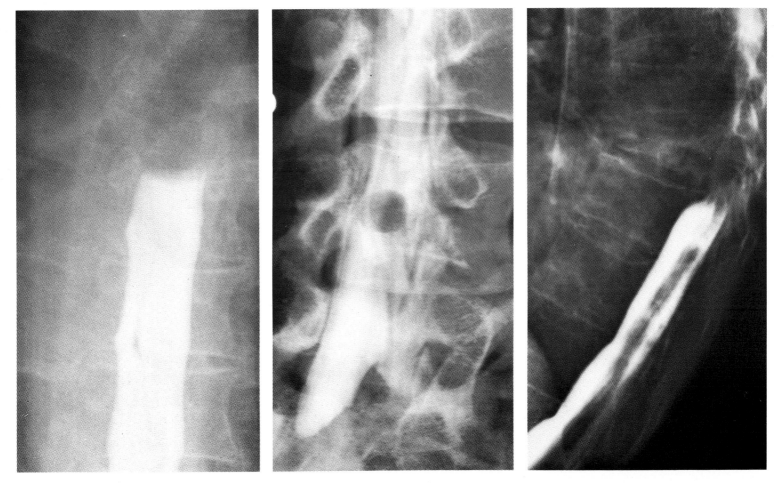

Fig. 11.28 Thoracic neurofibroma: myelography showing complete obstruction at the D6 level.

This 53 year old woman had a severe mid-thoracic pain for 3 years followed by lower limb weakness and ill-defined sensory symptoms spreading from the legs to the abdomen. Examination showed a spastic paraparesis with a sensory level at D7.

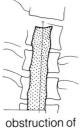

obstruction of
myodil column

Fig. 11.29 Lumbar neurofibroma: myelogram showing an intradural filling defect at the L4 level.

This 22 year old woman had a long history of left leg pain with weakness of the foot. On examination there was a café-au-lait patch on the left buttock and impaired pin prick over the lateral thigh and calf. A neurofibroma was excised.

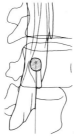

filling defect

Fig. 11.30 Extradural metastasis: myelogram showing a collapsed vertebral body with secondary obstruction of the theca due to a metastasis from a hypernephroma.

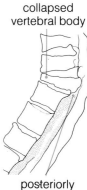

collapsed
vertebral body

posteriorly
displaced
spinal cord

Spinal Dysraphism

Failure of fusion of midline structures may affect the cranium or spinal column. In the cranium, if severe, anencephaly results; lesser degrees of fusion failure produce meningoencephalocoeles, particularly in the occipital region. In the spine, meningocoele or myelomeningocoele result, presenting in infancy, or spina bifida occulta may be detected radiologically without associated neurological deficit.

Some disorders of midline fusion may present with neurological disorders in adult life, including such diverse problems as splitting of the spinal cord, tethering of the cord and cauda equina and infiltration of the same structures by dermoid tumours or lipomata.

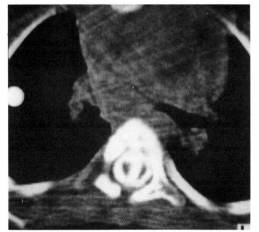

Fig. 11.31 Spinal dysraphism: CT scan showing split spinal cord.

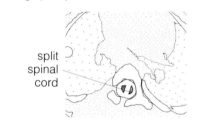

split spinal cord

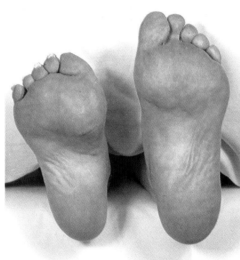

Fig. 11.32 Spinal dysraphism: shortening of the right foot with pes cavus.

This 40 year old woman had her right leg splinted as a child. The foot had always been clubbed with altered sensation in the toes, and she complained of urgency of

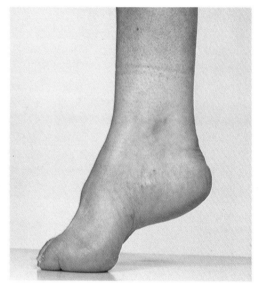

micturition. Examination showed atrophy of the right leg with pes cavus, absent ankle and right knee reflexes and reduced pin prick sensation over the right foot and toes. Lumbar radiographs showed an extensive failure of fusion.

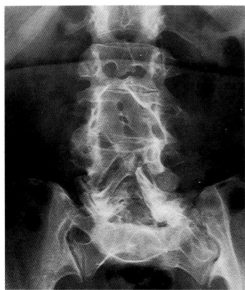

Fig. 11.33 Spinal dysraphism: lumbar radiograph showing extensive failure of fusion.

Same patient as in figure 11.32.

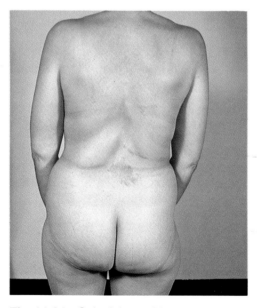

Fig. 11.34 Spinal dysraphism: naevus over the lumbar region (left) with wasting of the left leg (right).

This 36 year old woman had a history of left pes cavus with altered feeling in the foot,

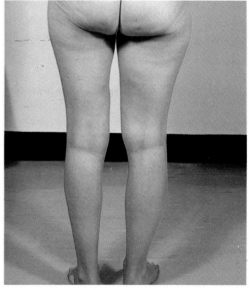

buttock, outer thigh and calf. Examination showed global wasting and weakness of the left leg, maximal distally, with an absent ankle jerk. Pin prick was reduced over the left S3-5 dermatomes, and there was a naevus over the lower lumbar spine.

Diastematomyelia refers to a split of the spinal cord by a spur extending posteriorly from the adjacent vertebral body (Fig. 11.31). Tethering of the cord or cauda equina presenting in adult life produces lower or upper motor neurone signs according to the structures involved, usually with alteration of sphincter control (Fig. 11.32). In some patients, a tuft of hair or naevus over the lumbosacral junction points to the presence of an underlying skeletal defect (Figs. 11.33 & 11.34). Lipomata overlying the lumbosacral spine have a similar connotation. Exploration of such lesions, where skeletal changes exist, usually reveals deep extension of the lipoma through the theca into the spinal canal. Neurological abnormalities frequently coexist (Figs. 11.35-11.37).

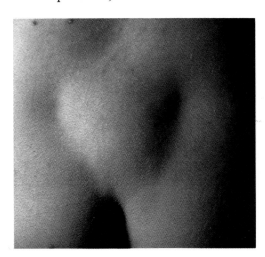

Fig. 11.35 Spinal dysraphism: lipoma overlying the lumbosacral junction.

This 18 year old girl had noticed a fatty swelling over the lumbosacral junction for several years. There were no neurological symptoms or signs. Lumbar radiographs showed a spina bifida occulta at S1.

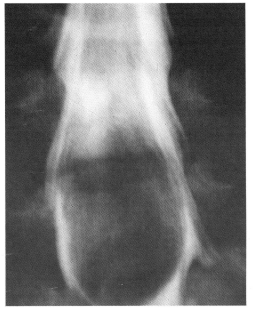

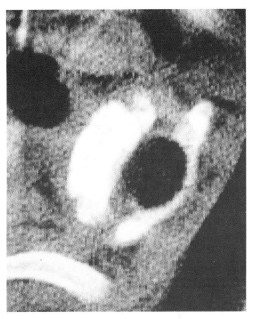

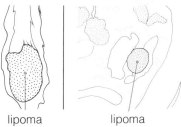

Fig. 11.36 Spinal dysraphism: myelogram (left) showing an intradural mass, also revealed by CT scan (right).

This 6 month old child had been noted to have a subcutaneous lipoma over the lumbosacral junction. Exploration of the lumbosacral subarachnoid space revealed an intradural fatty mass.

lipoma   lipoma

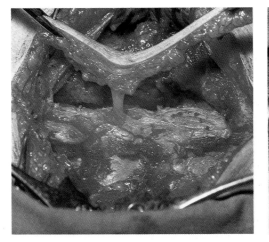

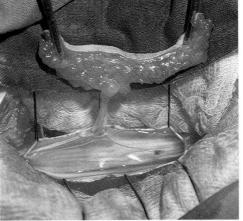

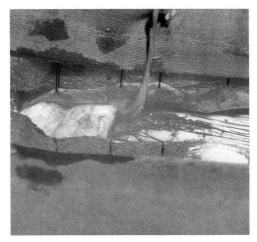

Fig. 11.37 Surgical photographs illustrating the extension of a tract from the skin to a dermoid lying within the conus.

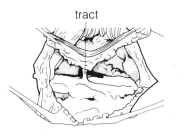

tract

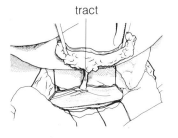

tract

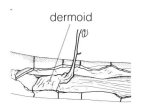

dermoid

Arachnoid Cysts

These are usually of no significance, being incidental findings at myelography, though on occasions they appear to be capable of causing spinal cord compression (Figs.11.38 & 11.39).

Syringomyelia

In this condition, cystic cavitation of the spinal cord occurs, most prominently in the cervical region, sometimes in association with cyst formation in the brain stem (syringobulbia) (Fig.11.40). There is a close association between the condition and a number of developmental anomalies at the foramen magnum, particularly the Type 1 Arnold-Chiari malformation. The condition sometimes follows spinal cord injury, and may occur in association with intramedullary tumours of the cord.

It has been suggested that, in the presence of outflow obstruction from the fourth ventricle, waves transmitted from choroid plexus pulsation are directed down the central canal of the cord with subsequent extravasation or

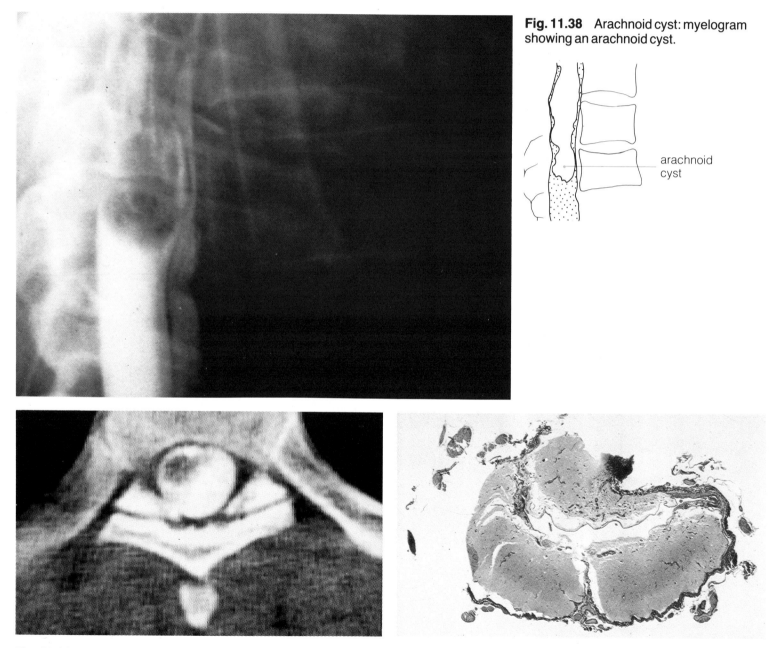

Fig. 11.38 Arachnoid cyst: myelogram showing an arachnoid cyst.

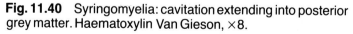
arachnoid cyst

Fig. 11.39 Arachnoid cyst: CT scan showing an arachnoid cyst partly displacing the spinal cord.

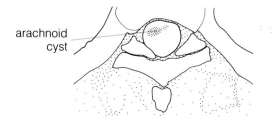
arachnoid cyst

Fig. 11.40 Syringomyelia: cavitation extending into posterior grey matter. Haematoxylin Van Gieson, ×8.

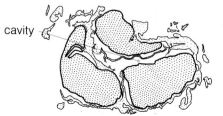
cavity

expansion with cyst formation. The hypothesis has not been universally accepted. An alternative idea is that cerebrospinal fluid (CSF) under increased pressure in the subarachnoid space, for example during coughing, is unable to move into the cranial cavity, and instead becomes displaced along the Virchow-Robin spaces of the cord.

Early symptoms of syringomyelia include stiffness or weakness of the lower limbs and altered sensation in one or both hands. Pain in the neck or upper limbs is not uncommon and symptoms due to an associated syringo-

bulbia may coexist. The neck may appear abnormally short. Typically there is wasting of the hands, upper limb areflexia and dissociated sensory loss over the hands or shoulders. Loss of pain and thermal sensation in the hands results in recurrent injuries (Fig.11.41). A Horner's syndrome may reflect either cord or brain stem involvement (Fig.11.42). If the cervical cord cavitation extends upwards to the midcervical region, wasting of the periscapular and shoulder muscles is likely to follow (Fig.11.43).

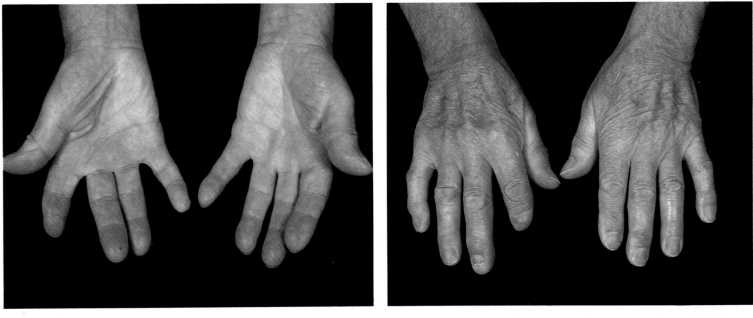

Fig. 11.41 Syringomyelia: wasting of the small hand muscles and loss of the terminal phalanx of the right index finger.

This 75 year old man had sensory symptoms in the hands for 20 years and was aware of loss of thermal sensation. The hands had been weak for many years. Examination showed a mild left

Horner's syndrome and fasciculation of the tongue margins. There was wasting of the spinati and small hand muscles with global upper limb weakness and areflexia. Pin prick was depressed from C2 to D4. The lower limbs were mildly spastic with depressed vibration sense.

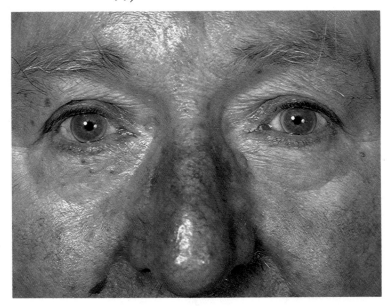

Fig. 11.42 Syringomyelia: narrowing of the left palpebral fissure.

Same patient as figure 11.41.

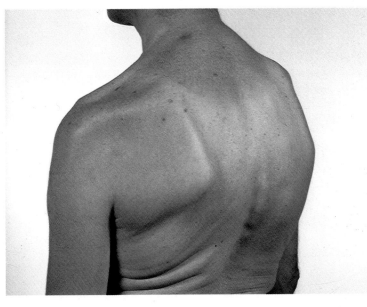

Fig. 11.43 Syringomyelia: wasting of the periscapular muscles.

Same patient as in figure 11.41.

Myelography reveals widening of the cord, maximal in the upper thoracic and lower cervical regions (Fig. 11.44). It may be possible, by the use of air as the contrast medium, to establish that the cystic cavitation of the cord communicates with the subarachnoid space. CT scanning, or MRI, indicate the density of the cavity within the cord (Fig. 11.45).

Subacute Combined Degeneration of the Spinal Cord

Studies in vitamin B_{12}-depleted animals suggest that demyelination predominates in this condition, with later axonal degeneration of a lesser degree. The end result is severe myelin and axonal degeneration with replacement gliosis. There is discoloration of the lateral and posterior columns of the spinal cord, predominantly in the mid- and upper thoracic regions (Fig.11.46). There are often associated degenerative changes in the optic nerves.

It has been suggested that the condition results from a failure to detoxify cyanide produced in the body. A more likely explanation might stem from the fact that vitamin B_{12} is a coenzyme in the methyl malonyl CoA mutase

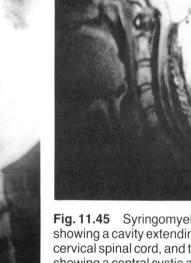

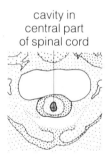

Fig. 11.45 Syringomyelia: MRI scan (left) showing a cavity extending throughout the cervical spinal cord, and the CT scan (right) showing a central cystic area within the spinal cord.

(Right) This 31 year old woman had a 2 year history of progressive weakness of the right leg. Cerebellar ectopia was present and foramen magnum decompression was performed.

cavity in
cervical
spinal cord

cavity in
central part
of spinal cord

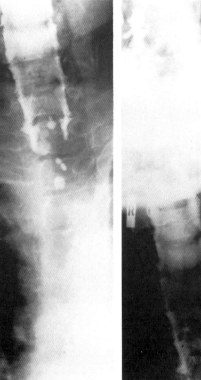

Fig. 11.44 Syringomyelia: myelogram showing diffuse expansion of the cervical cord.

Same patient as in figure 11.41.

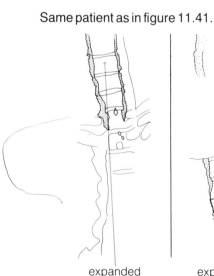

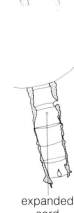

expanded cord

expanded cord

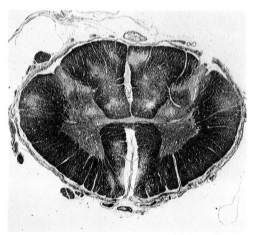

Fig. 11.46 Subacute combined degeneration. There is widespread myelin loss in the white matter. Weigert-Pal. ×6.

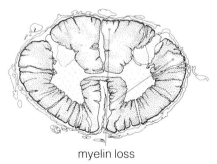

myelin loss

reaction. Interruption of this reaction produces a deficiency of unsaturated fatty acids in cerebral phospholipids.

Sensory symptoms are prominent with peripheral paraesthesiae affecting the legs more than the hands. Subsequently, weakness and stiffness of the legs appear and changes in mood and behaviour may be seen. Cutaneous changes include pallor, angular stomatitis, a smooth tongue and vitiligo (Figs. 11.47–11.49). Many patients show associated haematological changes, including anaemia, macrocytosis and a megaloblastic bone marrow (Fig.11.50).On occasions, however, these indices are entirely normal despite unequivocal neurological changes.

Fig. 11.47 Subacute combined degeneration: facial appearance.

This 67 year old woman had a long history of hypopituitarism. Anaemia with a megaloblastic bone marrow was first noted in 1972 and treated with vitamin B12 for 3 months only. From 1978 she complained of heaviness and numbness of the legs. Examination showed a pale woman with glossitis and angular stomatitis. There was lower limb wasting though with intact reflexes. Further investigation confirmed pernicious anaemia and her neurological symptoms improved with replacement therapy.

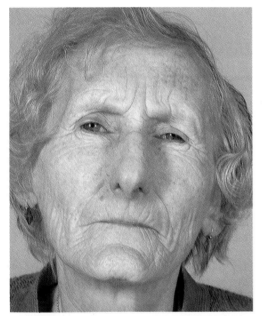

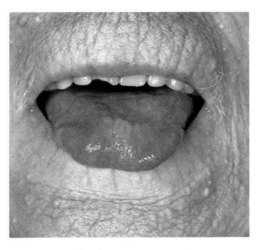

Fig. 11.48 Subacute combined degeneration: atrophy of the tongue.

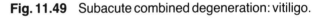

Fig. 11.49 Subacute combined degeneration: vitiligo.

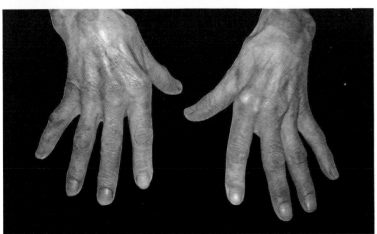

Fig. 11.50 Subacute combined degeneration: mean corpuscular volume (MCV) changes over a six year period.

Spinal Cord Angioma

This condition predominates in men, the diagnosis usually being established between the ages of 40 and 70 (Fig.11.51). The majority arise in the lower dorsal or dorsolumbar region. Symptoms include pain, sensory disturbances, weakness and alteration of sphincter function. Exercise or posture may aggravate or precipitate symptoms. Progress is usually gradual rather than abrupt. Examination often shows a mixture of upper and lower motor neurone signs with sensory change.

Myelography reveals tortuous filling defects (Fig.11.52). Selective angiography of feeding vessels confirms the diagnosis and, via embolisation, has been used as a method of treatment (Fig.11.53). Better results are achieved, however, with direct surgical excision of feeding vessels.

Arachnoiditis

This condition, probably a heterogeneous one, is associated with several disorders, including spinal cord angioma and spinal tumours. It may follow trauma to the spinal column, meningeal infection or be subsequent to myelography. Many years may elapse between the putative precipitating factor and the development of symptoms.

It predominates in the dorsal segment with thickened arachnoid bound to the dura, spinal cord and nerve roots. Cyst formation may occur. Typically it results in pain

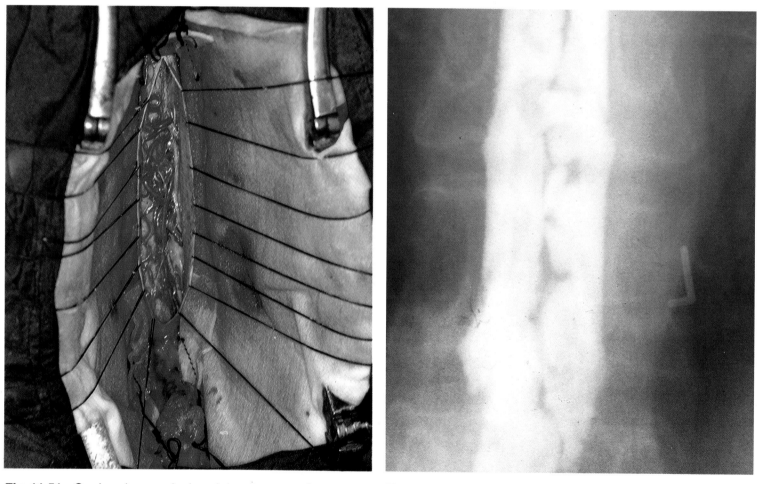

Fig. 11.51 Cord angioma: spinal cord showing an angiomatous malformation at the midcervical level.

Fig. 11.52 Cord angioma: myelogram showing the outline of tortuous vessels on the cord surface.

angioma

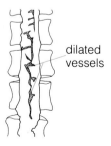

dilated vessels

followed by the features of spinal cord compression. Manometric block is sometimes seen, with a raised CSF protein concentration though usually with a normal cell count. Myelography reveals fragmentation of the contrast medium sometimes with complete block (Fig.11.54). There is no specific treatment.

Traumatic Lesions

Survival from spinal cord injury is better in younger patients, and in those with paraplegia rather than tetraplegia. Injuries of the spine can be conveniently divided into fracture dislocations, fractures alone and dislocations alone. The first of these is most common. Most vertebral injuries are at the levels of C1/2, C4/6 and T11/L2.

Short of complete transection, injury to the cord results in destruction of grey and white matter with haemorrhage. Severe injuries may result in profound loss of motor and sensory function with initial loss of reflex activity below the level of the lesion (spinal shock). This state rarely persists, and more commonly a slow recovery of intrinsic reflex function of the cord ensues.

Lateral radiographs of the spine establish the degree of vertebral injury. More sophisticated procedures may be necessary to demonstrate the existence of a traumatic meningocoele (Fig. 11.55) or secondary changes in the spinal cord (Fig. 11.56).

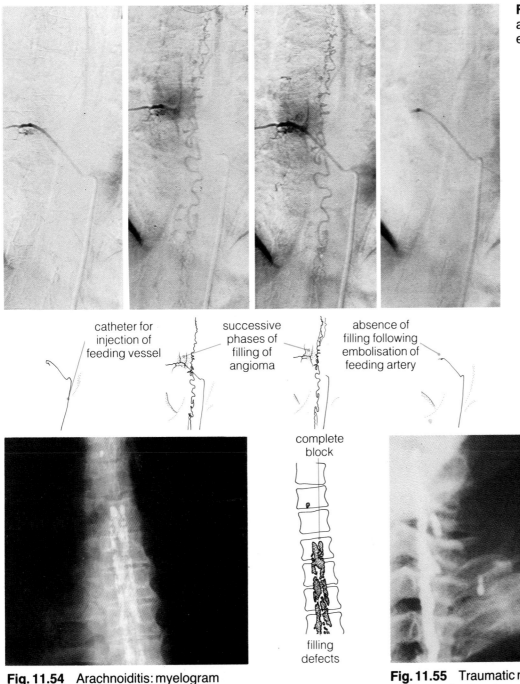

Fig. 11.53 Cord angioma: spinal angiography before (1-3) and after (4) embolisation of the feeding vessel.

catheter for injection of feeding vessel

successive phases of filling of angioma

absence of filling following embolisation of feeding artery

complete block

filling defects

Fig. 11.54 Arachnoiditis: myelogram showing multiple patchy filling defects due to tuberculous arachnoiditis.

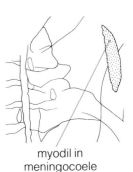

myodil in meningocoele

Fig. 11.55 Traumatic meningocoele: myelography showing contrast medium trapped in a large cervical meningocoele.

This 30 year old man developed a neck swelling after a motorcycle accident in which the left C5-T1 nerve roots had been avulsed.

11.19

Friedreich's Ataxia

This condition, usually inherited as a recessive, generally appears between the ages of 2 and 16, and only rarely presents after the age of 20. Pathological changes include loss of myelinated fibres in the corticospinal and spinocerebellar tracts and in the posterior columns (Fig.11.57). There is atrophy of dorsal root ganglia and frequently changes in some cranial nerve nuclei and the cerebellum. There is an associated cardiomyopathy.

Typical features include limb and gait ataxia and lower limb areflexia. Dysarthria is usual, as are extensor plantar responses and proprioceptive loss. Kyphoscoliosis and pes cavus are seen in the majority. Less conspicuous are optic atrophy and distal wasting. The responsible gene has been estimated to occur at a rate of 1 in 100 in the population.

Radiation Myelopathy

This has been reported after spinal cord irradiation in between 0.6 and 17.5% of cases. There is a transient form, with mild sensory symptoms and often a Lhermitte's sign where the cervical cord is involved; an acute form, thought to be associated with occlusion of spinal cord vessels; and finally a chronic, progressive type. In this third group, after a delay of up to 5 years, sensory symptoms, sometimes of a Brown-Séquard type develop, followed by paraplegia or tetraplegia, severe sensory loss and, frequently, sphincteric disturbance.

Pathological changes include necrosis of grey and white matter with prominent vascular changes including arteriolar necrosis and vessel occlusion. Limitation of the amount of spinal cord irradiation can prevent these changes.

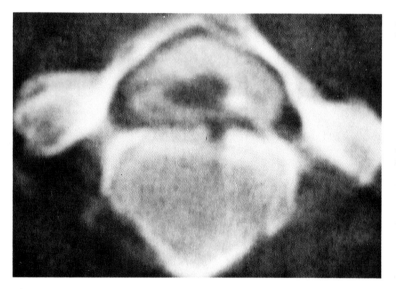

Fig. 11.56 Traumatic cord lesion: CT scan showing a flattened spinal cord.

This 26 year old man had developed a paraplegia after a blow on the neck.

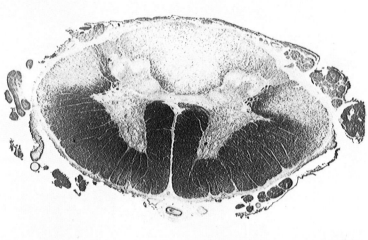

Fig. 11.57 Friedreich's ataxia: thoracic cord showing loss of myelinated fibres from the posterior and lateral columns. Weigert-Pal. ×10.

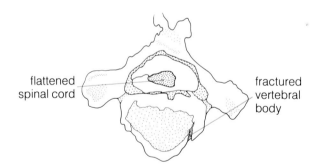

flattened spinal cord

fractured vertebral body

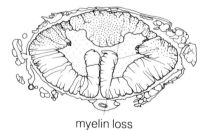

myelin loss

12. Cranial Nerve, Neuro-ophthalmological and Neuro-otological Syndromes

Cranial nerve syndromes may affect a single nerve or a combination, in which case the particular combination will suggest the location and nature of the causative lesion. Along with these, a number of neuro-ophthalmological syndromes, particularly those affecting the pupil and ocular movements, will be described.

First Cranial Nerve
Disturbances of olfaction are not commonly encountered in neurological practice. Alteration of smell and taste may follow head injury, or occur in isolation after a non-specific upper respiratory tract infection. With com-

pression of one olfactory nerve or bulb, unilateral anosmia results, and may serve to localise lesions such as subfrontal meningioma.

Second Cranial Nerve
A large number of conditions can produce optic atrophy with consequent changes in the appearance of the optic disc, including familial disorders, for example Leber's optic atrophy, primary demyelination followed by axonal degeneration of the nerve, as in multiple sclerosis and compression of the nerve. Typically, an optic nerve lesion produces a reduced visual acuity with depression of the

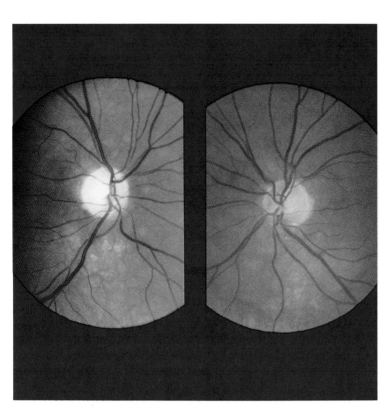

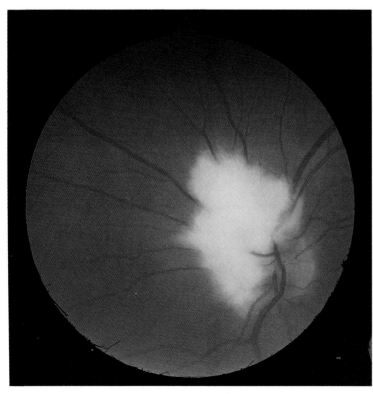

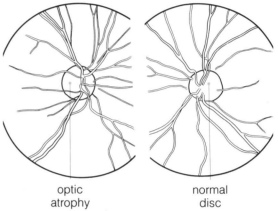

Fig. 12.1 Optic atrophy: fundus photograph showing atrophy of the right optic disc. The left optic disc is normal.

optic
atrophy

normal
disc

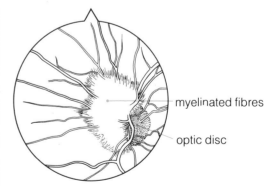

Fig. 12.2 Fundus photograph showing myelinated nerve fibres.

myelinated fibres

optic disc

light response, a central field defect and, usually, some degree of pallor of the optic disc, though this particular physical sign is notoriously subjective (Fig. 12.1). Myelinated nerve fibres surrounding the disc are often misinterpreted as representing a large, atrophic disc (Fig. 12.2).

Lesions compressing the optic nerve may be detected by their effects on adjacent structures. For example, optic chiasm glioma in children frequently produces widening of the optic canals which is visible radiologically (Fig. 12.3). Compression of one optic nerve by a subfrontal mass, with subsequent raised intracranial pressure, produces the Foster Kennedy syndrome, with unilateral optic atrophy and contralateral papilloedema (Fig. 12.4).

PUPILLARY SYNDROMES
Horner's Syndrome

The sympathetic fibres destined for the eye pursue a long, complex course which remains uncrossed. Interruption of the pathway produces ptosis with meiosis of varying degree. In the initial stages, the conjunctival vessels may be transiently dilated (Fig. 12.5). If the lesion is proximal to the carotid bifurcation, sympathetic fibres to the facial sweat glands are affected, leading to ipsilateral loss of facial sweating.

A number of pharmacological agents are used to further localise the site of a sympathetic lesion producing a Horner's syndrome, at least in terms of its pre- or post-ganglionic origin. 4% cocaine eye-drops dilate the normal

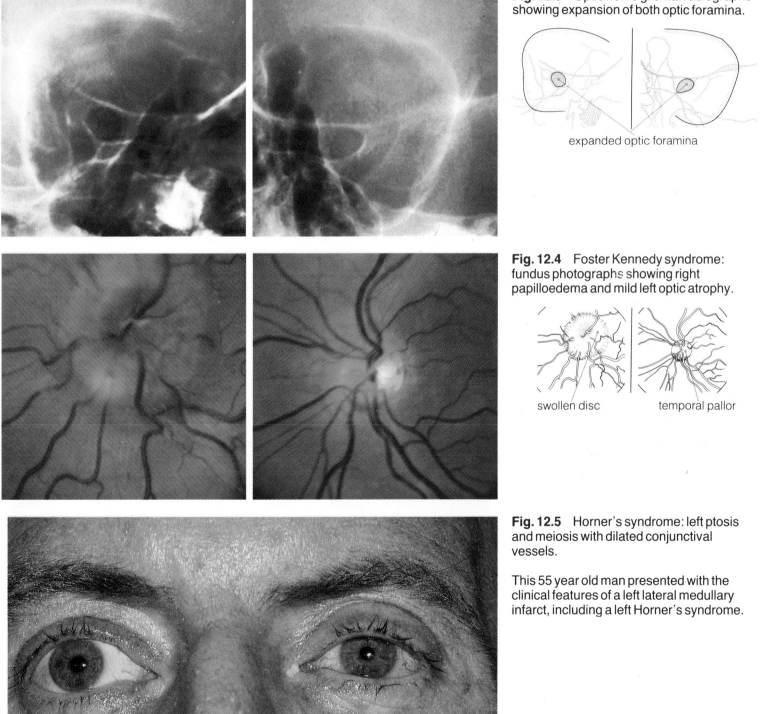

Fig. 12.3 Optic nerve glioma: radiographs showing expansion of both optic foramina.

expanded optic foramina

Fig. 12.4 Foster Kennedy syndrome: fundus photographs showing right papilloedema and mild left optic atrophy.

swollen disc   temporal pallor

Fig. 12.5 Horner's syndrome: left ptosis and meiosis with dilated conjunctival vessels.

This 55 year old man presented with the clinical features of a left lateral medullary infarct, including a left Horner's syndrome.

12.3

pupil, but fail to influence a Horner's pupil, irrespective of the site of the lesion (Figs. 12.6 & 12.7). 1% hydroxy-amphetamine releases noradrenaline at post-ganglionic nerve endings: therefore, a post-ganglionic Horner's pupil fails to dilate due to depletion of these stores, whilst a pre-ganglionic Horner's pupil will dilate normally (Fig. 12.8). Conversely, post-ganglionic sympathetic lesions produce denervation hypersensitivity, permitting the affected pupil to dilate with dilute (1:1000) adrenaline.

Tonic Pupil Syndrome

Typically, this produces unilateral, less commonly bi-lateral, pupillary dilatation. The pupil is fixed, or nearly so, to light and fails to dilate in the dark (Fig. 12.9). With a near effort, slow constriction of the pupil results, and an equally slow dilatation follows release of the stimulus (Figs. 12.10 & 12.11). Accommodation behaves in a simi-lar fashion. The pupil usually displays hypersensitivity to a weak parasympathomimetic agent, for example, 2.5% methacholine.

The condition predominates in women and tends to pre-sent between the ages of 20 and 50. It can follow an acute iridoplegia, orbital trauma or viral infection. In some in-stances, the condition is associated with depression of the deep tendon reflexes (Holmes-Adie syndrome).

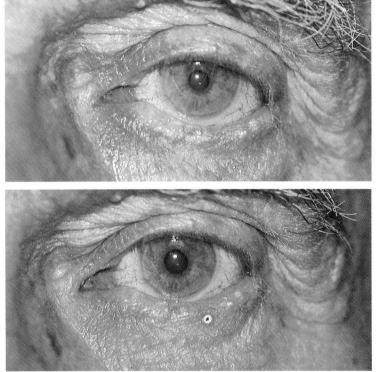

Fig. 12.6 Horner's syndrome: the normal, left pupil before (upper) and after (lower) instillation of 4% cocaine.

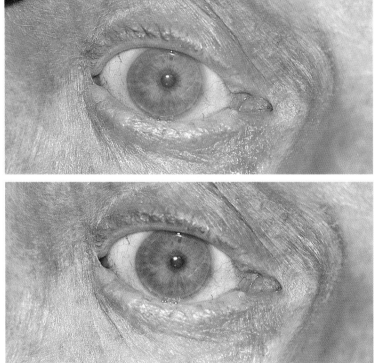

Fig. 12.7 Horner's syndrome: the affected, right pupil before (upper) and after (lower) instillation of 4% cocaine – there is no response. The upper lid has been retracted.

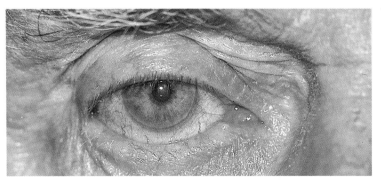

Fig. 12.8 Horner's syndrome: dilatation of the pupil after instillation of 1% hydroxyamphetamine.

Same patient as in Fig. 12.7.

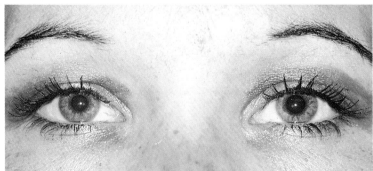

Fig. 12.9 Tonic pupil: the left pupil is dilated compared to the right.

This 31 year old woman had been aware of pupillary asymmetry for some time. She presented with left facial numbness, the aetiology of which was not established. It rapidly resolved. Examination showed a typical left tonic pupil. The triceps and ankle jerks were depressed.

12.4

Iridoplegia

An isolated iridoplegia, with a fixed dilated pupil unresponsive to a light or near stimulus, can result from an organic disturbance, most likely at the level of the ciliary ganglion, but it is more commonly due to accidental or deliberate installation of mydriatic eye-drops (Fig. 12.12).

Argyll Robertson Pupil

Typically both pupils (the condition is usually bilateral) are small and slightly irregular. The light reaction is absent or depressed with a more complete reaction to a near stimulus (Fig. 12.13). Iris atrophy is sometimes present. In this form, the condition is almost always due to tertiary syphilis of the central nervous system. The responsible lesion probably lies in the upper mid-brain, rostral to the oculomotor nucleus, interrupting the light reflex pathway together with descending, cortical, inhibitory fibres to the pupillary constrictor nucleus.

OPHTHALMOPLEGIA
Internuclear Ophthalmoplegia

This condition occurs when the pathway (medial longitudinal fasciculus) from one paramedian pontine lateral gaze centre to the contralateral medial rectus nucleus is interrupted. On lateral gaze, the medial rectus fails to fully adduct the eye (Fig. 12.14). There is usually nystagmus in

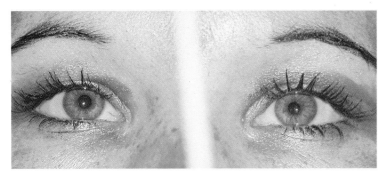

Fig. 12.10 Tonic pupil: after one minute's near effort, the previously dilated left pupil is now actually smaller than the right.

Same patient as in figure 12.9.

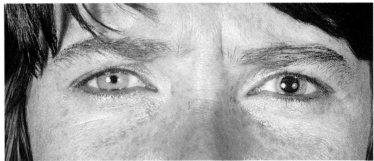

Fig. 12.12 Iridoplegia: dilated left pupil.

This 30 year old woman presented with a two month history of blurred vision followed by dilatation of the left pupil. Examination showed a dilated left pupil responding only slightly to light and near. She denied using eye drops.

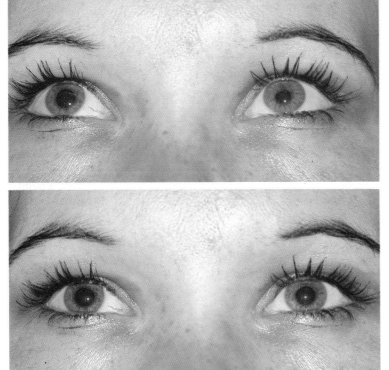

Fig. 12.11 Tonic pupil: gradual dilatation after release of the near stimulus, at 15 seconds (upper) and still incomplete at 60 seconds (lower).

Same patient as in figure 12.9.

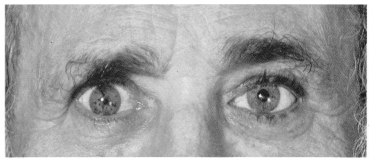

Fig. 12.13 Argyll Robertson pupil: the patient's right pupil was small, slightly irregular and fixed to light, though reacting to a near stimulus. The left eye is artificial.

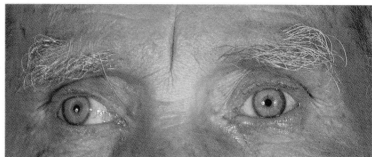

Fig. 12.14 Internuclear ophthalmoplegia: the patient is looking to the right and the left eye has failed to adduct.

the abducting eye. When bilateral the condition is accompanied by vertical nystagmus.

Bilateral internuclear ophthalmoplegia in young adults is most commonly due to multiple sclerosis, whereas it frequently has a vascular basis in the elderly.

If the lesion affecting the medial longitudinal fasciculus extends ventrally to the ipsilateral paramedian pontine lateral gaze centre, an internuclear ophthalmoplegia is accompanied by an ipsilateral horizontal gaze paresis, the so-called 'one-and-a-half syndrome' (Fig. 12.15). The syndrome most commonly derives from a vascular lesion.

Peri-aqueductal Syndrome

This syndrome, also termed the dorsal midbrain or Parinaud's syndrome, produces failure of upward gaze with preserved downward gaze. Attempts at upward gaze provoke convergence-retractory nystagmus. The pupils become fixed to light though not to a near stimulus. The condition is most commonly due to a pinealoma, but has been described with other disorders, including arteriovenous malformation (Figs. 12.16 & 12.17).

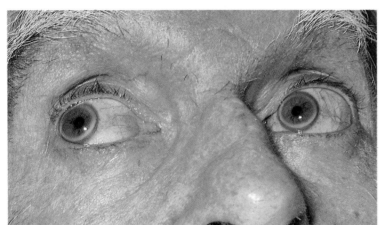

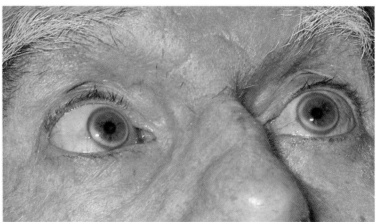

Fig. 12.15 'One-and-a-half syndrome': on looking to the right (left) the patient's left eye fails to adduct fully. On looking to the left (right) there is an incomplete left gaze paresis.

This 73 year old man gave a history of giddiness, diplopia and left facial numbness. Examination showed a left gaze paresis, a left internuclear ophthalmoplegia but no definite facial numbness. Assessment of his limbs was restricted by the effects of old poliomyelitis. The left plantar response was extensor.

Fig. 12.16 Peri-aqueductal syndrome: CT scan at two levels showing ventricular dilatation with aneurysmal dilatation of the vein of Galen. Pre-contrast (upper) and post-contrast (lower).

This 21 year old woman had had blurred vision for several months with chronic bifrontal headaches. She had noticed an increased frequency of micturition, weight gain and irregular periods. She was lethargic. Poor upward gaze was associated with convergence – retractory nystagmus. There was a suggestion of reduced adduction on lateral gaze. The light response was absent. Limb reflexes were brisk.

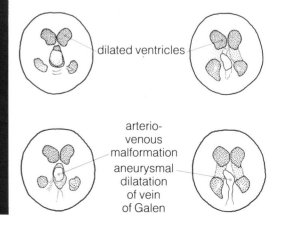

dilated ventricles

arterio-
venous
malformation
aneurysmal
dilatation
of vein
of Galen

Third Nerve Palsy

Lesions of this nerve may occur at any point along its course, from the nucleus to the orbit. Accompanying physical signs may serve to localise the site of the lesion, as may the character of the palsy itself. Nuclear lesions produce particular combinations of muscle weakness predictable from the disposition of the third nerve nuclear complex. When the nerve is affected within the brain stem, long tract signs are likely to be present. For example, in Benedikt's syndrome, a third nerve palsy, often incomplete, is accompanied by contralateral limb ataxia (Fig. 12.18). There are many causes of peripheral third nerve lesions. In diabetes, an acute painful paresis can occur, typically sparing the pupil. The responsible lesion is ischaemic, sparing the peripherally placed pupillomotor fibres (Fig. 12.19).

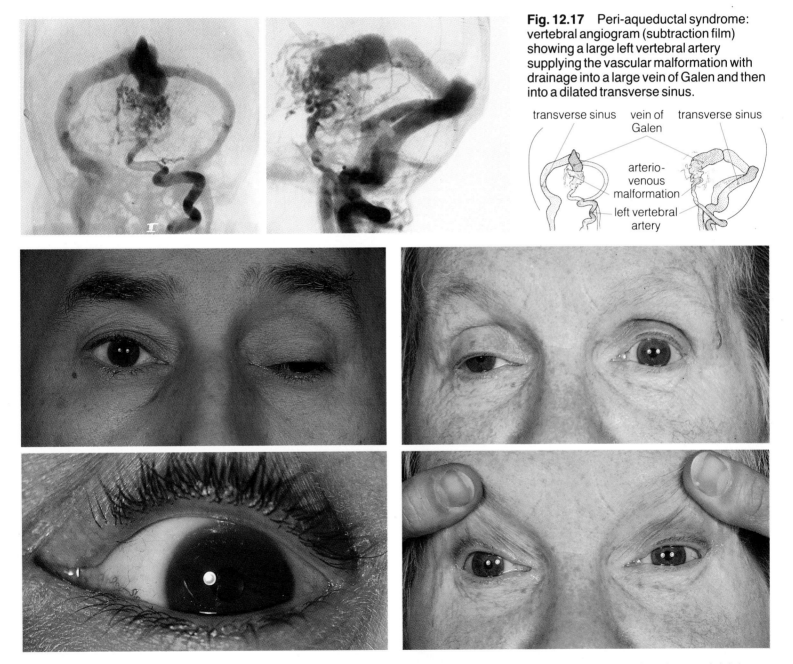

Fig. 12.17 Peri-aqueductal syndrome: vertebral angiogram (subtraction film) showing a large left vertebral artery supplying the vascular malformation with drainage into a large vein of Galen and then into a dilated transverse sinus.

transverse sinus   vein of Galen   transverse sinus

arterio-venous malformation

left vertebral artery

Fig. 12.18 Third nerve palsy in Benedikt's syndrome: left third nerve palsy with pupil sparing.

This 56 year old man had had a previous right hemiparesis. Four weeks earlier he had developed left ptosis and difficulty using the right arm. He had noticed diplopia. Examination showed a pupil-sparing third nerve paresis on the left, and marked right-sided cerebellar incoordination.

Fig. 12.19 Third nerve palsy in diabetes: there is a partial right ptosis with abduction and depression of the globe. The pupils were equal in size.

This 72 year old lady had a history of diabetes for 20 years. In 1973 she developed poor vision in the left eye. In 1982 she experienced pain above the right eye, followed by ptosis and diplopia. Examination showed a partial right third nerve paresis with pupil sparing. The paresis recovered.

Recovery is the rule, sometimes with evidence of aberrant reinnervation. Compression of the nerve by a posterior communicating aneurysm produces an ophthalmoplegia in which pupillary involvement is almost inevitable (Fig. 12.20). By the time of presentation, there are usually signs of subarachnoid haemorrhage as well (Fig. 12.21).

Fourth Nerve Palsy

This is an uncommon condition. The only muscle to be affected is the superior oblique, leading to diplopia on downward and inward gaze (Fig. 12.22). Some of the causes include head injury, vascular disease and diabetes, though often, the cause cannot be established.

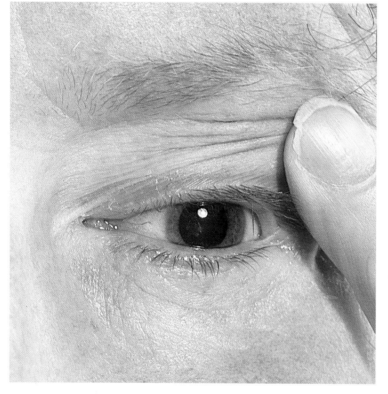

Fig. 12.20 Third nerve palsy: left eyelid elevated to show third nerve paresis with a dilated pupil.

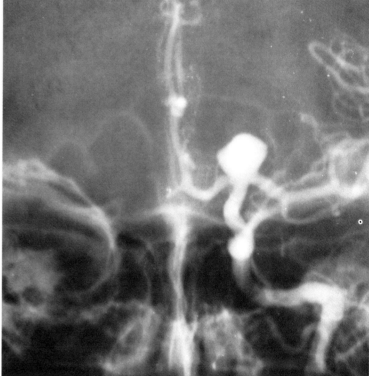

Fig. 12.21 Third nerve palsy: angiogram showing a posterior communicating aneurysm.

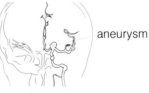

aneurysm

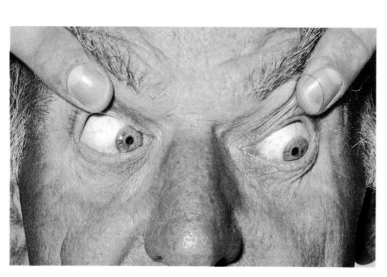

Fig. 12.22 Fourth nerve palsy:

This 65 year old man had developed diplopia with vertical image separation six months previously. Neurological examination showed reduced downward and inward gaze of the right eye but no other abnormalities. No basis for the problem was discovered.

Sixth Nerve Palsy

Lateral rectus weakness may result from myasthenia, orbital disease and dysthyroid eye disease in addition to lesions of the abducens nerve. Nuclear lesions produce a horizontal gaze paresis due to involvement of the adjacent pontine lateral gaze centre. Pontine lesions can affect the intramedullary part of the nerve, when coexisting fifth and seventh nerve lesions, together with a contralateral hemiparesis, are likely (Fig. 12.23). Peripherally, the nerve can be affected by nasopharyngeal carcinoma, chordoma, infection of the petrous temporal bone, cavernous aneurysm (Fig. 12.24), hypertension and diabetes. A sixth nerve palsy, either unilateral or bilateral, may also be a manifestation of raised intracranial pressure.

Parasellar Syndrome

Lesions within the cavernous sinus, for example, a carotid aneurysm, are likely to involve the third, fourth and sixth nerves, together with the first, second and, rarely, third component of the trigeminal nerve. Sympathetic involvement may lessen the degree of pupillary dilatation (Figs. 12.25-12.27).

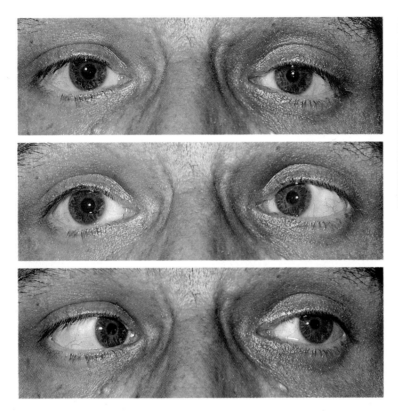

Fig. 12.23 Bilateral sixth nerve palsies: there is a tendency to convergence (upper), with incomplete abduction of the right (middle) and left (lower) eye.

This 24 year old man presented with intermittent diplopia. Initial examination suggested an isolated divergent paralysis. Later, sixth nerve palsies appeared along with gait ataxia and deteriorating mental status. CT and CSF examinations were normal but his visual evoked responses showed delayed potentials.

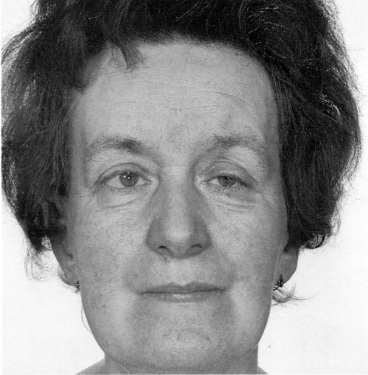

Fig. 12.24 Sixth nerve palsy: the right eye is deviated inwards due to unopposed action of medial rectus. The patient had a long standing left ptosis.

This 48 year old woman developed diplopia due to a sixth nerve palsy, followed by right visual failure and right facial numbness. Investigations established the presence of a transitional-cell carcinoma arising from the sphenoid sinus.

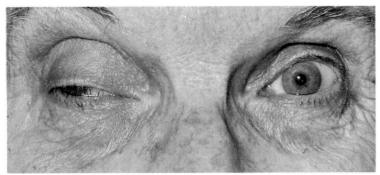

Fig. 12.25 Parasellar syndromes – cavernous aneurysm: severe right ptosis with abducted and depressed globe.

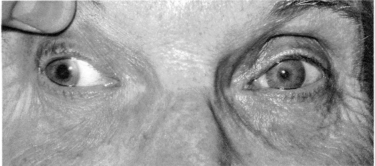

This 64 year old woman gave a three month history of ptosis. Examination showed hypertension and a total right third nerve paresis. The pupil was midposition in size and fixed to light. The CT scan established the presence of a cavernous aneurysm.

12.9

Occasionally such aneurysms merely cause a focal disturbance of neurological function (Fig. 12.28).

A caroticocavernous fistula is usually the result of trauma or a spontaneous event in an 'artherosclerotic' individual, producing gross congestion of feeding vessels to the cavernous sinus, including the superior ophthalmic and conjunctival veins. Typically, there is a pulsating exophthalmos in association with an orbital bruit,

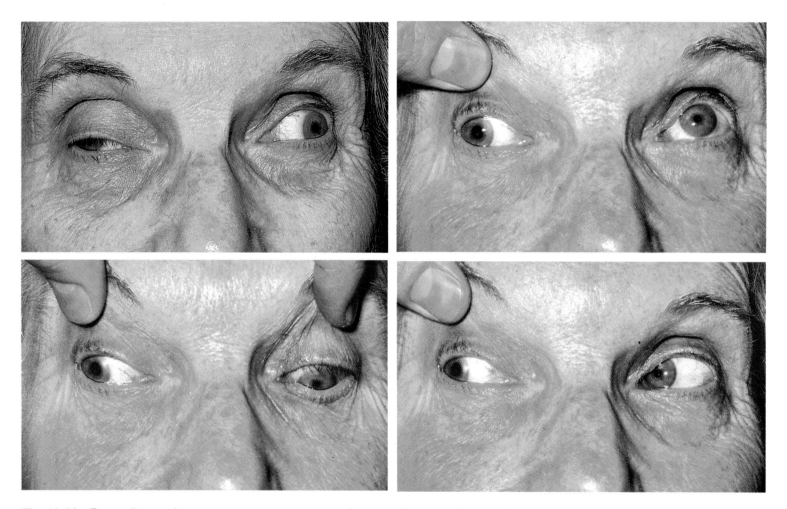

Fig. 12.26 Parasellar syndromes – cavernous aneurysm: the right eye fails to adduct (upper left), elevate (upper right), and depress (lower left) but abducts fully (lower right).

Same patient as in figure 12.25.

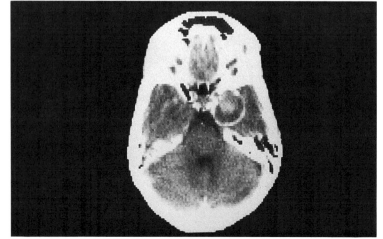

Fig. 12.27 Parasellar syndromes – cavernous aneurysm: CT scan showing the lesion.

Same patient as in figure 12.25.

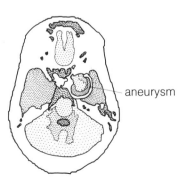

aneurysm

ophthalmoplegia, orbital pain and gross proptosis with oedema of the lids and conjunctivae (Fig. 12.29). There may be bilateral involvement due to interconnection between the two cavernous sinuses. Angiography confirms the diagnosis which may be suggested on the CT scan by proptosis, congestion of orbital contents and dilatation of the superior orbital vein (Fig. 12.30). Involvement of parasellar structures commonly occurs after invasion by

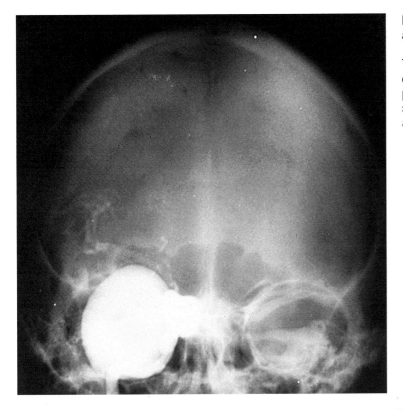

Fig. 12.28 Parasellar syndromes – cavernous aneurysm: carotid angiogram, showing filling of the aneurysm.

The patient, aged 45 years, presented with a six month history of diplopia. Examination showed bilateral exophthalmos (there was a past history of thyrotoxicosis) with weakness predominantly of right superior rectus. Angiography revealed a large cavernous aneurysm.

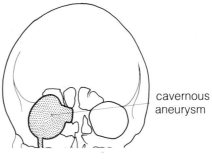

cavernous aneurysm

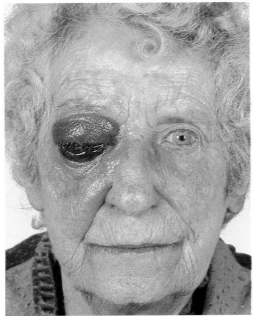

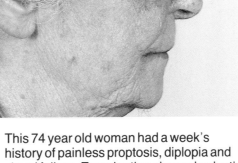

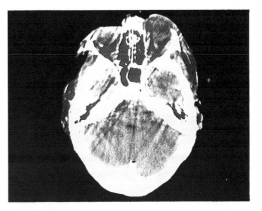

Fig. 12.30 Caroticocavernous fistula: CT scan showing right proptosis and a dilated superior ophthalmic vein.

Same patient as in figure 12.29.

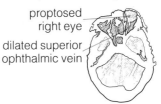

proptosed right eye

dilated superior ophthalmic vein

Fig. 12.29 Caroticocavernous fistula: right proptosis and gross oedema of lids and peri-orbital tissues.

This 74 year old woman had a week's history of painless proptosis, diplopia and visual failure. Examination showed pulsating exophthalmos without an orbital bruit.

nasopharyngeal carcinoma. Extension into the cranial cavity takes place through the floor of the middle cranial fossa (Fig. 12.31). Invasion of the orbit via the superior orbital fissure leads to proptosis and destruction of the bony walls of the orbit (Figs. 12.32 & 12.33).

Orbital Disease

Tumours within the orbit include optic nerve sheath meningioma, primary tumours of skeletal muscle and metastases (Fig. 12.34). Orbital meningiomas arise in relatively young individuals and generally produce a combination of proptosis and insidious visual failure. Orbital pseudotumour is a curious condition in which pain and

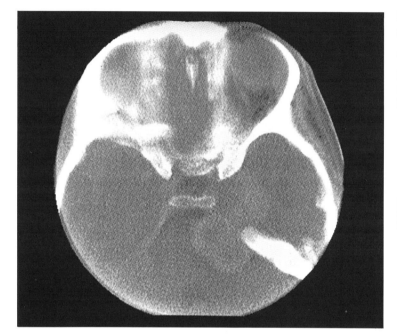

Fig. 12.31 Parasellar syndromes: CT scan showing a mass adjacent to the right cavernous sinus.

This 3 year old child presented with a short history of right ptosis. A restricted examination suggested a complete ophthalmoplegia. At craniotomy an extradural mass was found. Biopsy revealed a tumour of neuro-ectodermal origin.

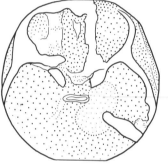

parasellar mass

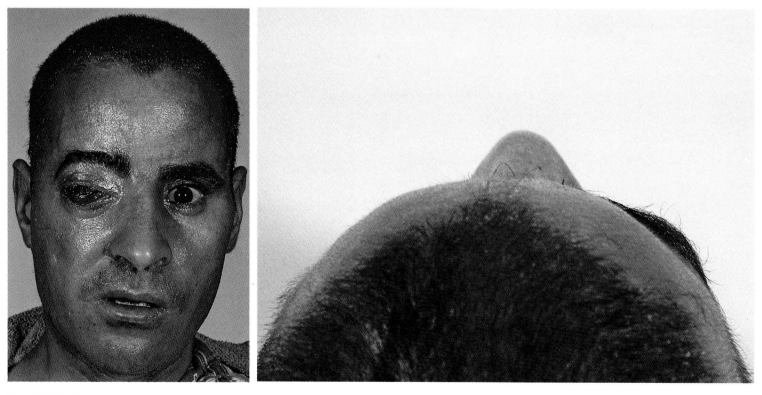

Fig. 12.32 Parasellar syndrome: nasopharyngeal carcinoma with severe right proptosis.

12.12

ophthalmoplegia are accompanied by proptosis. The condition has an association with the collagen vascular diseases.

Dysthyroid Eye Disease

This is a frequent, though often unappreciated, cause of diplopia in the adult. The condition may be suggested by the presence of lid retraction and lag sometimes with conjunctival oedema. Characteristically, upward gaze is restricted, due to fibrotic shortening of the inferior rectus muscle (Fig. 12.35). Sometimes thyroid function tests are normal in these patients though the T_3 suppression test is said to be abnormal in the majority.

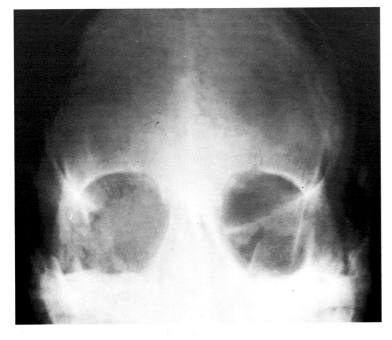

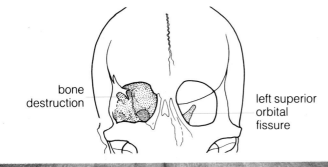

Fig. 12.33 Parasellar syndrome: nasopharyngeal carcinoma. This skull radiograph shows destruction of the walls of the right superior orbital fissure.

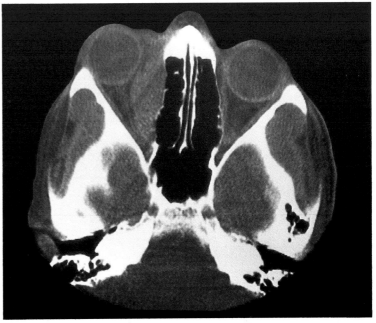

Fig. 12.34 Orbital disease: CT scan showing a left orbital mass.

This 22 year old woman with a known breast rhabdomyosarcoma developed proptosis with impaired vision in the left eye. Examination showed proptosis, periorbital oedema and a palpable mass along the medial wall of the orbit.

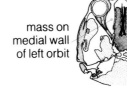

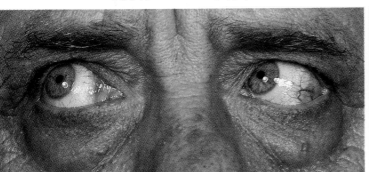

Fig. 12.35 Dysthyroid eye disease: normal dextro-elevation of the left eye with depressed laevo-elevation and concomitant lid retraction.

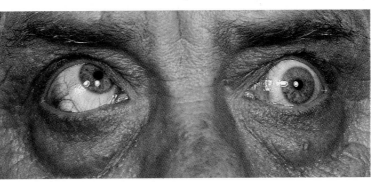

This 52 year old man gave a two month history of diplopia. Examination showed failure of elevation of the left eye, particularly to the left. There was bilateral lid lag. Thyroid function tests were normal.

Trigeminal Lesion

The fifth cranial nerve has both sensory and motor components. The sensory fibres supply the skin from the vertex to the angle of the jaw apart from an area over the angle innervated by the C 2 dermatome. Other structures supplied include the cornea, mucosa of the paranasal sinuses and nasal cavity, mouth and tongue, together with the teeth, gums and hard and soft palates. The motor component supplies the muscles of mastication, that is the ptery-goids, masseter and temporalis, together with mylohyoid, anterior belly of digastric, tensor tympani and tensor veli palatini.

The fifth nerve may be affected within the brain stem, for example, in brain stem vascular disease or syringobulbia, or in any part of its peripheral course. Motor involvement produces weakness in jaw opening and closure. The jaw deviates to the paralysed side and atrophy may be detectable in the masseter or temporalis muscles (Figs.

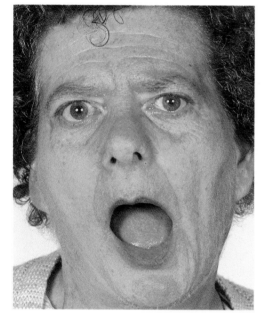

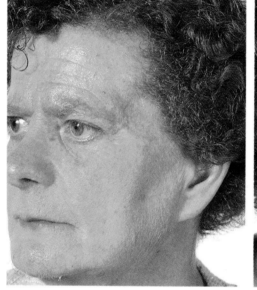

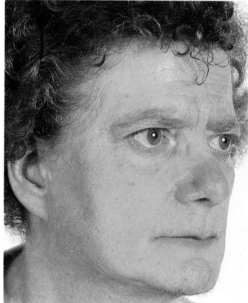

Fig. 12.36 Trigeminal lesion: deviation of the jaw to the left due to unopposed action of the right pterygoids.

This 57 year old woman had had a cerebellar astrocytoma excised at the age of 17. Examination showed nystagmus, a left trigeminal lesion and predominant left limb ataxia, all of long-standing.

Fig. 12.37 Trigeminal lesion: wasting of left temporalis (left) compared to normal (right).

Same patient as in figure 12.36.

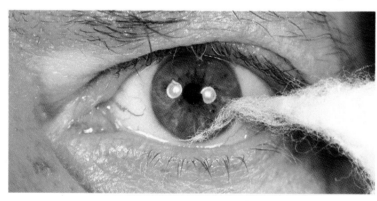

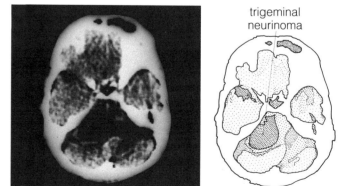

Fig. 12.38 Trigeminal lesion: depressed left corneal response. Same patient as in figure 12.36.

Fig. 12.39 Trigeminal lesion: CT scan showing a trigeminal neurinoma.

This 74 year old woman gave a two year history of altered balance and left facial numbness. Examination showed nystagmus, a depressed left corneal response and left-sided cerebellar signs together with gait ataxia. At operation a partially cystic neurinoma was found arising from the trigeminal nerve.

12.36 & 12.37). Sensory loss includes depression of the corneal response (Fig. 12.38).

Trigeminal neurinoma is rare. It produces facial pain or paraesthesiae with facial sensory loss and long tract signs secondary to compression of brain stem structures (Fig. 12.39). Involvement of the gasserian ganglion by tumour is typically painful. Causative lesions include nasopharyngeal carcinoma, tumours of the sphenoid sinus and metastatic disease (Fig. 12.40). Sixth nerve involvement is common in such instances (Fig. 12.41).

Trigeminal sensory neuropathy is a rare disorder in which progressive disturbance of trigeminal sensory function occurs, usually unilaterally, with sparing of motor function.

Seventh Nerve Lesions

The seventh cranial nerve is predominantly motor, supplying the muscles of facial expression, together with buccinator, stylohyoid, the posterior belly of digastric and

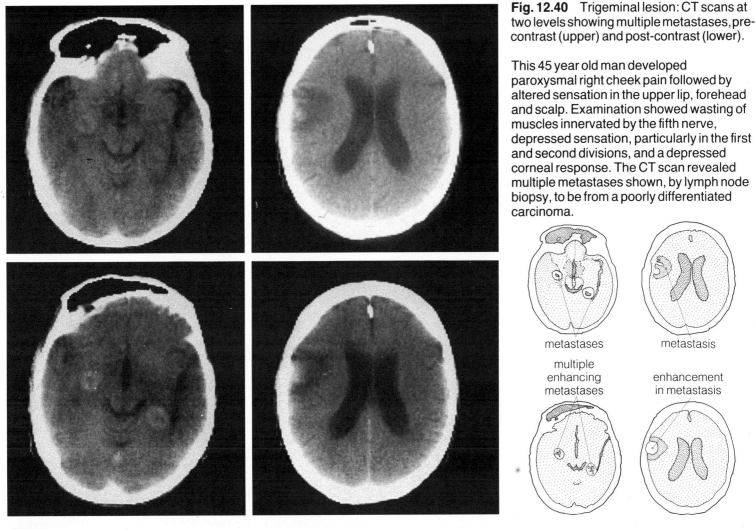

Fig. 12.40 Trigeminal lesion: CT scans at two levels showing multiple metastases, pre-contrast (upper) and post-contrast (lower).

This 45 year old man developed paroxysmal right cheek pain followed by altered sensation in the upper lip, forehead and scalp. Examination showed wasting of muscles innervated by the fifth nerve, depressed sensation, particularly in the first and second divisions, and a depressed corneal response. The CT scan revealed multiple metastases shown, by lymph node biopsy, to be from a poorly differentiated carcinoma.

metastases   metastasis

multiple
enhancing
metastases   enhancement
                  in metastasis

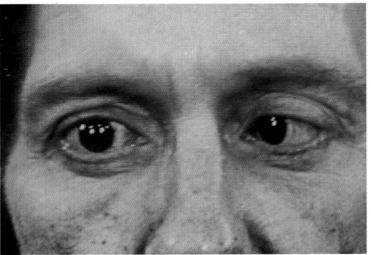

Fig. 12.41 Trigeminal lesion: an associated sixth nerve palsy producing failure of abduction of the right eye. (Taken from a television recording.)

Same patient as in figure 12.40.

stapedius. Its chorda tympani branch contains taste fibres from the anterior two-thirds of the tongue and secreto-motor fibres to the submaxillary and submandibular glands. Secretomotor fibres to the lacrimal gland reach it from the geniculate ganglion via the greater superficial petrosal nerve and the sphenopalatine ganglion. There are a small number of somatic sensory fibres in the facial nerve, conveying impulses from an area behind the ear.

Upper motor neurone facial weakness relatively spares the upper face, due to its bilateral cortical representation (Fig. 12.42). With nuclear and infranuclear lesions, all facial fibres are equally affected, unless the involvement is particularly distal. Leprosy commonly affects the facial nerve, often bilaterally (Fig. 12.43). Bell's palsy is an acute lower motor neurone facial weakness of unknown aetiology. It is often preceded by pain in or around the ear, and may be associated with loss of taste and hyperacusis if chorda tympani and the nerve to stapedius, respectively, are involved (Fig. 12.44). In the Ramsay Hunt syndrome, or geniculate zoster, there is a lower motor neurone facial weakness with vesicles in or around the pinna. If denervation of facial muscle occurs, reinnervation of one part of the face may take place with fibres originally destined for another. Typically in such cases, weakness of orbicularis oris may disappear when peri-ocular muscles are contracted (Fig.·12.45). Another example of the process produces aberrant reinnervation of the lacrimal gland leading to lacrimation when the patient salivates.

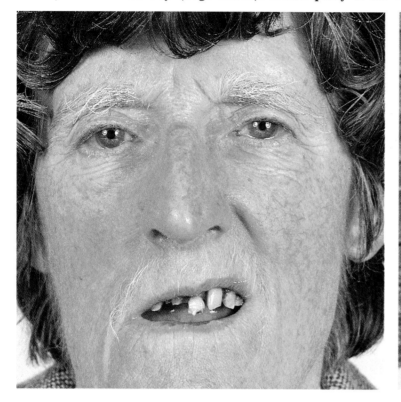

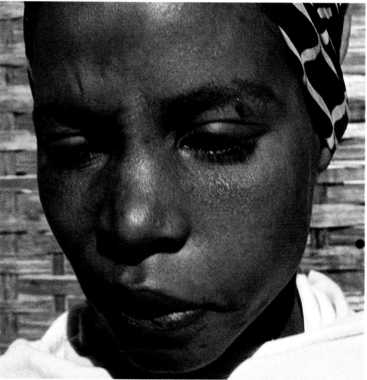

Fig. 12.42 Seventh nerve lesion: the patient has been asked to bare her teeth. There is an upper motor neurone facial weakness mainly affecting the lower part of the face.

Fig. 12.43 Seventh nerve lesion: a severe left lower motor neurone facial weakness due to leprosy.

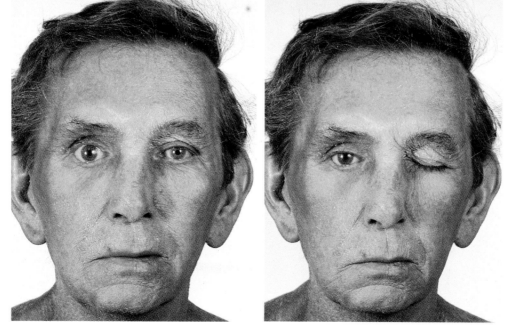

Fig. 12.44 Seventh nerve lesion: Bell's palsy. At rest (left) there is widening of the right palpebral fissure and drooping of the angle of the mouth. With eye closure (right) there is failure of contraction of orbicularis oculi.

This 64 year old man with haemochromatosis had a one month history of right facial weakness without loss of taste. Examination showed a virtually complete right lower motor neurone facial weakness. His right eye is artificial.

12.16

Hemifacial Spasm

Hemifacial spasm is characterised by intermittent contraction of the muscles supplied by one facial nerve (Fig. 12.46). The distribution of affected muscle fibres tends to vary from spasm to spasm. Eventually a lower motor nuerone facial weakness supervenes. The condition is sometimes due to compression of the facial nerve in the posterior fossa by meningioma, aneurysm or an atheromatous vessel.

Facial and Palatal Myoclonus

This is associated with a number of brain stem disorders, particularly cerebrovascular disease. The myoclonus usually appears some months after the initiating process and tends to persist. It produces a rhythmic contraction of muscle, most commonly between 30 and 300 Hz and it imparts a characteristic flutter to the voice. Electromyographic analysis reveals a regularly discharging complex (Fig. 12.47).

Facial Myokymia

This produces a fine, continuous flickering of muscle in part, or in the whole, of the distribution of the facial nerve (Fig. 12.48). It is most commonly benign, but can occur in multiple sclerosis and other intramedullary disorders as well as extramedullary lesions. It usually remits after a few weeks.

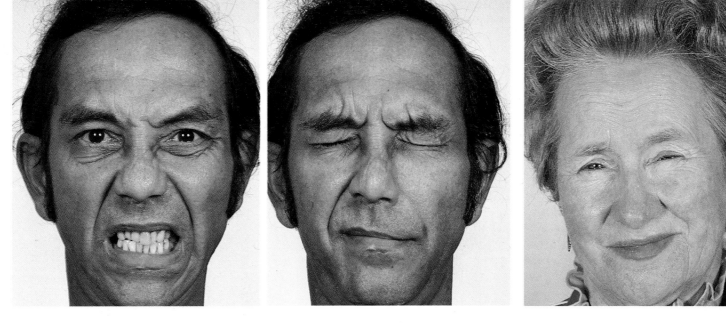

Fig. 12.45 Seventh nerve lesions: previous Bell's palsy and recent upper motor neurone facial weakness. Attempts at retraction of the mouth (left) reveal a lower facial weakness on the right. With eye closure (right) there is paradoxical contraction of the angle of the mouth.

Fig. 12.46 Hemifacial spasm: left-sided spasm, causing narrowing of the palpebral fissure and elevation of the angle of the mouth.

This 56 year old woman had had spasms of contraction of the left facial muscles for 16 years. Examination showed a frequent left hemifacial spasm in association with a lower motor neurone facial weakness.

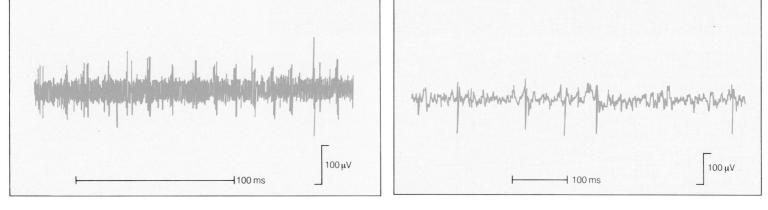

Fig. 12.47 Facial myoclonus: EMG trace showing discharging complexes.

This 31 year old woman had suffered brain stem damage following a road traffic accident. Some time later left-sided facial and palatal myoclonus appeared.

Fig. 12.48 Facial myokymia: EMG trace showing discharging units.

Eighth Nerve Lesions

It has been estimated that approximately 10% of unilateral hearing loss is due to an acoustic neuroma. These neuromas account for some 8% of all intracranial tumours. The tumours usually arise within the internal auditory meatus, most commonly from the superior vestibular nerve. They are slightly more common in women, and most commonly present between the ages of 30 and 60.

As the tumour expands, it protrudes into the cerebello-pontine angle, causing compression of the brainstem and, later, the cerebellum (Fig. 12.49).

The usual presentation is with unilateral hearing loss,

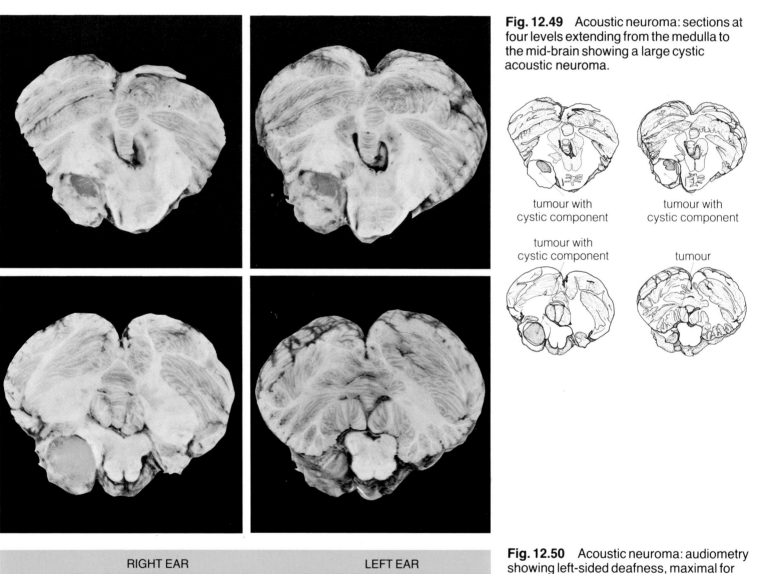

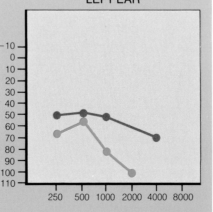

Fig. 12.49 Acoustic neuroma: sections at four levels extending from the medulla to the mid-brain showing a large cystic acoustic neuroma.

tumour with cystic component

tumour with cystic component

tumour with cystic component

tumour

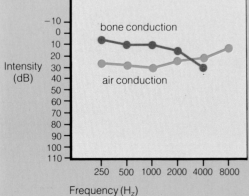

Fig. 12.50 Acoustic neuroma: audiometry showing left-sided deafness, maximal for high tones.

RIGHT EAR

LEFT EAR

bone conduction

air conduction

Intensity (dB)

Frequency (Hz)

occasionally of acute onset, in association with tinnitus. Vertigo is less common. Later there may be facial pain and numbness, facial weakness and ipsilateral cerebellar signs. Pain in the ear or more generalised headaches can occur, though not necessarily due to obstructive hydrocephalus.

Audiometry is not specific, though it usually shows a high tone loss. Rarely, deafness is not demonstrable.

Loudness recruitment is almost always absent, and the caloric responses are typically depressed or absent (Figs. 12.50 & 12.51). Widening of the internal auditory meatus, with or without bone erosion, is found in at least 70% of cases (Fig. 12.52). Before the introduction of CT scanning, further radiological investigation usually involved air encephalography (Fig. 12.53) or myodil cister-

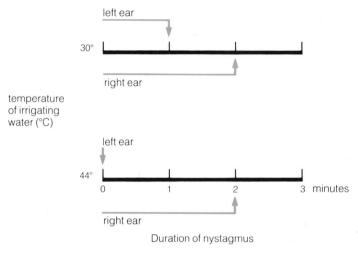
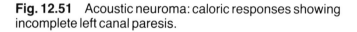

Fig. 12.51 Acoustic neuroma: caloric responses showing incomplete left canal paresis.

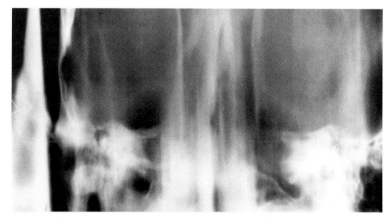

Fig. 12.52 Acoustic neuroma: tomography showing widening of the right internal auditory meatus.

Same patient as in figure 12.50.

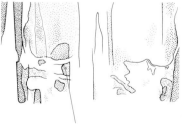

expanded right internal auditory meatus

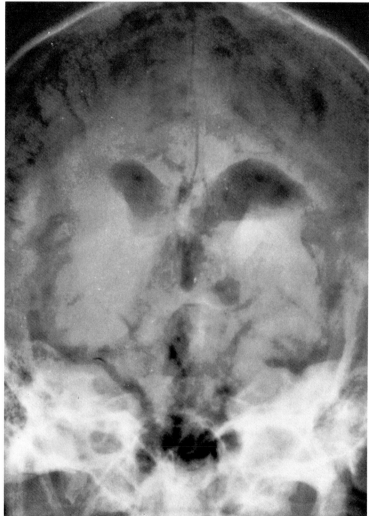

Fig. 12.53 Acoustic neuroma: air encephalogram showing a mass in the left cerebellopontine angle.

Same patient as in figure 12.50.

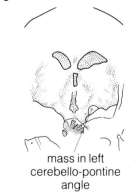

mass in left cerebello-pontine angle

12.19

nography, the latter procedure being capable of detecting small intracanalicular tumours. Vertebral angiography may be necessary to assess the degree and distribution of the tumour's blood supply (Fig. 12.54).

CT scanning has largely displaced these diagnostic procedures. Pre-contrast scans show a low or isodense mass with uniform or, rarely, ring enhancement (Fig. 12.55). Other lesions may arise at this site, including menin-

gioma, cholesteatoma, epidermoids, metastatic tumours and tumours extending from the cerebellum. Acoustic neuromas, however, account for some 80% of all masses occurring at this site. Surgical removal of the tumour may be followed by facial paralysis, the effect of which can be partially offset by faciohypoglossal anastomosis (Figs. 12.56 & 12.57). The complication has been less since the introduction of microsurgical techniques.

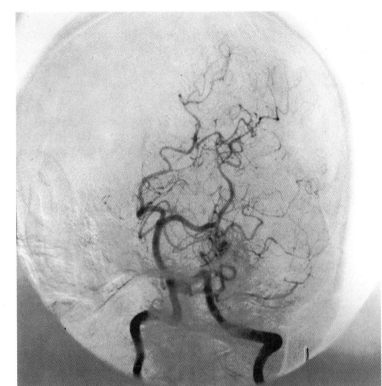

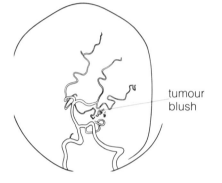

Fig. 12.54 Acoustic neuroma: vertebral angiogram showing the tumour's blood supply.

Same patient as in figure 12.50.

tumour blush

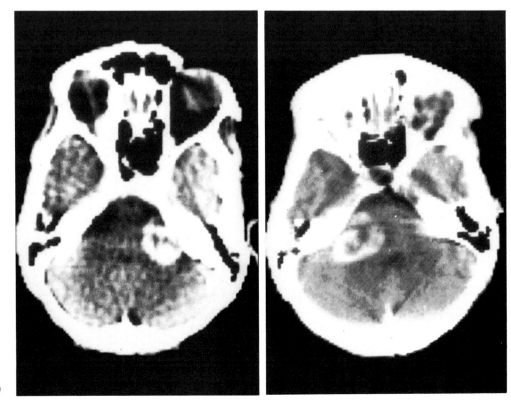

Fig. 12.55 Acoustic neuroma: CT scans showing a uniformly enhancing mass in the right cerebellopontine angle (left) and ring enhancement of a left cerebellopontine mass (right).

(Left). This 68 year old woman presented with a five month history, initially of facial pain and numbness, followed by deafness and tinnitus. Her balance had deteriorated. Examination showed nystagmus, and right fifth, seventh and eighth nerve palsies. (Right). This 69 year old woman had been aware of left-sided deafness for several months. Her balance had been altered and she had developed pressure sensations in the temples. She had nystagmus, left deafness and slight gait ataxia.

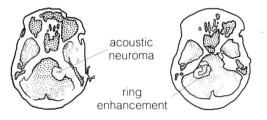

acoustic neuroma

ring enhancement

Lower Cranial Nerve Syndromes

These are rarely encountered in neurological practice. The jugular foramen syndrome produces alteration in function in the ninth, tenth and eleventh cranial nerves, all of which traverse the foramen. Examination of the ninth cranial nerve is difficult, but it is most readily assessed by testing sensation in the region of the tonsillar fossa. With involvement of the vagus nerve, the palate deviates to the non-paralysed side and there is unilateral paralysis of the vocal cord (Fig. 12.58). Eleventh cranial nerve

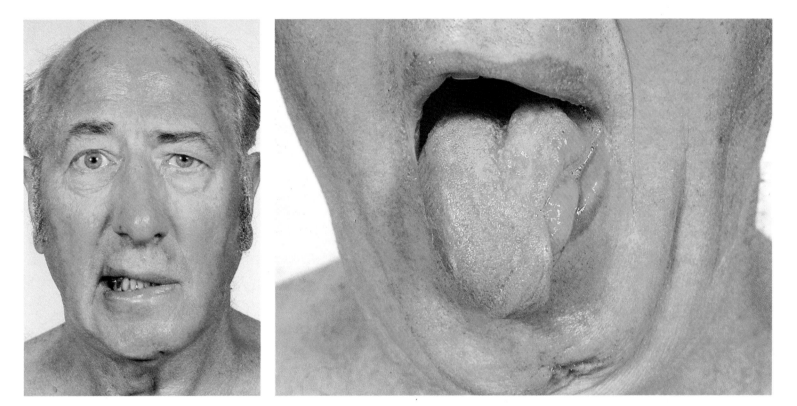

Fig. 12.56 Acoustic neuroma: facial palsy following removal of a left acoustic neuroma.

Same patient as in figure 12.50.

Fig. 12.57 Acoustic neuroma: atrophy of the left side of the tongue following a faciohypoglossal anastomosis.

Same patient as in figure 12.50.

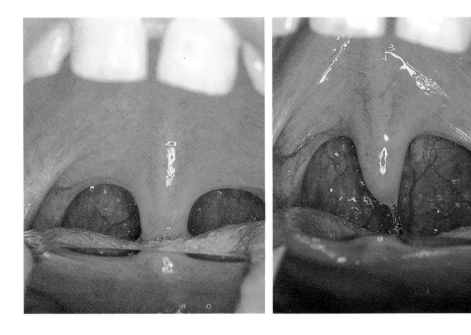

Fig. 12.58 Jugular foramen syndrome: palatal palsy showing the midline position of the uvula at rest (left) and deviation to the right on phonation (right).

This 42 year old man, with a history of hypertension, developed pain in the left side of the neck, followed by difficulty in swallowing. Examination showed questionable blunting of sensation in the left tonsillar fossa, and definite involvement of the tenth and eleventh cranial nerves. The aetiology was not established and the condition gradually recovered.

damage results in weakness, with or without wasting, of sternomastoid and the upper fibres of the trapezius (Fig. 12.59). The jugular foramen syndrome may be due to a tumour within the cranial cavity, for example a neurinoma, meningioma or cholesteatoma. Lesions at or astride the foramen are liable to damage fibres of the twelfth nerve emerging through the anterior condylar canal, leading to atrophy of the tongue and deviation to the affected side on protrusion (Fig. 12.60). Lesions at this site include carotid body tumours.

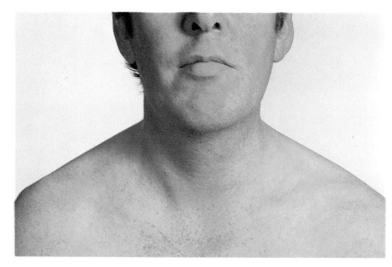

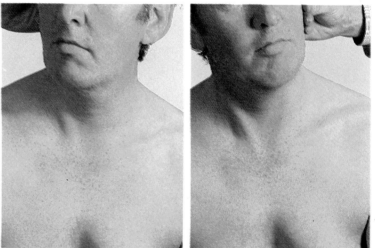

Fig. 12.59 Jugular foramen syndrome: wasting of the left sternomastoid, evident at rest (left) and when the patient attempts to rotate his head to the right (right).

Same patient as in figure 12.58.

Fig. 12.60 Hypoglossal lesions: unilateral twelfth nerve palsy, producing wasting of the left side of the tongue.

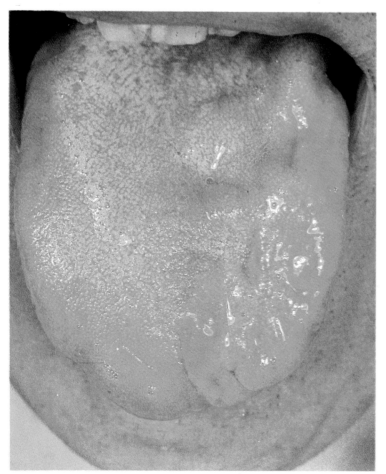

13. Non-Metastatic Neurological Syndromes and Neurological Complications of Systemic Disease

It has been estimated that approximately 20% of patients with cancer will, at some time, develop a substantial neurological disturbance. Most of these are due to metastases, but some result from the treatment used and a small number are examples of the non-metastatic syndromes associated with malignancy.

NON-METASTATIC SYNDROMES

Polioencephalomyelitis

Here the pathological processes include encephalitis affecting the brain stem or limbic system, and myelitis (Figs. 13.1 & 13.2). A subacute cerebellar degeneration may be associated with these, in which the patient develops ataxia, usually both for gait and limb movement, and dysarthria. Nystagmus is often absent. Pathologically there is a diffuse loss of Purkinje cells in the cerebellar cortex (Fig. 13.3). The condition is most commonly associated with carcinoma of the lung and ovary.

Fig. 13.1 Polioencephalitis: perivascular lymphocytic cuffing at the junction of cortex and white matter in the right temporal lobe. H&E stain, × 150.

The patient, aged 79, presented with a confusional state leading to signs of dementia in association with an extrapyramidal syndrome. Post-mortem showed an undifferentiated bronchial carcinoma.

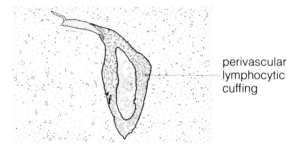

perivascular lymphocytic cuffing

Fig. 13.2 Polioencephalitis: microglial nodule in the left temporal cortex. H&E stain, × 130.

Same patient as in figure 13.1.

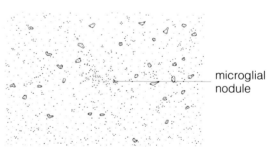

microglial nodule

Fig. 13.3 Subacute cerebellar degeneration: almost total absence of Purkinje cells in the cerebellar hemisphere (left, cresyl violet stain, × 80). A normal control is shown (right, luxol fast blue with cresyl violet counterstain stain, × 70).

This woman developed ataxia and dysarthria at the age of 43, followed by right hemiparesis and incontinence. She died four years later. By then there were widespread metastases from an ovarian carcinoma.

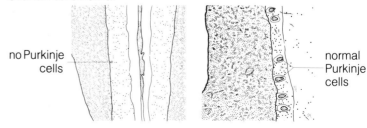

no Purkinje cells

normal Purkinje cells

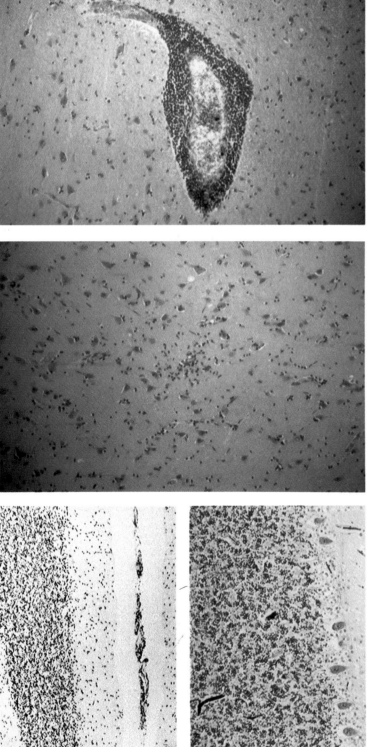

Neuropathy

In pure sensory neuropathy, the patient complains of paraesthesiae, numbness and ataxia due to loss of proprioceptive information. The condition is usually progressive and mainly tends to affect the lower limbs. Loss of digital proprioception produces purposeless, involuntary movement of the fingers with the eyes closed (Fig. 13.4).

Pathologically, destruction of dorsal root ganglia is found, with an inflammatory reaction and secondary degeneration of the posterior columns (Figs. 13.5 & 13.6). It most often complicates oat cell carcinoma of the lung.

A mixed neuropathy, embracing motor and sensory components, is less certainly associated with cancer and may be more a reflection of the patient's nutritional status. Osteosclerotic myeloma, however, is definitely associated with a peripheral neuropathy.

Motor neurone disease

A picture resembling amyotrophic lateral sclerosis has been reported in cancer patients, but an association has not been established.

Eaton-Lambert syndrome

This has been discussed previously (see Figs. 3.34 & 3.35). It can also arise in the absence of an underlying carcinoma.

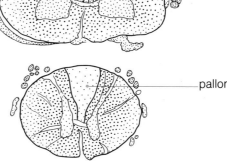

Fig. 13.4 Sensory neuropathy: involuntary movement of the fingers exacerbated by eye closure.

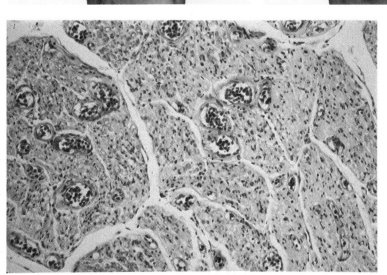

Fig. 13.5 Sensory neuropathy: dorsal root section showing inflammatory cell infiltration. H&E stain, × 120.

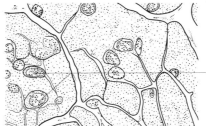

inflammatory cell infiltration

Fig. 13.6 Sensory neuropathy: sections of the cervical (upper) and the thoracic (lower) cord showing pallor of the posterior columns, mainly cuneatus. Luxol fast blue stain.

This patient developed a non-Hodgkin's lymphoma at the age of 59. Within a few months, she had developed ataxia and lower limb weakness. Examination showed weakness, areflexia and impairment of sensation.

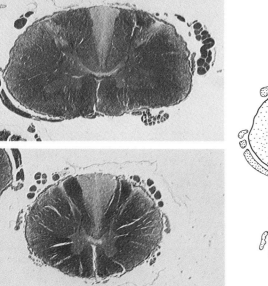

pallor

pallor

Primary muscle disease

A condition occurs which combines neuropathic features, for example depressed reflexes, with proximal muscle weakness. The EMG and muscle biopsy suggest a myopathic component. This neuromyopathic syndrome has been described with varying frequency in cancer patients.

Polymyositis and dermatomyositis are also associated with proximal muscle weakness, often with pain and tenderness. The association with cancer is most convincingly established for cases of dermatomyositis.

NERVOUS SYSTEM INFECTION IN CANCER PATIENTS

Progressive multifocal leucoencephalopathy is most commonly associated with leukaemia and lymphoma, but may arise in cancer, or with certain other diseases. The patient presents with alteration of mood and behaviour followed by focal neurological deficits including weakness, visual loss and speech disturbance. Involvement of the spinal cord is uncommon. The majority of patients die within a few months. The EEG may show diffuse, slow wave activity but the CSF is usually normal.

Pathologically the condition consists of multiple areas of demyelination in the cerebrum and cerebellum (Fig. 13.7). Giant astrocytes are found together with cells contining viral particles, at the periphery of the plaques (Fig. 13.8). Papovavirus has been isolated from these lesions.

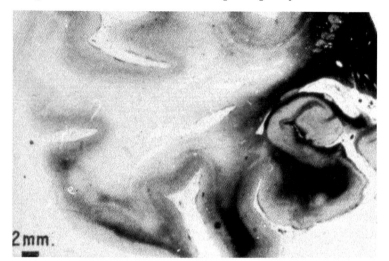

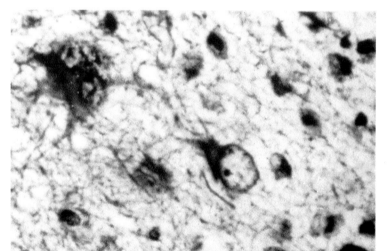

Fig. 13.7 Progressive multifocal leucoencephalopathy: demyelination in the right temporal lobe becoming confluent at the periphery. Woelcke-Heidenhain stain.

This 74-year-old man had presented with malaise, at which time lymphadenopathy was detected. A diagnosis of lymphatic leukaemia was established. He subsequently became dysphasic and withdrawn. His left arm was found to be weak and he later became comatose.

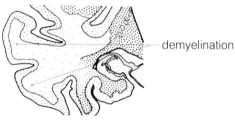

Fig. 13.8 Progressive multifocal leucoencephalopathy: plaque of demyelination with a multinucleate astrocyte (upper, Mallory's phosphotungstic acid haematoxylin stain, × 1000) and a section showing a giant astrocytic nucleus (lower, H&E stain, × 300).

This 63-year-old man with a history of diabetes and vascular disease presented with difficulty in swallowing and alteration of personality. He became anarthric, and had weakness of the face, tongue and palate. He died after inhalation of fluid. No carcinoma was found at post-mortem.

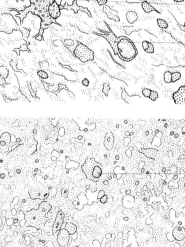

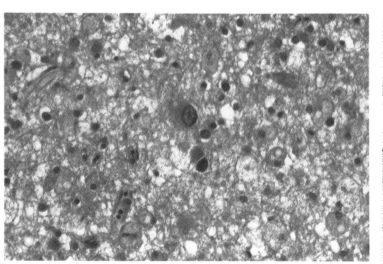

Herpes zoster infection

This is the most frequent infection of the nervous system in patients with cancer. The most frequent manifestation results from involvement of the dorsal root ganglia, but cranial nerve ganglia, particularly the gasserian, may also be affected (Fig. 13.9). Rarely, a generalised infection with the virus may result. Other infections encountered in cancer patients include bacterial and fungal meningitis and viral and toxoplasmic encephalitis.

NEUROLOGICAL COMPLICATIONS OF SYSTEMIC DISEASE

Previous sections of this atlas have demonstrated the overlap between general medical and neurological disorders.

Rather than repeat this material, a brief discussion of the neurological manifestations of endocrine disease will serve to illustrate the connection.

Thyroid disease

Thyrotoxicosis may present with proximal weakness (Fig. 13.10 and see also Fig. 3.26), and usually the upper limbs are more severely affected. Rarely, bulbar and extra-ocular muscles are involved. Myasthenia gravis and the syndrome of periodic paralysis are associated with thyrotoxicosis. Some patients with thyrotoxicosis display choreiform movements which subside when they become euthyroid. Dysthyroid eye disease may be associated with biochemical evidence of thyroid dysfunction.

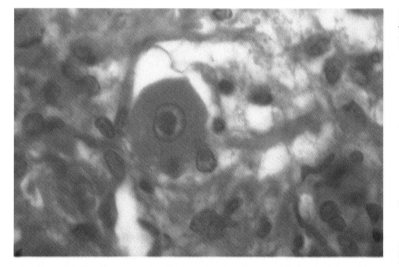

Fig. 13.9 Trigeminal herpes zoster: Cowdry type A inclusions in the nucleus of a ganglion cell and a satellite cell in a patient with Hodgkin's disease. H&E stain, × 1300.

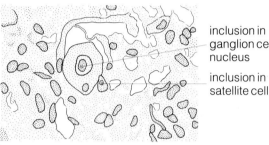

inclusion in ganglion cell nucleus

inclusion in satellite cell

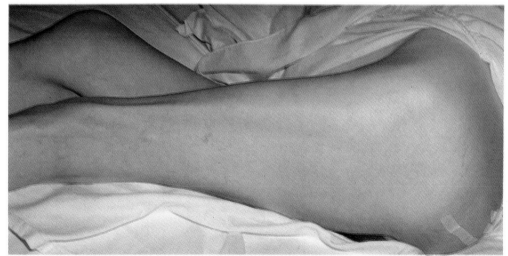

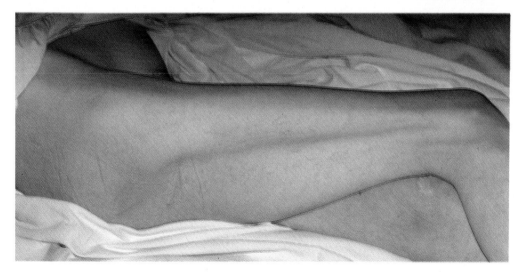

Fig. 13.10 Thyrotoxic myopathy: proximal lower limb wasting.

This 60-year-old patient had been admitted following a myocardial infarct. Severe proximal weakness became apparent during her admission. Examination showed mild deltoid weakness but more substantial proximal weakness, with wasting, in the lower limbs. She had slight lid lag and a retrosternal goitre. The T4 level was grossly elevated.

13.5

Myxoedema can cause proximal muscle stiffness with slowness of contraction. Both a proximal myopathy and a neuropathy may occur. Some patients present with carpal tunnel syndrome, and deafness, dementia and cerebellar ataxia have also been described. The changes in facial configuration following treatment are often dramatic (Fig. 13.11). The counterpart to the low voltage ECG is an almost iso-electric EEG (Fig. 13.12).

Pituitary disorders

The effect of pituitary tumours on the visual pathway has already been considered (see 'Headache Syndromes and Cerebral Tumours'). With massive suprasellar extension, obstruction of the third ventricle may result, with consequent hydrocephalus. The presence of a tumour which is secreting growth hormone is usually declared by the patient's facial appearance (Fig. 13.13) and the configuration of the hands and feet (Fig. 13.14). Neurological complications of acromegaly include carpal tunnel syndrome, a generalised neuropathy and muscle weakness sometimes amounting to a frank myopathy.

Adrenal disorders

Though muscle weakness is prominent in Addison's disease, specific pathological changes in the muscle tissue have not been described. Proximal myopathy may complicate Cushing's disease and can follow corticosteroid therapy, particularly with triamcinolone. The myopathy reverses when therapy is withdrawn.

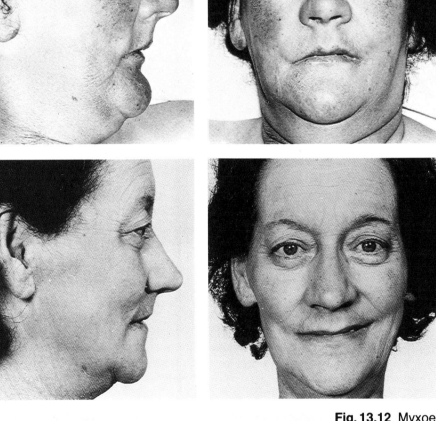

Fig. 13.11 Myxoedema: facial appearance before (upper) and after (lower) initiating treatment.

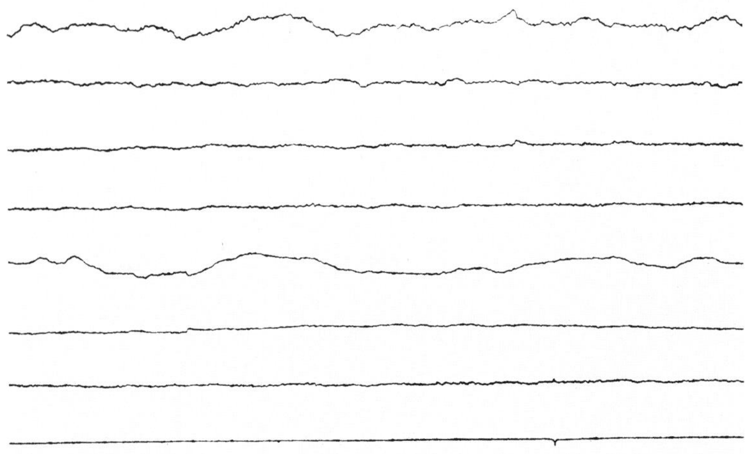

Fig. 13.12 Myxoedema: EEG recording (Channels 1-8, position 2) showing low voltage.

Parathyroid disorders

Behavioural disturbances are found with the hypercalcaemia secondary to hyperparathyroidism, and proximal myopathy sometimes occurs. Hypoparathyroidism results in hypocalcaemia, complicated sometimes by tetany or generalised convulsions.

Islet cell tumours

These are notoriously difficult to diagnose. They may present to the neurologist as a behavioural problem, as epilepsy or, rarely, with distal muscle wasting consequent to profound hypoglycaemia.

SYMPTOMS DUE TO NON-NEUROLOGICAL DISEASE

Not infrequently, patients whose symptoms appear to be neurologically based have a disorder of some other system. Examples include some patients with headache or limb pain.

Headache due to sinus infection

Chronic sinus infection is often suggested as a cause of headache and facial pain, but there is little evidence that radiological abnormalities of the sinuses, for example mucosal thickening, are more common in a 'headache population'. Acute sinus infection is painful, but most patients with this condition will not be seen in a neurological clinic (Fig. 13.15).

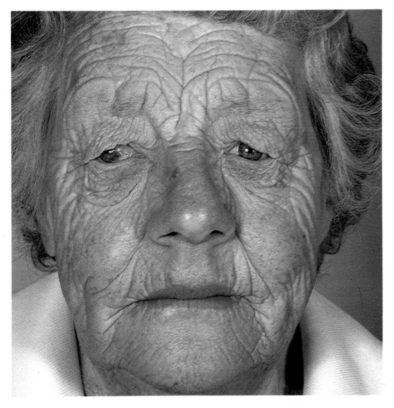

Fig. 13.13 Acromegaly: facial appearance.

This 60-year-old woman had poor vision in the right eye for several years following an injury. Subsequently the vision of the left eye deteriorated though assessment was complicated by the presence of macular degeneration. CT scan confirmed suprasellar extension of a pituitary tumour.

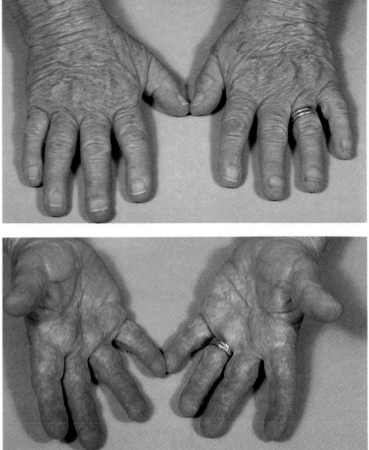

Fig. 13.14 Acromegaly: appearance of the hands.

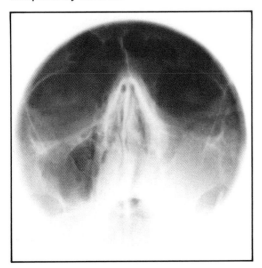

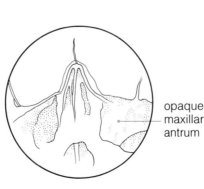

opaque left maxillary antrum

Fig. 13.15 Acute sinusitis: skull radiograph showing an opaque left maxillary antrum.

This 19-year-old male gave a week's history of pain around the left eye extending into the cheek. He had had a purulent discharge from the left nostril. The left maxillary antrum was tender. A rapid recovery resulted with antibiotic therapy.

13.7

Non-neurological causes of limb pain

There are many neurological causes of limb pain, including the entrapment neuropathies and referred root pain from the cervical and lumbar regions. Bone disease may be confused with these conditions, particularly if wasting local to the site of the pain has occurred. Osteoid osteoma most commonly arises in one of the leg bones, usually between the ages of 10 and 30. The pain is predominantly nocturnal and is relieved by salicylates. Radiographs generally reveal an area of bony sclerosis surrounding a central radiolucent core but the characteristic appearance may take some months to develop (Fig. 13.16). Primary bone tumours may present in a similar fashion, and where there is focal wasting, confusion with a neurological disorder becomes likely (Figs. 13.17 & 13.18). Osteomalacia results in bone pain and tenderness, usually scattered throughout the skeleton, and often associated with a proximal myopathy. It is sometimes secondary to chronic administration of anti-convulsant medication via an effect on increased liver metabolism of vitamin D (Fig. 13.19).

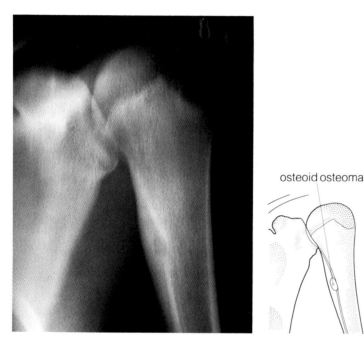

osteoid osteoma

Fig. 13.16 Osteoid osteoma: radiograph of the left humerus.

This 17-year-old male gave a one year history of left arm pain, most apparent at night. Examination showed a long-standing mild left hemi-atrophy. Radiographs of the humerus were reported as normal but failed to include the upper quarter. Further views suggested an osteoid osteoma which was excised.

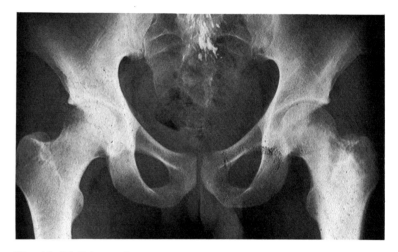

Fig. 13.17 Primary bone tumour: radiograph of the pelvis showing a lytic lesion in the neck of the femur.

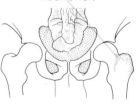

lytic lesion in neck of left

This 24-year-old man presented with a ten month history of left thigh pain. Examination showed wasting of the left buttock and thigh with depression of the left knee jerk. Myelography failed to reveal a root lesion. Radiographs of the femur showed a lytic lesion in the neck which was found to be a Ewing's sarcoma.

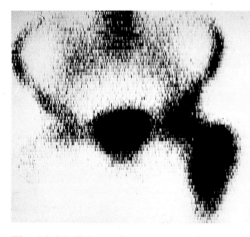

Fig. 13.18 Primary bone tumour: bone scan showing increased uptake in the head of the left femur.

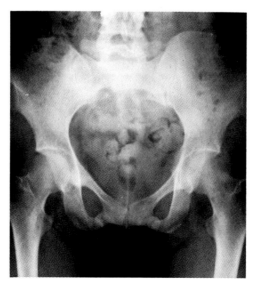

Fig. 13.19 Osteomalacia: radiograph showing a Looser's zone in the pelvis.

This 17-year-old girl had a long history of epilepsy. For a year she had increasing difficulty in walking and climbing stairs, together with pelvic pain. There was biochemical and radiological evidence of osteomalacia which reversed with vitamin D treatment.

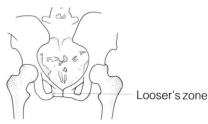

Looser's zone

Index